Gun Violence and Mental Illness

Gun Violence and Mental Illness

Edited by

Liza H. Gold, M.D.

Robert I. Simon, M.D., Co-editor

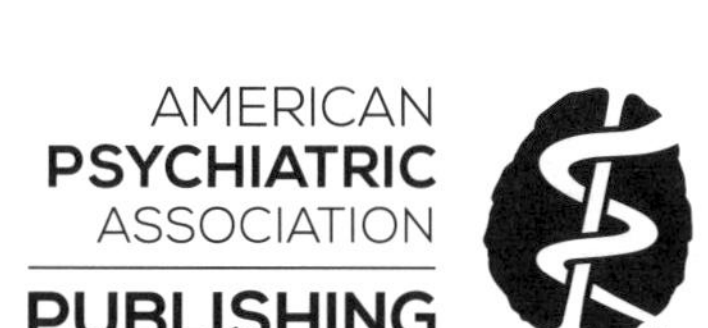

Note: The authors have worked to ensure that all information in this book is accurate at the time of publication and consistent with general psychiatric and medical standards, and that information concerning drug dosages, schedules, and routes of administration is accurate at the time of publication and consistent with standards set by the U.S. Food and Drug Administration and the general medical community. As medical research and practice continue to advance, however, therapeutic standards may change. Moreover, specific situations may require a specific therapeutic response not included in this book. For these reasons and because human and mechanical errors sometimes occur, we recommend that readers follow the advice of physicians directly involved in their care or the care of a member of their family.

Books published by American Psychiatric Association Publishing represent the findings, conclusions, and views of the individual authors and do not necessarily represent the policies and opinions of American Psychiatric Association Publishing or the American Psychiatric Association.

If you wish to buy 50 or more copies of the same title, please go to www.appi.org/specialdiscounts for more information.

Copyright © 2016 American Psychiatric Association
ALL RIGHTS RESERVED

Manufactured in the United States of America on acid-free paper
19 18 17 16 15 5 4 3 2 1
First Edition

Typeset in Minion Pro and Vectora LT

American Psychiatric Association Publishing
1000 Wilson Boulevard
Arlington, VA 22209-3901
www.appi.org

Library of Congress Cataloging-in-Publication Data
Gun violence and mental illness / edited by Liza H. Gold ; coedited by Robert I. Simon. — First edition.
p. ; cm.
Includes bibliographical references and index.
ISBN 978-1-58562-498-0 (pbk. : alk. paper)
I. Gold, Liza H., 1958– , editor. II. Simon, Robert I., editor. III. American Psychiatric Association, issuing body.
[DNLM: 1. Firearms—legislation & jurisprudence—United States. 2. Mentally Ill Persons—United States. 3. Mental Disorders—psychology—United States. 4. Risk Assessment—methods—United States. 5. Suicide—United States. 6. Violence—United States. WM 29.5]
HV7436
363.33087′4—dc23

2015034835

British Library Cataloguing in Publication Data
A CIP record is available from the British Library.

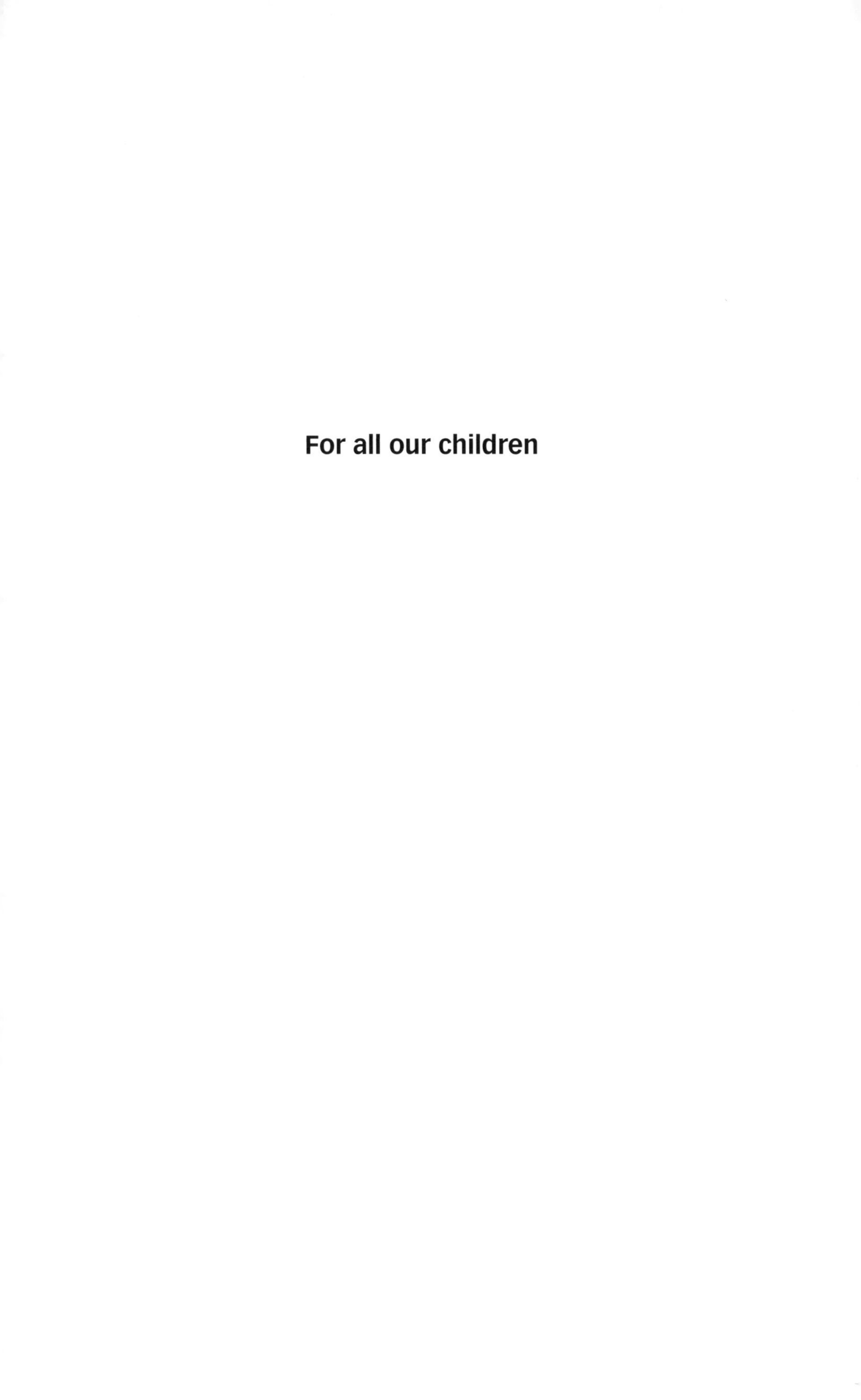

For all our children

Contents

Contributors

George D. Annas, M.D., M.P.H.
Deputy Director of Forensic Psychiatry and Assistant Professor of Psychiatry, SUNY Upstate Medical University, Syracuse, New York

Peter Ash, M.D.
Professor, Department of Psychiatry and Behavioral Sciences, Emory University, Atlanta, Georgia

Deborah Azrael, Ph.D.
Bouvé College of Health Sciences, Northeastern University; Co-Director, Harvard Injury Control Research Center, Boston, Massachusetts

Catherine Barber, M.P.A.
Harvard Injury Control Research Center, Boston, Massachusetts

Carl C. Bell, M.D., DLFAPA
Professor of Psychiatry and Public Health (ret.), University of Illinois at Chicago; Director, Institute for Juvenile Research (ret.), Jackson Park Hospital, Chicago, Illinois

Renée Binder, M.D.
Distinguished Professor of Psychiatry, University of California San Francisco School of Medicine, San Francisco, California

Shani A. L. Buggs, M.P.H.
Research Assistant, The Johns Hopkins Bloomberg School of Public Health Center for Gun Policy and Research, Baltimore, Maryland

Eric Y. Drogin, J.D., Ph.D., ABPP (Forensic)
Department of Psychiatry, Harvard Medical School, Boston, Massachusetts

Shannon Frattaroli, Ph.D., M.P.H.
Associate Professor, The Johns Hopkins Bloomberg School of Public Health Center for Gun Policy and Research, Baltimore, Maryland

Liza H. Gold, M.D.
Clinical Professor of Psychiatry, Georgetown University School of Medicine, Washington, D.C.

Anna Grilley, M.S.P.H.
Educational Fund to Stop Gun Violence, Washington, D.C.

Josh Horwitz, J.D.
Executive Director, Educational Fund to Stop Gun Violence, Washington, D.C.; Visiting Scholar, Department of Health Policy & Management, Johns Hopkins Bloomberg School of Public Health, Baltimore, Maryland

James L. Knoll IV, M.D.
Director of Forensic Psychiatry and Professor of Psychiatry, SUNY Upstate Medical University, Syracuse, New York

Emma E. McGinty, Ph.D., M.S.
Assistant Professor, Department of Health Policy and Management, Center for Mental Health and Addiction Policy Research, Center for Gun Policy & Research, Johns Hopkins Bloomberg School of Public Health, Baltimore, Maryland

Matthew Miller, M.D., M.P.H., Sc.D.
Professor of Health Sciences and Epidemiology; Director, Undergraduate Program in Health Sciences, Department of Health Sciences, Bouvé College of Health Sciences, Northeastern University; Co-Director, Harvard Injury Control Research Center, Boston, Massachusetts

Daniel C. Murrie, Ph.D.
Director of Psychology, Institute of Law, Psychiatry, and Public Policy; Professor of Psychiatry and Neurobehavioral Sciences, University of Virginia School of Medicine, Charlottesville, Virginia

Donna M. Norris, M.D.
Assistant Clinical Professor, Department of Psychiatry, Harvard Medical School, Boston, Massachusetts

Debra A. Pinals, M.D.
Assistant Commissioner, Forensic Services, Massachusetts Department of Mental Health, Boston; Associate Professor of Psychiatry, Law and Psychiatry Program, Department of Psychiatry, University of Massachusetts Medical School, Worcester, Massachusetts

Marilyn Price, M.D., C.M.
Assistant Professor, Department of Psychiatry, Harvard Medical School; Law and Psychiatry Service, Massachusetts General Hospital, Boston, Massachusetts

Patricia R. Recupero, J.D., M.D.
Clinical Professor of Psychiatry, Warren Alpert Medical School of Brown University; Senior Vice President Education and Training, Care New England, Providence, Rhode Island

Robert I. Simon, M.D.
Clinical Professor of Psychiatry, Georgetown University School of Medicine, Washington, D.C.; Chairman Emeritus, Department of Psychiatry, Suburban Hospital, Bethesda, Maryland

Carol Spaderna, L.L.B. (Hons.)
Department of Psychology, Aberystwtyth University, Ceredigion, United Kingdom

Robert L. Trestman, Ph.D., M.D.
Professor of Medicine, Psychiatry, and Nursing, and Executive Director, Correctional Managed Health Care, University of Connecticut Health Center, Farmington, Connecticut

Donna Vanderpool, M.B.A., J.D.
Vice President, Risk Management Professional Risk Management Services, Inc., Arlington, Virginia

Fred R. Volkmar, M.D.
Irving B. Harris Professor of Child Study Center, Yale University School of Medicine, New Haven, Connecticut; Editor in Chief, *Journal of Autism and Developmental Disorders*

Kelly Ward, J.D.
Educational Fund to Stop Gun Violence, Washington, D.C.

Daniel W. Webster, Sc.D., M.P.H.
Director, Johns Hopkins Center for Gun Policy & Research, Deputy Director for Research, Johns Hopkins Center for the Prevention of Youth Violence; Professor of Health Policy and Management, Johns Hopkins Bloomberg School of Public Health, Baltimore, Maryland

Disclosure of Competing Interests

The chapter authors have no competing interests to report.

Foreword

Renée Binder, M.D.

The December 2012 Sandy Hook Elementary School shootings, in which 20 children and six teachers and educators in Newtown, Connecticut, were killed, were a national tragedy. This shooting and the shootings in Aurora, Colorado; at the Washington Navy Yard in Washington, D.C.; at Fort Hood, Texas; at Virginia Tech in Blacksburg, Virginia; in Isla Vista, California; in Charleston, South Carolina; and others have focused the attention of the media and the nation on the intersection between gun violence and mental health. People with serious mental illness are stigmatized as being the perpetrators of these types of crimes, and this has resulted in efforts to keep guns out of the hands of individuals with mental illness.

The statistics regarding gun violence, however, suggest that a different focus is needed to reduce the morbidity and mortality due to firearms. Approximately 30,000 people per year, or about 80 per day, die from gun violence in the United States (Centers for Disease Control and Prevention 2015; Wintemute 2015). Most do not die in a mass murder rampage committed by an individual with mental illness. Mass shootings account for less than 1% of deaths and injuries each year due to gun violence (Overberg et al. 2013). In contrast, suicide, which is associated with mental illness, accounts for about 65% of firearm deaths (American Association of Suicidology 2015).

Although the database is limited, the number of people with serious mental illness who use firearms to kill strangers is minute. Only 3%–5% of all violent acts are committed by people with serious mental illness (Fazel and Grann 2006), and about 1% of all violence appears to be committed by people with serious mental illness using firearms to kill strangers (Swanson et al. 2015). Therefore, even if guns were removed from all individuals with serious mental disorders, hardly a dent would be made in the number of firearm homicides, including mass shootings.

Why is there so much misunderstanding about the relationship between mental illness and violence? Focusing attention on those with mental illness and their access to firearms makes it appear that action is being taken "to do something about gun violence." Our federal firearm laws refer to people with mental illness as "mental defectives" (Gun Control Act of 1968, 18 U.S.C. § 922[d][4]) and bar some of them from gun ownership in the mistaken belief that this makes us safer. One of the destructive outcomes of the focus on people with mental illness is the increase in stigma—stigma that is activated and reinforced every time a mass shooting occurs, often even before any information regarding the shooter's mental health history becomes available.

This book is a timely analysis of the complicated issues associated with gun violence and mental illness. It brings together a diverse group of professionals who define the issues, discuss evidence-based research regarding mental illness and firearm violence, and propose the revision and extension of public policy mechanisms to address these problems. The contributors to the book, in addition to providing analysis, discuss the implementation of new policies and mechanisms to prevent and mitigate gun violence and to address the individual and social burdens of serious mental illness.

In February 2015, an interdisciplinary, interprofessional group of leaders of eight national health professional organizations, including the American Psychiatric Association, and the American Bar Association addressed gun violence as a public health problem (Weinberger et al. 2015). Considering gun violence to be a public health problem is not a novel idea, but it is an idea whose time has come. New perspectives are needed that suggest innovative and effective approaches to reducing gun violence, including the incidence of firearm suicide, that do not stigmatize individuals with mental illness.

This outstanding book, edited by Liza Gold, M.D., and coedited by Robert I. Simon, M.D., provides a resource for mental health professionals, general physicians, public health professionals, and others in understanding the problems of gun violence and developing novel interventions to decrease the number of deaths from gun violence, including suicide, each year. The chapter authors address obstacles to the development of effective policy regarding both mental illness and gun violence. They provide a comprehensive description of the problems from many angles, templates for solutions, and indicators of future work that needs to be done.

References

American Association of Suicidology: Facts and statistics. Available at: http://www.suicidology.org/resources/facts-statistics. Accessed January 13, 2015.

Centers for Disease Control and Prevention: Injury prevention and control: data and statistics. Available at: http://www.cdc.gov/injury/wisqars/index.html. Accessed February 11, 2015.

Fazel S, Grann M: The population impact of severe mental illness on violent crime. Am J Psychiatry 163(8):1397–1403, 2006 16877653

Overberg P, Hoyer M, Hannan M, et al.: Explore the data on U.S. mass killings since 2006. Gannett Digital, 2013. Available at: http://www.usatoday.com/story/news/nation/2013/09/16/mass-killings-data-map/2820423/. Accessed March 1, 2015.

Swanson JW, Sampson NA, Petukhova MV, et al: Guns, impulsive angry behavior, and mental disorders: results from the National Comorbidity Survey Replication (NCS-R). Behav Sci Law 33(2–3):199–212, 2015 25850688

Weinberger SE, Hoyt DB, Lawrence HC, et al: Firearm-related injury and death in the United States: a call to action from 8 health professional organizations and the American Bar Association. Ann Intern Med 162(7):513–516, 2015 25706470

Wintemute GJ: The epidemiology of firearm violence in the twenty-first century United States. Annu Rev Public Health 36: 5–19, 2015 25533263

Introduction

Liza H. Gold, M.D.

Columbine, Virginia Tech, Aurora, and Newtown: these names immediately bring to mind the all-too-familiar images of death, fear, panic, and grief that accompany the heartbreaking mass shootings that make headlines across the country. Every firearm death or injury, whether to a child or to an adult and whether by homicide, suicide, or unintentional accident, is a tragedy for the victims, their families, their communities, and our society. The pain and loss experienced by those whose lives are shattered by gun violence cannot be overstated.

Media coverage of mass shootings typically include images of the perpetrators, who are often wild-eyed, dazed, or bizarre-looking young men. These images are inevitably accompanied by speculation that the perpetrators were mentally ill and that their mental illnesses caused their deadly attacks. When available, menacing images of perpetrators posing with firearms also accompany media coverage, stoking fears that any of us could become victims of these crazed mass murderers.

Sensationalized mass shootings bring gun violence and mental illness into national discussion, if only for a limited number of news cycles. These events and their media coverage reinforce the common belief that individuals with serious mental illness are violent and dangerous, especially if they have access to firearms. Such assertions are easy to believe, especially after mass shootings: who but a madman would commit such heinous crimes? Indeed, one survey found that the top perceived cause of gun violence (80% of people polled) is failure of the mental health system to identify individuals who are a danger to others (Saad 2013). Another survey found that 80% of Americans support laws to prevent individuals with mental illness from purchasing guns (Pew Research Center 2013), in the belief that such laws will keep all of us safer from irrational and unpredictable gun violence.

Mental illness and gun violence are complex public health problems that do in fact overlap, but not primarily—or even significantly—in the tragic but fortunately rare phenomenon of mass shootings. Although of little comfort to grieving families, survivors, and shattered communities, mass shootings are not the primary link between mental illness and firearm deaths and injuries. As horrific as mass shootings are, their sensational nature unfortunately obscures our view of the real associations between gun violence and mental illness. Until we understand the nature of the relationship between these two major problems, we are not likely to be able to decrease the devastating toll that each takes on our society.

The Database: Firearm Death and Injury and Mental Illness

Anyone who dies from firearm violence has died from a preventable injury. Nevertheless, firearm injury is a leading cause of morbidity and mortality in the United States (Table 1). The number of people killed in mass shootings each year represents less than 1% of all firearm homicides (Table 2) (Blair and Schweit 2014; Follman et al. 2013; Overberg et al. 2015). Approximately two-thirds of all people who die by firearms each year have committed suicide; the great majority of homicides, the bulk of the remaining one-third of firearm deaths, are related to interpersonal violence. Most people who commit suicide have a significant psychiatric disorder. Most people who commit homicide do not.

Since 2002, approximately 30,000 people each year have died by firearms and more than 70,000 have been injured (Table 2). From 2001 through 2013, more than 400,000 people died from firearm injuries (Centers for Disease Control and Prevention 2015). From 2002 to 2012, an average of 82.3 people a day died from firearm violence. Of these deaths, 32.5 were homicides and 49.8 were suicides (Wintemute 2015). Deaths due to firearms exceeded motor vehicle deaths in 10 states in 2009; in 12 states and the District of Columbia in 2010; and in 14 states and the District of Columbia in 2011. More than 90 percent of American households own a car, while little more than a third of American households have a gun. Americans' exposure to motor vehicles vastly outweighs their exposure to firearms. Yet in 2011, there were 32,351 gun deaths and 35,543 motor vehicle deaths nationwide (Violence Policy Center 2015a, 2015b, 2015c).

Firearm suicides consistently claim nearly twice as many lives as firearm homicides every year (Table 2). From 1999 through 2013, firearm suicides were the leading cause of violence-related injury deaths in the United States for all age groups combined (34.4%); firearm homicides (22.2%) were the second (Table 1). Since 2008, suicide has become, overall, the tenth leading cause of death for all age groups combined (Centers for Disease Control and Prevention 2015).

Firearms are by far the most lethal means of suicide; 90% of firearm suicide attempts result in death (Miller et al. 2004). Between 30,000 and 40,000 people commit suicide each year, and over 50% of these individuals use firearms to kill themselves. Between 2000 and 2013, firearm suicide was the third leading cause

TABLE 1. Leading causes of all violence-related injury deaths, by age group, 1999–2013

Rank	All ages	5–9	10–14	15–24	25–34	35–44	45–54	55–64	65+
1	Suicide, firearm: 34.4%	Homicide, firearm: 38.6%	Suicide, suffocation: 35.6%	Homicide, firearm: 44.3%	Homicide, firearm: 34.5%	Suicide, firearm: 30.2%	Suicide, firearm: 37.3%	Suicide, firearm: 47.1%	Suicide, firearm: 62.7%
2	Homicide, firearm: 22.2%	Homicide, unspecified: 11.3%	Homicide, firearm: 28.8%	Suicide, firearm: 22.2%	Suicide, firearm: 24.9%	Homicide, firearm: 19.6%	Suicide, poisoning:** 18.5%	Suicide, poisoning: 17.2%	Suicide, poisoning: 9.6%
3	Suicide, suffocation:* 15.0%	Homicide, suffocation: 8.8%	Suicide, firearm: 17.8%	Suicide, suffocation: 16.1%	Suicide, suffocation: 16.8%	Suicide, suffocation: 17.6%	Suicide, suffocation: 15.4%	Suicide, suffocation: 12.4%	Suicide, suffocation: 9.0%

*Hanging deaths are recorded as suffocation injuries.

**Overdose deaths are recorded as poisoning injuries.

Source. Adapted from Centers for Disease Control and Prevention: WISQARS Leading Causes of Death Reports, National and Regional, 1999–2013. Available at: http://webappa.cdc.gov/sasweb/ncipc/leadcaus10_us.html. Accessed August 4, 2015.

TABLE 2. Firearm-related fatal injuries

Year	Total firearm fatalities[a]	Total suicides	Firearm suicides	Total homicides[b]	Firearm homicides[b]	Number of people killed in public mass shootings[c]	Mass shooting deaths as percentage of total firearm homicides
2013	33,636	41,149	21,175	16,121	11,208	27	0.24
2012	33,563	40,600	20,666	16,668	11,622	63	0.54
2011	32,351	39,518	19,990	16,238	11,068	23	0.21
2010	31,672	38,364	19,392	16,259	11,078	12	0.11
2009	31,347	36,909	18,735	16,799	11,493	34	0.30
2008	31,593	36,035	18,223	17,826	12,179	26	0.21
2007	31,224	34,598	17,352	18,361	12,632	37	0.29
2006	30,896	33,300	16,883	18,573	12,791	22	0.17
2005	30,694	32,637	17,002	18,124	12,352	17	0.14
2004	29,569	32,439	16,750	17,357	11,624	5	0.04
2003	30,136	31,484	16,907	17,732	11,920	7	0.06
2002	30,242	31,655	17,108	17,638	11,829	0	0.00
2001	29,573	30,622	16,869	20,308	11,348	5	0.04
2000	28,663	29,350	16,586	16,765	10,801	7	0.04

[a]Includes unintentional and undetermined fatal injuries.

[b]Not including law enforcement/justice–related homicides; data are from Centers for Disease Control and Prevention 2015.

[c]2000–2005 data are from Follman et al. 2013, and 2006–2013 data are from Overberg et al. 2015.

of death overall for children and young adults ages 10–24 and the second leading cause for adults ages 25–34; and, as noted above, the leading cause of violence-related injury deaths for people 35 and older (Table 1) (Centers for Disease Control and Prevention 2015).

Homicide occurs at lower rates than suicide but still claims far too many lives (Table 2). Although rates of homicide overall have decreased by nearly 50% since 1992, firearms are still the most commonly used homicide weapons, and the percentage of those killed by firearms has remained stable (Cooper and Smith 2013). In 2011, firearms were involved in 68% of murders (Cooper and Smith 2013). Sadly, firearm homicide is the leading cause of violence-related injury death for children ages 5–9 and the second leading cause for children and young adolescents ages 10–14; it is the leading cause of violence-related injury death for older adolescents and adults ages 15–34 (Table 1) (Centers for Disease Control and Prevention 2015).

The risk of firearm mortality is not evenly distributed, raising troubling issues of gender, race, and culture (e.g., Metzl and MacLeish 2015). Overall, firearm mortality is highest among Caucasian males ages 35–64; in 2012, of all firearm deaths in this age group, 89.2% were suicides (Wintemute 2015). In contrast, in the same year, overall firearm mortality among African Americans was highest between ages 15 and 44; of these deaths, 88.7% were homicides (Wintemute 2015). Other demographic disparities have also been identified. For example, men are more likely than women to die from either firearm suicide or homicide (Centers for Disease Control and Prevention 2015); firearm suicide is more common in rural areas, whereas firearm homicide is more common in more highly populated urban areas (Centers for Disease Control and Prevention 2015; Wintemute 2015).

Owning a gun for lawful reasons is a constitutional right (*District of Columbia v. Heller*, Vol. 554 U.S. 570, 2008). The two most common, legitimate reasons given for owning firearms are protection (48%) and hunting (32%) (Pew Research Center 2013). Notably, civilian ownership of firearms is by far higher in the United States than in any other country in the world (Karp 2011). Although data on levels of gun ownership in the United States have not been systematically or definitively collected, a Congressional Research Service report indicates that in 2007, Americans owned approximately 310 million firearms (Krouse 2012). Per capita firearm ownership in the United States now exceeds one (W.J. Krouse, personal communication, February 2015). Ownership of guns is reported in 34% of homes, and many households own more than one firearm (Pew Research Center 2013).

In both firearm suicide and homicide groups (Richardson and Hemenway 2011; Siegel et al. 2013), the most substantial and significant correlation with mortality is access to firearms. Given the rates of civilian firearm ownership, the finding that U.S. firearm death rates are the highest in the world is not surprising.

In 2003, the firearm death rate in the United States was more than seven times higher than in 22 other comparable high-income countries (Richardson and Hemenway 2011). Of all firearm deaths in the countries evaluated, 80% occurred in the United States. Of all women killed by firearms in the 23 countries, 86% were American; 87% of all children ages 0–14 killed by firearms were American.

Compared with other countries, the United States carries a disproportionate burden of firearm homicides and suicides as well as unintentional firearm fatalities (Richardson and Hemenway 2011). Additional analyses of statistics from the 23 countries examined demonstrate that compared with other high-income countries:

- Overall homicide firearm rates in the United States were 19.5 times higher.
- Firearm homicide rates for individuals ages 15–24 in the United States were 42.7 times higher.
- Firearm suicide rates in the United States were 5.8 times higher.
- Unintentional firearm death rates in the United States were 5.5 times higher.

Despite these elevated rates of firearm death and injury, individuals with serious mental illness account for only 3%–5% of all violent incidents in the United States. Furthermore, only a small fraction of these involve firearms (Fazel and Grann 2006; Van Dorn et al. 2012). Recent analysis of data from the MacArthur Violence Risk Assessment Study (Monahan et al. 2001) found that in this groundbreaking study's population, only 1% of gun violence perpetrated against strangers was committed by individuals with mental illness (Steadman et al. 2015). This finding is consistent with data from another study showing a significant and robust relationship between gun ownership and nonstranger homicides but no statistically significant relationship between gun ownership and stranger firearm homicide rates (Siegel et al. 2014).

As observed by Appelbaum (2013), even if all violence, not just gun violence, accounted for by mental disorders could somehow be eliminated, 90%–97% of violent behavior would continue to occur. Most violent behavior, including firearm violence, is associated with factors other than serious mental illness; the most significant of these factors is substance abuse (Elbogen and Johnson 2009; Swanson et al. 2013, 2015; Van Dorn et al. 2012). Moreover, when individuals with serious mental illness become violent, those individuals most at risk are family members, not strangers (Estroff et al. 1998; Nordström and Kullgren 2003; Steadman et al. 1998). In fact, individuals with serious mental illness are more likely to be victims than to be perpetrators of violence (Desmarais et al. 2014; Roy et al. 2014).

Individuals with mental illness are much more likely to present a danger to themselves than to others. In stark contrast to the lack of direct association between mental illness and violence, the strong direct association between suicide and mental illness has been repeatedly demonstrated. As the authors of one literature review concluded, "The presence of a psychiatric disorder is among the most consistently reported risk factors for suicidal behavior. Psychological autopsy studies reveal that 90–95 percent of the people who die by suicide had a diagnosable psychiatric disorder at the time of the suicide" (Nock et al. 2008, p. 145).

Gun Violence and the Stigma of Mental Illness

Attempts at constructive discussion of the complex problems of gun violence and mental illness present numerous challenges. The all-too-familiar comments made by politicians and pundits in the wake of mass shootings are often tainted by the stigma and negative stereotypes associated with mental illness and influenced by the political pressures and social passions that accompany discussion of firearms. In addition, the common misconception that serious mental illness is a major cause of gun violence toward others presents significant obstacles to the discussion of effective interventions to address both serious public health problems.

The mistaken belief that mental illness is the primary cause of gun violence results in repeated calls from all sides of the debate regarding firearm regulation, particularly after a mass shooting, to "keep guns out of the hands of the mentally ill and criminals." For example, in 2013, Michael Bloomberg, one of the founders of the organization Mayors Against Illegal Guns (now Everytown for Gun Safety) and a gun control advocate, stated, "[T]he vast majority of American people favor basic steps that would help keep guns out of the hands of the mentally ill, criminals, and other dangerous people" (Bloomberg 2013). Similarly, Wayne LaPierre, CEO of the National Rifle Association (NRA) since 1991 and perhaps the most widely known guns rights advocate, has called the government's failure to prosecute "violent felons, gang members and the mentally ill who possess firearms" "unacceptable" (LaPierre 2013). Such statements suggest a misleading and stigmatizing parity between mental illness and criminal behavior.

In contrast to comments such as these, which typically follow a mass shooting, public discussion of gun violence that occurs on a daily basis rarely includes speculation regarding mental illness as a causative factor. In fact, national discussion does not regularly address the daily occurrence of firearm death and injury at all. Our complacency with the much higher rates of nonsensational firearm death is puzzling. One author has suggested that levels of firearm violence have transitioned from an *epidemic* condition, where numbers are steadily increasing, to an *endemic* condition, which is always present and exacts an ongoing toll but in which trends have plateaued. Therefore, firearm violence only grabs our attention when distinguishable—as mass shootings are—from the "routine" gun violence in which we typically lack interest (Christoffel 2007).

Certainly, debates regarding firearm legislation reform following a mass shooting ascribed to a “madman” are not intended to address the endemic levels of gun violence and suicide in our society. Moreover, legislation based on misconceptions regarding mental illness and firearm violence, such as New York’s 2013 Secure Ammunition and Firearms Enforcement (SAFE) Act, proposed and passed within weeks after the 2012 Sandy Hook shootings, is unlikely to prevent the few individuals with serious mental illness who do commit mass shootings from perpetrating these crimes. As observed by Swanson (2013), such debates and legislation focus on “people control,” which inevitably leads to a misplaced focus on mental illness as “a presumed vector of gun violence and a categorical prohibitor of gun access” (p. 1233).

Calls to do something about people with mental illness as a means of addressing the problem of gun violence play to popular misconceptions; legislative initiatives directed toward identifying the “dangerously mentally ill” are politically expedient. Nevertheless, such approaches are not feasible for practical reasons and are not likely to be effective (Swanson et al. 2015). Examining data from the National Comorbidity Survey Replication, Swanson et al. (2015) found that only 8%–10% of individuals for whom there was evidence of psychopathology and impulsive angry behavior and who carried firearms have ever been psychiatrically hospitalized, and only a small fraction of those were involuntarily hospitalized. Only individuals who have been involuntarily committed are subject to current firearm restrictions. Therefore, demands for a “national database of lunatics” (Curry 2012) and to get “homicidal maniacs” who are “going to kill” off the streets (Associated Press 2013; NBC Meet the Press 2012) reflect and contribute to negative stereotypes regarding mental illness and gun violence; they do little to address either public health problem.

Such statements also reflect the equally erroneous misconception that mental health professionals should be able to predict which of their patients will commit mass shootings and to take steps to protect the public from these patients. The assumption is that if psychiatrists and psychologists fail to do so, they must not be doing their jobs right. These beliefs are also not supported by evidence.

Although perpetrators of mass shootings often share certain demographic features (Bjelopera et al. 2013), a profile that would assist in identifying those few individuals, with or without mental illness, who go on to commit mass shootings does not exist. Moreover, the development of such a profile is unlikely (Swanson 2011). Because mass shootings are relatively uncommon events, epidemiological data cannot be reliably gathered; research is limited by common problems associated with statistically infrequent events, such as small effect size and rare outcomes (Swanson 2011).

That said, those who call the mental health system in this country “broken” (Associated Press 2013; LaPierre 2013) are not wrong. Although no evidence indicates that even the best mental health care system would prevent mass shootings, accessing mental health care in the United States is difficult and sometimes impossible, even when a person's situation meets the strict legal criteria for involuntary commitment. The present availability of acute inpatient psychiatric beds has decreased to levels similar to those in the mid-nineteenth century, when the social activist Dorothea Dix mobilized political and economic resources to provide humane care for individuals with mental illness (Torrey et al. 2012). Access to outpatient services is limited by availability of resources, funding, ability to pay for services, and by fragmentation of mental health and supporting social services. Many individuals with serious mental illness are in effect denied care because they are unable to navigate a bureaucratic labyrinth that even individuals without mental illness find confusing and difficult. As a result, many people with serious mental illness cycle between the streets, homeless shelters, emergency rooms, and jails and prisons.

The pervasive negative stereotypes of individuals with mental illness, which have been increasing over recent decades (Frank and Glied 2006; McGinty et al. 2013; Yang et al. 2013), needs no additional reinforcement from the media, politicians, and leaders of advocacy groups. For example, federal legislation prohibiting people with certain histories of mental illness from possessing firearms has codified the offensive term "mental defective" (Gun Control Act of 1968, 18 U.S.C. § 922[d][4]). This term is a vestige of the horrific eugenics movement (Linker 2013), which led to practices such as forced sterilization of individuals with mental illness. The Bureau of Alcohol, Tobacco, Firearms and Explosives acknowledged in 2014 that the term was "outdated" (Department of Justice, Bureau of Alcohol, Tobacco, Firearms, and Explosives 2014, p. 744). Nevertheless, use of this term cannot be amended by regulation; federal legislation is required in order to do away with this statutory terminology.

Nowhere is the stigma associated with mental illness more evident than in the beliefs regarding mental illness and violent behavior in general, and mass shootings in particular. Individual and institutional stigmatization of mental illness contribute to the multiple obstacles in accessing mental health care. Perhaps the most tragic consequence of stigma and misconceptions about gun violence and mental illness is their ultimate result: an inability to design effective policies to decrease the morbidity and mortality associated with each of these devastating problems.

Moving Forward: New Perspectives on Gun Violence and Mental Illness

A comprehensive analysis of the reasons for the misperceptions surrounding gun violence and mental illness is a challenging undertaking. Such a review raises issues of civil rights, the law, firearm regulation, the availability of and access to mental health care, insurance and social programs that pay for this care, the prison system, and the role of government in addressing issues of public health, in addition to issues related to the stigma associated with mental illness.

Nevertheless, the goal of this volume is to begin just such a discussion. To our knowledge, this is the first text to utilize evidence-based, public health, and multidisciplinary perspectives to examine gun violence and mental illness in conjunction. The chapter authors are leading mental health clinicians, legal scholars, and public health professionals and researchers, tasked with defining these complex issues and suggesting interventions based on best available evidence.

Importantly, we asked chapter authors to put aside their political biases regarding firearms and to address gun violence and mental illness as public health problems subject to multiple interventions on individual and collective levels. All contributors rose to this challenge. We believe their work has resulted in a unique and dispassionate review of the misconceptions that influence the national discussions regarding gun violence and mental illness; existing evidence regarding these phenomena; and evidence supporting new and, it is hoped, more effective interventions. We believe that only this approach can move the discussion of these volatile and divisive issues forward with more light and less heat.

Considering mental illness as a public health problem is not particularly controversial; in contrast, characterization of gun violence as a public health issue could not be more controversial. Many "pro-gun" advocates believe that the words "public health," when used in relation to firearms, are medical code words for gun control. These arguments are used to invalidate and silence the public health perspectives in debates regarding firearm regulation reform.

This political dynamic played out publicly after President Obama nominated Dr. Vivek Murthy for the position of surgeon general in 2013. In October 2012, Dr. Murthy had voiced the opinion that guns and gun violence are a health care issue. The NRA vigorously opposed Dr. Murthy's confirmation, stating, "[U]nder the guise of public health research, confirmation of Dr. Murthy would pose a serious threat to the rights of gun owners" (National Rifle Association Institute for Legislative Action 2014). Murthy's confirmation was initially blocked, as one senator stated, because "President Obama, instead of nominating a health professional, . . . nominated an anti-gun activist" (Carroll 2014).

A Public Health Model to Decrease the Morbidity and Mortality of Firearms

Public health approaches to firearm violence are not, as some believe, attempts on the part of the medical profession to assist purported government restriction or confiscation of firearms. The field of public health focuses on problems associated with significant levels of morbidity and mortality (Institute of Medicine and National Research Council 2013). Public health professionals are interested in devising broad strategies to prevent or ameliorate injury and disease (Gostin

2010). A public health approach involves addressing complex problems systematically and developing multiple types of interventions, with a focus on the following (Hemenway and Miller 2013; Institute of Medicine and National Research Council 2013):

1. Prevention (as far upstream as possible)
2. Scientific methodology to identify risk and patterns
3. Multidisciplinary, broad, and inclusive collaboration

Public health approaches emphasize cooperation and mutually shared obligation in pursuit of the greatest good for the greatest number of people. The goal of public health interventions is not to find fault or assign blame but to eliminate preventable causes of death or injury "before something bad happens" (Hemenway 2009, p. 1). An approach that prioritizes shared responsibility facilitates prevention of disease or injury (Hemenway and Miller 2013). Individuals of course have a responsibility to behave in ways that promote their own health and safety and those of others. However, some health needs—for example, water sanitation and road safety—cannot be addressed on an individual level. These require organized collaboration, infrastructure, regulation, and shared resources (Hemenway 2009).

Government intervention and regulation are often required when an inherently dangerous product might affect the health of large numbers of people; firearms are legal products that are inherently dangerous. Defining firearm violence as a public health concern is not "anti-gun" or "anti-gun-owner" (Hemenway 2009). Such mischaracterizations oversimplify the legitimate interests of all stakeholders concerned with gun violence in our country.

Public health approaches to problems that affect large numbers of people offer the hope of effecting changes from which everybody benefits. Risk factors, trends, and causes of health problems—the epidemiological cornerstones of public health—inform public health analyses. This information can be used to design effective interventions at as many levels of a problem as can be identified, some of which may include government regulation, in the hopes of changing social norms and decreasing morbidity and mortality.

The problem of deaths and injuries due to motor vehicle accidents is a less controversial example of a problem affecting large numbers of people and involving a legal but inherently dangerous product (although owning a car, obviously, is not a constitutional right). As a result of legal and social interventions designed on a public health model to make motor vehicles and roads safer (Mozaffarian et al. 2013), many of which involved government regulation, vehicle mortality rates have fallen by nearly 25% since 2004 (National Highway Traffic Safety Administration 2014). The public health model addressing motor vehicle deaths and injuries has never been characterized as "anti-car."

Despite the successful reduction of motor vehicle morbidity and mortality, we all understand that not every motor vehicle fatality or injury can be prevented; people still die every day in car accidents. The success of the public health analysis and approach to decreasing motor vehicle morbidity and mortality rates lies in ensuring that fewer car accidents occur and that when they do happen, fewer people are killed or injured. The list of public health successes, as defined by decreasing rates of death and injury, include childproof caps on medication bottles, increased use of smoke detectors in homes, improved child safety in playgrounds, decreased morbidity and mortality from tobacco use, and many others (Hemenway 2009; Mozaffarian et al. 2013).

Ultimately, the mission of public health is to unite diverse groups of people with the goal of improving health and the conditions that promote health for everyone (Hemenway 2004). Despite significant areas of disagreement between "pro-gun" and "anti-gun" groups, common ground that can form the basis for collaboration does exist. For example, in a 2013 survey, 79% of gun owners, 86% of people living in gun-owning households, and 85% of people in non-gun-owning households supported making private gun sales and sales at gun shows subject to background checks. Sixty-seven percent of Americans supported maintaining a federal database to track gun sales (Pew Research Center 2013).

We believe that as a society, we can agree that more than 30,000 deaths a year from firearm injuries, many of them involving children and young adults, is unacceptable. We believe we can agree that too many individuals with mental illness revolve through the mental health and criminal justice systems without receiving the social support and lifesaving treatment they need. We believe we can agree that perspectives that suggest new and potentially effective approaches to reducing gun violence that do not stigmatize those with mental illness are a social good from which we all can benefit.

The complete eradication of firearm violence and elimination of the burdens of mental illness are not practical goals and are not likely to be achieved. However, the success of a public health approach to these problems is calculated by considering every life saved from firearm suicide, homicide, or injury, and by considering every life improved by ameliorating the pain and dysfunction associated with mental illness. A public health approach to the problems of gun violence and mental illness offers the hope of just such successes.

Public health interventions are directed toward achieving a high level of health throughout society for the many, rather than the best possible health for the few (Gostin 2010). Unfortunately, interventions that serve the public health may not serve the best interests of any given individual. The inherent tension between public health policy and its intrusions into individuals' lives can at times create dilemmas for physicians and other health professionals.

Laws and regulations designed to increase public safety but that intrude into and potentially damage the physician-patient relationship, even if they benefit society as a whole, must be carefully weighed and considered. Physicians are obligated to look after the good of the person who consults them for care, not the public at large, although exceptions to this rule do exist. In medical and mental health care, intrusions into patients' autonomy and privacy raise issues not easily reconciled with clinicians' obligations to protect their patients' privacy and confidentiality. As a result, mental health professionals, as well as other physicians, tend to oppose government intrusion into the doctor-patient relationship. Legal arguments for exceptions to patient confidentiality are controversial and can result in appeals to the highest state and federal courts (e.g., *Jaffee v. Redmond,* 518 U.S. 1, 1996; *Tarasoff v. Regents of the University of California* 17 Cal. 3d 425, 1976).

Certainly, when benefits to public health are likely to be negligible, policies that mandate intrusions that violate confidentiality, such as New York's SAFE Act, are difficult to justify. Such legislation represents unreasonable and unfair intrusions of public health concerns based on negative stereotypes into the confidentiality and privacy of the physician-patient relationship. As Metzl and MacLeish (2015) noted, rather than physicians and mental health professionals being mandated to report on patients, "psychiatric expertise might be put to better use by enhancing U.S. discourse about the complex anxieties, social and economic formations, and blind assumptions that make people fear each other in the first place" (p. 246).

Physicians, Firearm Violence, and Public Health

In addition to having ethical obligations to patients, physicians and mental health professionals also have ethical obligations to safeguard public health. Physicians have played major roles in improving public health since the mid-nineteenth century, when Dr. John Snow demonstrated that cholera could be prevented by avoiding contaminated water. The American Medical Association (2015) has observed, "Physicians are uniquely suited to advocate for the improvement of the public's health." Medical ethical guidelines include statements about physicians' public health obligations. For example, the American Psychiatric Association's (APA's) *Principles of Medical Ethics With Annotations Especially Applicable to Psychiatry* state, "A physician shall recognize a responsibility to participate in activities contributing to the improvement of the community and the betterment of public health. Psychiatrists should foster the cooperation of those legitimately concerned with the medical, psychological, social, and legal aspects of mental health and illness" (American Psychiatric Association 2013, p. 9).

Public health professionals and researchers have called on physicians to take a leadership role in addressing firearm violence as a problem that affects many patients (Frattaroli et al. 2013). In a position paper on reducing firearm-related injuries and deaths (Butkus et al. 2014), the American College of Physicians stated, "The medical profession has a special responsibility to speak out on prevention of firearm-related injuries and deaths, just as physicians have spoken out on other public health issues" (p. 859), and recommended a public health approach to prevent firearm violence.

Most recently, eight interdisciplinary medical professional organizations, including the APA, have issued a joint "call to action," stating that firearm violence "is not just a criminal violence issue but also a major public health problem" (Weinberger et al. 2015, p. 513). The obligation of mental health professionals and physicians is twofold in that firearm suicide, which accounts for more than half of all suicides every year (Table 2), is both preventable and strongly associated with mental illness.

Nevertheless, the APA has also recognized the potential for political advocacy to appear cloaked as professional opinion and thereby carry an authority to which it is not entitled. The APA's ethical principles therefore also advise psychiatrists to be mindful of and clarify for themselves and others the distinction between their personal opinions and their professional authority, and to differentiate between their roles as private citizens and as psychiatric experts (American Psychiatric Association 2013).

The intent of this volume is to find a way to fulfill our obligations to promote public health and safety without compromising our obligations to safeguard patients' privacy and confidentiality and without exploiting our professional authority to support personal political advocacy. As physicians, researchers, mental health professionals, and "stewards of the public health" (Selker et al. 2013, p. 601), psychiatrists serve both our patients and society by educating the public and suggesting interventions to reduce the morbidity and mortality of both gun violence and mental illness. Doing so in conjunction with public health experts, public policy experts, and legal experts is consistent with professional ethics as well as our duties to our patients.

Only active participation at a public health level will allow mental health professionals to have a voice in designing policy that balances public health interests with responsibilities to patients and that calls out the individual and institutional stigmatization of mental illness in current firearm regulation debates and policies. The discussions presented here are neither partisan polemics nor apologies for adopting a public health model to discuss the problems of gun violence and mental illness. This volume is provided in the hopes of moving the national discussion away from nonproductive debate and toward effective interventions to reduce the morbidity and mortality of gun violence that do not stigmatize individuals with mental illness.

Firearm Violence and Mental Illness: Defining the Problems

In Part I, "Defining the Problems," the chapter authors tease apart the complicated relationship between gun violence and mental illness. In Chapter 1, McGinty and Webster address the common misconception that serious mental illness is a risk factor for violence generally and for firearm violence specifically. Mental illness is only marginally associated with increased rates of violence, and much of that increase is mediated by other variables, such as substance use and a history of violence. These factors are strongly associated with violent behavior, with or without mental illness. Small subgroups of individuals with serious mental illness are at elevated risk of committing violence (Choe et al. 2008), and some mass shootings have been committed by psychotic individuals. Nevertheless, links between serious mental illness and violence generally, especially firearm violence, are weak and typically mediated by other factors (Swanson et al. 2015).

As discussed by Miller and colleagues in Chapter 2, research has consistently found a strong link between access to firearms and suicide. In addition, and in contrast to acts of violence toward others, suicide is highly associated with mental illness. Firearms are by far the most lethal means used in suicide, and suicide attempts with firearms are more likely to be fatal than suicide attempts by any other means. The chapter authors discuss the evidence showing that restricting access to firearms during times of crisis for individuals struggling with thoughts of suicide can be lifesaving.

As reviewed by Bell in Chapter 3, urban firearm homicide victims are predominantly young African American men. The myths that these deaths are related primarily to crime have obscured the profoundly interpersonal nature of most urban violence. For example, according to the Firearm and Injury Center at Penn (2011), the Federal Bureau of Investigation reported in 2009 that only 16% of firearm homicides occurred in connection with a known or suspected felony; 46% occurred under nonfelony circumstances such as arguments and gang conflicts. Dr. Bell also discusses the evidence indicating that the morbidity and mortality of gun violence in highly vulnerable and predominantly African American urban populations can be decreased by a variety of interventions, many of which involve strengthening interpersonal and community bonds and involvement.

Knoll and Annas in Chapter 4 and Ash in Chapter 5 explore, respectively, the mass shootings and school shootings that make headlines and whose perpetrators are commonly assumed or believed to have mental illness. As the authors of these chapters discuss, most perpetrators do not have a serious mental illness, and the authors provide salient discussions of the evidence regarding mass shooters and review possible interventions along a spectrum of public health options to avert "downstream" violence by providing services and support "upstream," as well as approaches to maintaining safety in public places.

In Chapter 6, Price and colleagues address the issues raised by the use of categorical mental health prohibitions and reporting requirements regarding a history of mental illness in the National Instant Criminal Background Check System. Federal law and most states' laws prohibit the sale or possession of firearms to individuals with certain mental health histories. These authors review the evolution of categorical mental health prohibitions and discuss the evidence regarding their efficacy.

Notably, many people who meet the federal and state mental health prohibitions have not exhibited any indications that owning or possessing a firearm would place them or the public in danger. Conversely, very few of the mass shooters in the past decade have met criteria that would have legally prohibited them from possessing firearms. Evaluation of data from the National Comorbidity Survey Replication demonstrated that only a small number of individuals in a high-risk category of having histories of impulsive angry behavior combined with gun access had ever been hospitalized for a mental health problem (Swanson et al. 2015). Moreover, the potential of such legislation to increase the stigma to which individuals with mental illness are already vulnerable and to increase the government's intrusions into the physician-patient relationship cannot be ignored.

Assuming for the sake of argument that mental health professionals could consistently and reliably identify the very few "dangerously mentally ill" individuals prior to their committing an act of violence, the options for intervention are limited. As Drogin and Spaderna review in Chapter 7, the criteria for involuntary psychiatric commitment have narrowed over the past decades. Once primarily a medical decision, involuntary commitment to a psychiatric institution is now primarily a legal determination, based on meeting a burden of proof and narrowly defined criteria and fulfilling a requirement for due process. The presence of acute mental illness alone, even psychosis, is not enough to meet criteria for involuntary commitment in any state.

Finally, in Chapter 8, Trestman and colleagues examine the mental health system in the United States. Even when an individual's situation has met the narrow criteria for involuntary psychiatric commitment, the availability of resources nationwide is such that finding an available inpatient bed is sometimes impossible. Physicians often face an untenable choice between violating an individual's rights by holding him or her involuntarily beyond the legally specified time limit or letting the individual go despite the elevated risks of violence or suicide. Although unrelated to the phenomenon of mass shootings, evaluation of the public health crisis involving mental illness clearly indicates that more resources need to be made available.

Where We Go From Here: Evidence-Based Interventions

In Part II, "Moving Forward," the chapter authors examine the efficacy of past interventions and propose evidence-based clinical and public policy interventions, addressing the problems of both mental illness and gun violence as defined in Part I. Chapter authors also indicate additional areas for research that could provide the basis for future evidence-based interventions or policy reforms.

No single intervention or simple solution will "solve" the problems of gun violence and mental illness. A variety of evidence-based interventions to decrease the toll of gun violence and mental illness must be designed and implemented. Framing both issues as public health problems allows stakeholders to identify the multiple factors that contribute to each and, therefore, the multiple levels of potential interventions. When evidence is lacking, interventions can be extrapolated on the basis of available data and additional research can be designed. Proposed interventions, if implemented, can be assessed for their efficacy and improved or altered as evidence indicates.

Part II of this volume stresses certain common themes in considering how to address the dual problems of gun violence and mental illness. First, interventions to decrease morbidity and mortality due to firearms need to move from discriminatory, non-evidenced-based categories of firearm prohibition to restricting firearm access based on individualized assessments of dangerousness or risk, with or without mental illness. Second, policy and treatment approaches to mental illness need to emphasize access and engagement, and not simply coercion. Third, those concerned with designing effective interventions need more research both on exploring relevant factors in firearms injury and death and on engaging and treating individuals with serious mental illness. The development of resources to create multiple opportunities for treatment engagement for individuals with mental illness—and, similarly, multiple opportunities to prevent firearm injury and death—is imperative. These approaches may or may not prevent the rare mass shooting committed by an individual with serious mental illness. However, such approaches are likely to do more for many more people, including decreasing the rates of firearm suicide, which is strongly associated with mental illness, and decreasing the rates of firearm homicide and injury, which are not.

The first two chapters of Part II, Chapters 9 and 10, focus on individualized mental health risk assessments. These chapters emphasize the potential to reduce risk on an individual basis by separating at-risk individuals from firearms, even temporarily, so treatment interventions can be provided before death or injury occurs. In Chapter 9, Murrie discusses individualized violence risk assessment and its role in the prevention of gun violence. He reviews the strengths and limitations of violence risk assessments, and discusses how they might be used to make decisions regarding mental health treatment or access to firearms when clinical or legal decision making is required. In Chapter 10, Simon and Gold review suicide risk assessments in mental health treatment, with particular attention to assessment and interventions involving firearms.

In Chapter 11, Pinals examines problems in accessing mental health treatment and discusses strategies to improve access on systems and individual levels. Increasing the numbers of individuals involuntarily committed, even if legally permissible, is not necessarily an effective strategy to decrease the morbidity and mortality of mental illness. In addition to suicide, the problems of those with serious mental illness include homelessness, substance abuse, and repeated involvement with the criminal justice system, leading to repeated episodes of incarceration. Pinals discusses interventions to decrease the toll these problems take both on individuals with serious mental illness and on our society.

In Chapter 12, Horwitz and colleagues discuss a promising and innovative policy initiative for decreasing access to firearms for individuals, with or without mental illness, who are at increased risk of harming themselves or others with firearms. This proposed legal intervention, a gun violence restraining order (GVRO), is modeled on the success of domestic violence restraining orders in decreasing the mortality of women due to firearm use by intimate partners. The GVRO allows for temporary removal of firearms at times of crisis, initiated by family members or law enforcement and based on individualized assessment and due legal process. A GVRO law was passed in California in 2015, largely in response to the 2014 Isla Vista mass shootings.

In Chapter 13, Gold and Vanderpool explore and discuss "relief from disabilities"—that is, restoration of firearm rights—a relatively unfamiliar but increasingly common feature in the intersecting worlds of firearm regulation and mental illness. Many individuals who have been prohibited from purchasing or possessing firearms because of a history of involuntary psychiatric commitment are able to legally petition to have their firearm rights restored. However, very few statutes require that restoration hearings include mental health evidence other than the records related to the original prohibiting event. Gold and Vanderpool propose that restoration hearings include a mental health evaluation and suggest a model that could be used or adapted to conduct restoration evaluations.

In Chapter 14, the closing chapter of the volume, Frattaroli and Buggs examine some of the larger social and public health interventions designed to decrease the toll of firearm violence. The authors describe how these interventions fit into a public health model and can be evidence based without stigmatizing any individuals or groups, such as those with mental illness. This chapter reminds readers of the many levels of potential public health interventions—individual, family, institutional, community, and policy—and describes how these can be identified, supported, and evaluated by research to achieve the goals of reducing the morbidity and mortality of firearm violence. This discussion also allows readers to consider where the preceding chapters fit in a public health model.

The State of Firearm Research

More research is clearly needed on every level in regard to effective interventions to decrease the toll of mental illness and firearm violence. Unfortunately, active research, particularly in the area of gun violence, is not robust. In 1996, under pressure from the NRA (Rosenberg 2013), Congress included language in an appropriations bill stating that "none of the funds made available for injury prevention and control at the Centers for Disease Control and Prevention [CDC] may be used to advocate or promote gun control" (Jamieson 2013). As a result, federal support for firearm injury prevention essentially ceased (Kellermann and Rivara 2013). Lack of funding resulted in lack of trained firearm researchers. Wintemute (2015), one of the foremost investigators in this field, estimates that the United States has no more than a dozen active, experienced investigators whose careers have been focused on firearms research (Wintemute 2013).

Hopefully, research efforts will be renewed. In January 2013, in the wake of the December 2012 Newtown shootings, President Obama directed the CDC and other federal agencies "to immediately begin identifying the most pressing firearm-related violence research problems" (Institute of Medicine and National Research Council 2013, p. 2). In response, the Institute of Medicine and National Research Council (2013) produced a 100-page report identifying multiple areas of research based on a public health approach.

President Obama's proposed budgets since 2012 have included requests that Congress appropriate $10 million for the CDC to conduct gun violence research (Frankel 2015). Congress has continued to deny this dedicated funding, and the CDC has been characterized as continuing to be "terrified" of gun research (Frankel 2015). Fortunately, other federal agencies and some private foundations are less reticent (Frankel 2015). As the benefits of firearm research become evident in its application toward effective interventions, we hope that the federal government will also begin to appropriate funding for firearm research.

Mental health resources are woefully underfunded. Increased funding for these resources is always welcomed, and commitments to increase and improve access to mental health have been made. For example, in 2014, the Department of Health and Human Services (HHS) awarded $99 million to train new youth mental health providers and increase youth access to mental health services (U.S. Department of Health & Human Services 2014). Bills to reform and fund mental health services have been introduced in Congress, in both the House of Representatives (e.g., Representative Tim Murphy's proposed Helping Families in Mental Health Crisis Act, H.R. 3717, proposed in 2013, amended and reproposed in 2015 as H.R. 2646) and the Senate (e.g., Senators Cassidy and Chris Murphy's 2015 proposed Mental Health Reform Act, S. 1893).

Nevertheless, such funding and reform is expressly linked to highly publicized incidents gun violence and mass shootings, reinforcing the misperception that those with mental illness are dangerously violent. HHS's grant awards were explicitly associated with President Obama's initiatives announced following the 2012 Sandy Hook shootings (The White House 2013). Although Senator Chris Murphy stated he was "certainly nervous about equating mental illness with violence" (Alpert 2015), he also stated that "his bill is 'part of a response' to a string of mass shootings across the country...including the Newtown shooting in 2012..." (Cirisano 2015). Calls for increased funding for and reform of mental health resources, however well intentioned, are exploiting a negative stereotype of those with mental illness that is not supported by research evidence. Moreover, improved mental health care, although desperately needed, will not measurably impact the type of gun violence at which such legislation is directed and is not a substitute for directly addressing the morbidity and mortality of gun violence.

What This Book Does Not Address

A discussion of each and every possible intervention regarding firearm violence and mental illness would require many more authors and volumes. We have not, for example, addressed issues specific to improving the safety of firearms through technology, such as personalizing firearms, or initiatives such as challenging the immunity of firearm manufacturers from product liability. We have not discussed the efficacy of different types of treatment for mental illness or addressed which of these are more effective in decreasing violent behavior. We also have not addressed pediatric issues or perspectives, although we recognize that accidental firearm injuries are the second leading cause of death for children in the United States (Centers for Disease Control and Prevention 2015).

Additionally, we recognize that the issues of mental illness and firearm violence, particularly firearm suicide, are nowhere more acute than in military and veteran communities, where suicide rates have risen dramatically over the past decade (Ursano et al. 2015). However, we have not specifically addressed the issues unique to veterans related to suicide, mental illness, access to firearms, and access to mental health treatment. We also have chosen not to address the psychological issues related to gun ownership—neither those issues associated with individuals nor those associated with advocacy groups. Finally, although we recognize the tragic toll that gun violence takes on those who are injured, or those whose loved ones are killed or injured, we do not address the psychiatric aftermath of firearm trauma.

Chapter Format and Content

Each chapter begins with several common misconceptions regarding gun violence and mental illness specific to the chapter's topic. These are followed by corresponding evidence-based facts related to the misconceptions. Each chapter ends with recommendations for interventions, based on the evidence reviewed and the discussion in the body of the chapter. The appendix to this volume is a list of resources that we hope will assist individuals, communities, and policy makers in addressing and we hope mitigating the tolls from gun violence and mental illness in the United States. This list is not intended to be comprehensive; rather, we hope it will give those interested a place to start their inquiries.

Finally, a few words regarding content: An edited volume will inevitably include some repetition of material across chapters. We have tried to limit this as much as possible without interrupting the flow of a chapter's arguments or discussion, but we recognize that some information is reviewed or provided in more than one chapter. We hope this serves to reinforce the significance of this information. In addition, even when presented more than once, the information is typically presented from different perspectives, which we hope will stimulate additional thought.

In conclusion, we hope this volume helps refocus discussions of mental illness and gun violence. Although individuals, with or without mental illness, who perpetrate mass shootings cause inestimable harm, their actions represent the least statistically significant type of gun violence. Individuals with mental illness who become violent rarely use firearms. When they do, they most often kill themselves rather than others. By adopting policies that broaden access to and engagement in mental health treatment and limiting access to firearms at times of crisis, we can potentially decrease rates of firearm suicide. By focusing on individuals in crisis, whether or not they suffer from mental illness, such policies may also help avert interpersonal firearm homicides and injuries, including those from mass shootings.

References

Alpert B: Sens. Cassidy and Murphy disagree on gun control, but unify for better mental health treatment. The Times-Picayune, August 4, 2015. Available at http://www.nola.com/politics/index.ssf/2015/08/sens_cassidy_and_murphy_disagr.html. Accessed August 5, 2015.

American Medical Association: Public Health Improvement. 2015. Available at: http://www.ama-assn.org/ama/pub/advocacy/state-advocacy-arc/state-advocacy-campaigns/public-health-improvement.page. Accessed February 11, 2015.

American Psychiatric Association: American Psychiatric Association Principles of Medical Ethics With Annotations Especially Applicable to Psychiatry. Washington, DC, American Psychiatric Association, 2013

Appelbaum PS: Public safety, mental disorders, and guns. JAMA Psychiatry 70(6):565–566, 2013 23553282

Associated Press: NRA: get "homicidal maniacs" off streets. USA Today, September 22, 2013

Bjelopera JP, Bagalman E, Caldwell SW, et al: Public Mass Shootings in the United States: Selected Implications for Federal Public Health and Safety Policy. Washington, DC, Congressional Research Service, 2013

Blair JP, Schweit KW: A Study of Active Shooter Incidents 2000–2013. Washington, DC, Federal Bureau of Investigation, U.S. Department of Justice, 2014

Bloomberg M: Statement of Mayor Bloomberg on Upcoming Anniversary of Newtown Massacre and Latest Report From Mayors Against Illegal Guns. New York, New York City Office of the Mayor, 2013. Available at: http://www1.nyc.gov/office-of-the-mayor/news/399-13/statement-mayor-bloomberg-upcoming-anniversary-newtown-massacre-latest-report-from. Accessed August 4, 2015.

Butkus R, Doherty R, Daniel H, et al: Reducing firearm-related injuries and deaths in the United States: executive summary of a policy position paper from the American College of Physicians. Ann Intern Med 160(12):858–860, 2014 24722815

Carroll L: Cruz: Obama's surgeon general pick is not a "health professional." Politifact, October 23, 2014

Centers for Disease Control and Prevention: Injury Prevention & Control: Data & Statistics. Atlanta, GA, Centers for Disease Control and Prevention, 2015. Available at: http://www.cdc.gov/injury/wisqars/index.html. Accessed February 11, 2015.

Choe JY, Teplin LA, Abram KM: Perpetration of violence, violent victimization, and severe mental illness: balancing public health concerns. Psychiatr Serv 59(2):153–164, 2008 18245157

Christoffel KK: Firearm injuries: epidemic then, endemic now. Am J Public Health 97(4):626–629, 2007 17329653

Cirisano T: Murphy proposes package of mental health reforms. CT Post, August 4, 2015. Available at: http://www.ctpost.com/news/article/Murphy-proposes-package-of-mental-health-reforms-6424754.php. Accessed August 5, 2015.

Cooper A, Smith EL: Homicide in the U.S. Known to Law Enforcement, 2011. Washington, DC, Bureau of Justice Statistics, 2013

Curry T: NRA chief: if putting armed police in schools is crazy, "then call me crazy." NBC News, December 23, 2012

Department of Justice, Bureau of Alcohol, Tobacco, Firearms and Explosives: Amended Definition of "Adjudicated as a Mental Defective" and "Committed to a Mental Institution" (2010R-21P). Fed Regist 79(4):744–747, 2014

Desmarais SL, Van Dorn RA, Johnson KL, et al: Community violence perpetration and victimization among adults with mental illnesses. Am J Public Health 104(12):2342–2349, 2014 24524530

Elbogen EB, Johnson SC: The intricate link between violence and mental disorder: results from the National Epidemiologic Survey on Alcohol and Related Conditions. Arch Gen Psychiatry 66(2):152–161, 2009 19188537

Estroff SE, Swanson JW, Lachicotte WS, et al: Risk reconsidered: targets of violence in the social networks of people with serious psychiatric disorders. Soc Psychiatry Psychiatr Epidemiol 33 (suppl 1):S95–S101, 1998 9857786

Fazel S, Grann M: The population impact of severe mental illness on violent crime. Am J Psychiatry 163(8):1397–1403, 2006 16877653

Firearm and Injury Center at Penn: Firearm Injury in the United States. Philadelphia, PA, Firearm and Injury Center at Penn, 2011

Follman M, Aronsen G, Pan D, et al: US mass shootings, 1982–2012 (2013 update). Mother Jones, September 16, 2013. Available at: http://www.motherjones.com/politics/2012/12/mass-shootings-mother-jones-full-data. Accessed January 5, 2015.

Frank RG, Glied SA: Better but Not Well: Mental Health Policy in the United States Since 1950. Baltimore, MD, Johns Hopkins University Press, 2006

Frankel TC: Why the CDC still isn't researching gun violence, despite the ban being lifted two years ago. The Washington Post, January 14, 2015

Frattaroli S, Webster DW, Wintemute GJ: Implementing a public health approach to gun violence prevention: the importance of physician engagement. Ann Intern Med 158(9):697–698, 2013 23400374

Gostin LO (ed): Public Health, Law and Ethics, 2nd Edition. Berkeley, University of California Press, 2010

Hemenway D: Private Guns, Public Health. Ann Arbor, University of Michigan Press, 2004

Hemenway D: While We Were Sleeping: Success Stories in Injury and Violence Prevention. Berkeley, University of California Press, 2009

Hemenway D, Miller M: Public health approach to the prevention of gun violence. N Engl J Med 368(21):2033–2035, 2013 23581254

Institute of Medicine and National Research Council: Priorities for Research to Reduce the Threat of Firearm-Related Violence. Washington, DC, National Academies Press, 2013

Jamieson C: Gun violence research: history of the federal funding freeze. Psychological Science Agenda, February 2013. Available at: http://www.apa.org/science/about/psa/2013/02/gun-violence.aspx. Accessed March 1, 2015.

Karp A: Estimating Civilian Owned Firearms. Geneva, Switzerland, Small Arms Survey, 2011

Kellermann AL, Rivara FP: Silencing the science on gun research. JAMA 309(6):549–550, 2013 23262635

Krouse WJ: Gun Control Legislation. Washington, DC, Congressional Research Service, 2012

LaPierre W: Testimony of Wayne LaPierre, Executive Vice President, National Rifle Association of America, before the U.S. Senate Committee on the Judiciary hearing on "What Should America Do About Gun Violence?" Washington, DC, National Rifle Association, Institute for Legislative Action, January 30, 2013. Available at: https://www.nraila.org/articles/20130130/testimony-of-wayne-lapierre-before-the-us-senate-committee-on-the-judiciary-hearing-on-what-should-america-do-about-gun-violence. Accessed August 4, 2015.

Linker B: On the borderland of medical and disability history: a survey of the fields. Bull Hist Med 87(4):499–535, 2013 24362272

McGinty EE, Webster DW, Barry CL: Effects of news media messages about mass shootings on attitudes toward persons with serious mental illness and public support for gun control policies. Am J Psychiatry 170(5):494–501, 2013 23511486

Metzl JM, MacLeish KT: Mental illness, mass shootings, and the politics of American firearms. Am J Public Health 105(2):240–249, 2015 25496006

Miller M, Azrael D, Hemenway D: The epidemiology of case fatality rates for suicide in the northeast. Ann Emerg Med 43(6):723–730, 2004 15159703

Monahan J, Steadman HJ, Silver E, et al: Rethinking Risk Assessment: The MacArthur Study of Mental Disorder and Violence. New York, Oxford University Press, 2001

Mozaffarian D, Hemenway D, Ludwig DS: Curbing gun violence: lessons from public health successes. JAMA 309(6):551–552, 2013 23295618

National Highway Traffic Safety Administration: U.S. Department of Transportation announces decline in traffic fatalities in 2013. National Highway Traffic Safety Administration, December 19, 2014. Available at: http://www.nhtsa.gov/About+NHTSA/Press+Releases/2014/traffic-deaths-decline-in-2013. Accessed February 11, 2015.

National Rifle Association Institute for Legislative Action: Bad medicine for gun owners: confirmation vote looms for Obama's anti-gun surgeon general nominee. NRA-ILA, December 12, 2014. Available at: https://www.nraila.org/articles/20141212/bad-medicine-for-gun-owners-confirmation-vote-looms-for-obamas-anti-gun-surgeon-general-nominee. Accessed February 10, 2015.

NBC Meet the Press: December 23: Wayne LaPierre, Chuck Schumer, Lindsey Graham, Jason Chaffetz, Harold Ford Jr., Andrea Mitchell, Chuck Todd. Transcripts on Meet the Press, 2012

Nock MK, Borges G, Bromet EJ, et al: Suicide and suicidal behavior. Epidemiol Rev 30:133–154, 2008 18653727

Nordström A, Kullgren G: Victim relations and victim gender in violent crimes committed by offenders with schizophrenia. Soc Psychiatry Psychiatr Epidemiol 38(6):326–330, 2003 12799783

Overberg P, Hoyer M, Hannan M, et al: Explore the data on U.S. mass killings since 2006. USA Today, posted December 2, 2013, updated 2015. Available at: http://www.usatoday.com/story/news/nation/2013/09/16/mass-killings-data-map/2820423/. Accessed March 1, 2015.

Pew Research Center: Why own a gun? Protection is now top reason. PewResearch.org, Washington, DC, May 9, 2013. Available at: http://www.pewresearch.org/daily-number/why-own-a-gun-protection-is-now-top-reason. Accessed January 6, 2015.

Richardson EG, Hemenway D: Homicide, suicide, and unintentional firearm fatality: comparing the United States with other high-income countries, 2003. J Trauma 70(1):238–243, 2011 20571454

Rosenberg ML: Firearm injuries and death: the cost of shooting in the dark. JAMA Psychiatry 70(10):1007–1008, 2013 23925927

Roy L, Crocker AG, Nicholls TL, et al: Criminal behavior and victimization among homeless individuals with severe mental illness: a systematic review. Psychiatr Serv 65(6):739–750, 2014 24535245

Saad L: Americans fault mental health system most for gun violence. Gallup, September 20, 2013. Available at: http://www.gallup.com/poll/164507/americans-fault-mental-health-system-gun-violence.aspx. Accessed March 20, 2015.

Selker HP, Selker KM, Schwartz MD: Gun violence is a health crisis: physicians' responsibilities. J Gen Intern Med 28(5):601–602, 2013 23558774

Siegel M, Ross CS, King C 3rd: The relationship between gun ownership and firearm homicide rates in the United States, 1981–2010. Am J Public Health 103(11):2098–2105, 2013 24028252

Siegel M, Negussie Y, Vanture S, et al: The relationship between gun ownership and stranger and nonstranger firearm homicide rates in the United States, 1981–2010. Am J Public Health 104(10):1912–1919, 2014 25121817

Steadman HJ, Mulvey EP, Monahan J, et al: Violence by people discharged from acute psychiatric inpatient facilities and by others in the same neighborhoods. Arch Gen Psychiatry 55(5):393–401, 1998 9596041

Steadman HJ, Monahan J, Pinals DA, et al: Gun violence and victimization of strangers by persons with a mental illness: data from the MacArthur Violence Risk Assessment Study. Psychiatr Serv Jun 15, 2015 26073414 [Epub ahead of print]

Swanson JW: Explaining rare acts of violence: the limits of evidence from population research. Psychiatr Serv 62(11):1369–1371, 2011 22211218

Swanson J: Mental illness and new gun law reforms: the promise and peril of crisis-driven policy. JAMA 309(12):1233–1234, 2013 23392291

Swanson JW, Robertson AG, Frisman LK, et al: Preventing gun violence involving people with serious mental illness, in Reducing Gun Violence in America: Informing Policy With Evidence and Analysis. Edited by Webster DW, Vernick JS. Baltimore, MD, Johns Hopkins University Press, 2013, pp 33–51

Swanson JW, Sampson NA, Petukhova MV, et al: Guns, impulsive angry behavior, and mental disorders: results from the National Comorbidity Survey Replication (NCS-R). Behav Sci Law, Apr 8, 2015 25850688 (Epub ahead of print)

Torrey EF, Fuller DA, Geller MD, et al: No Room at the Inn: Trends and Consequences of Closing Public Psychiatric Hospitals, 2005–2010. Arlington, VA, Treatment Advocacy Center, 2012

Ursano RJ, Kessler RC, Stein MD, et al: Suicide attempts in the US Army during the wars in Afghanistan and Iraq, 2004-2009. JAMA Psychiatry. July 8, 2015; doi: 10.1001/jamapsychiatry.2015.0987. Accessed August 5, 2015.

U.S. Department of Health and Human Services: HHS announces $99 million in new grants to improve mental health services for young people. HHS.gov, September 22, 2014. Available at: http://www.hhs.gov/news/press/2014pres/09/20140922a.html. Accessed March 2, 2015.

Van Dorn R, Volavka J, Johnson N: Mental disorder and violence: is there a relationship beyond substance use? Soc Psychiatry Psychiatr Epidemiol 47(3):487–503, 2012 21359532

Violence Policy Center: Gun deaths outpace motor vehicle deaths in 10 states in 2009 new analysis shows. Available at: http://www.vpc.org/press/1205gunsvscars.htm. Accessed August 20, 2015a.

Violence Policy Center: Gun deaths outpace motor vehicle deaths in 12 states and the District of Columbia in 2010. Available at: http://www.vpc.org/studies/gunsvscars13.pdf. Accessed August 20, 2015b.

Violence Policy Center: Gun deaths outpace motor vehicle deaths in 14 states and the District of Columbia in 2011. Available at: http://www.vpc.org/press/1407cars.htm. Accessed August 20, 2015c.

Weinberger SE, Hoyt DB, Lawrence HC, et al: Firearm-related injury and death in the United States: a call to action from 8 health professional organizations and the American Bar Association. Ann Intern Med 162(7):513–516, 2015 25706470

The White House: Now Is the Time: The President's Plan to Protect Our Children and Our Communities by Reducing Gun Violence. Washington, DC, The White House, January 16, 2013. Available at: http://www.whitehouse.gov/sites/default/files/docs/wh_now_is_the_time_full.pdf. Accessed March 2, 2015.

Wintemute GJ: Responding to the crisis of firearm violence in the United States: comment on "Firearm legislation and firearm-related fatalities in the United States." JAMA Intern Med 173(9):740–741, 2013 23467768

Wintemute GJ: The epidemiology of firearm violence in the twenty-first century United States. Annu Rev Public Health 36:5–19, 2015 25533263

Yang LH, Anglin DM, Wonpat-Borja AJ, et al: Public stigma associated with psychosis risk syndrome in a college population: implications for peer intervention. Psychiatr Serv 64(3):284–288, 2013 23450386

Acknowledgments

Writing and editing this volume has been a fascinating journey, and many people have provided assistance or support along the way. My thanks go first to Robert I. Simon, M.D., for his assistance with this book, as well as the many other books and projects I have had the privilege to share with him. I also thank him for his friendship and invaluable mentorship. I also thank Robert E. Hales, M.D., Rebecca Rinehart, John McDuffie, and American Psychiatric Association Publishing for their enthusiasm and support for this project.

This volume would not have been possible without the contributions of the chapter authors. They have my profound gratitude for being willing to think outside the box and for their patience with the editing process. Special thanks go to my former chief resident, Marilyn Price, M.D., for her help, support, and years of friendship.

I thank Josh Horwitz, J.D., executive director of the Educational Fund to Stop Gun Violence, for inviting me to join the Johns Hopkins Bloomberg School of Public Health Consortium for Risk-Based Firearm Policy. Josh and other members of the Consortium, as well as friends and colleagues in the American Academy of Psychiatry and the Law and the American Psychiatric Association, helped deepen my understanding of some of the complex issues discussed in this text. Special thanks and recognition go to Paul Appelbaum, M.D., Renée Binder, M.D., and Richard Bonnie, LL.B., for their responsiveness in answering my many questions. Jeffrey Swanson, Ph.D., has my gratitude for his exceptional tolerance of my many, many inquiries and his detailed responses.

I thank Jill Chmelik, my executive editorial manager, for her organizational support and constant encouragement; Charles Scott Dorris, MLIS, digital information services librarian at the Georgetown University Medical Center Dahlgren Memorial Library, for helping me navigate the technological mysteries of a twenty-first-century library; and William Krouse of the Congressional Research Service, for his time in discussing some of the statistical issues involved in firearm research. I thank Thomas G. Gutheil, M.D., and Jonathan Gold, Ph.D., for their support.

Finally, I'd like to thank Ian Jeff Nyden, Ph.D., always my first and best editor, for his constructive criticism, wisdom, and endless support, and Joshua and Alix Nyden for their encouragement.

Liza H. Gold, M.D.

PART I

Defining the Problems

1

Gun Violence and Serious Mental Illness

Emma E. McGinty, Ph.D., M.S.
Daniel W. Webster, Sc.D., M.P.H.

Common Misperceptions

☒ Most persons with serious mental illnesses, such as schizophrenia or bipolar disorder, are at high risk of committing violence toward others.

☒ Serious mental illness is one of the primary causes of gun violence in the United States.

☒ People with serious mental illness are more likely to perpetrate violent crime than to be victims of violent crime.

Evidence-Based Facts

☑ Most persons with serious mental illness are never violent. However, small subgroups of persons with serious mental illness are at increased risk of violence during certain high-risk periods, such as during a first episode of psychosis and the period surrounding inpatient psychiatric hospitalization.

☑ People with serious mental illness are rarely violent. Only 3%–5% of all violence, including but not limited to firearm violence, is attributable to serious mental illness. The large majority of gun violence toward others is not caused by mental illness.

☑ People with serious mental illness are far more likely to be the victims of violence, including but not limited to firearm violence, than the perpetrators of violent acts. Rates of violent crime victimization are 12 times higher among the population of persons with serious mental illness than among the overall U.S. population.

Gun violence is a critical public health problem in the United States. Of the 31,672 deaths in 2010 by firearms, 11,078 (35%) were homicides; 19,392 (61%) were suicides; and 1,202 (4%) were accidents, the result of legal intervention (e.g., a death in the course of an arrest), or deaths of undetermined intent (National Center for Injury Prevention and Control 2010). Across all age groups, firearm suicide and homicide are the fourth and fifth leading causes of injury-related death in the United States. Firearms are a leading cause of death among young people: firearm homicide is the second leading cause of injury-related death among those ages 15–24 and the third leading cause of injury-related death among adults ages 25–34, and firearm suicide is the fourth leading cause of injury-related death among these same age groups (National Center for Injury Prevention and Control 2014). In addition to this staggering death toll, in 2012 in the United States, more than 81,000 persons were treated in hospital emergency departments for nonfatal gunshot wounds, the bulk of which resulted from criminal assaults (National Center for Injury Prevention and Control 2012).

Although rare compared with other forms of gun violence, mass shootings receive extensive, nationwide news coverage (McGinty et al. 2014b) and capture the public's attention in a way that "everyday" gun violence does not. Some of the highest-profile mass shootings are those that occurred in 2007 at Virginia Tech (33 dead, including the shooter, and 17 wounded); in 2011 in Tucson, Arizona (6 dead and 13 wounded); in 2012 in Aurora, Colorado (12 dead and 70 wounded); in 2012 in Newtown, Connecticut (28 dead, including the shooter); in 2014 at Fort Hood, Texas (4 dead, including the shooter, and 16 wounded), and in Isla Vista, California (7 dead, including the shooter, and 7 wounded); and in 2015 in Charleston, South Carolina (9 dead and 1 wounded).

Although the United States has experienced far too many of these events, mass shootings are comparatively rare and represent only a small fraction of firearm deaths in the United States (Swanson et al. 2015). Nevertheless, mass shootings play an important role in Americans' understanding of the causes of and support for policy responses to gun violence (McGinty et al. 2014a). High-profile mass shootings heighten public attention to the problem of gun violence generally, and the issue of gun violence and mental illness in particular.

Serious mental illness, which includes conditions such as schizophrenia and bipolar disorder (Department of Health and Mental Hygiene and the Judiciary

2008), seems to have played a role in several mass shootings. The Virginia Tech (Friedman 2009), Tucson (Santos 2012), and Aurora (Sallinger 2012) shooters appear to have had serious mental illness, and the perpetrator of the 2014 Fort Hood shooting also had a history of mental illness (Sanchez and Brumfield 2014), although it is unclear what role mental illness played in his actions. The family of the Newtown shooter reported that he had an autism spectrum disorder and obsessive-compulsive disorder, but neither of these conditions is associated with increased risk of violence and there is no evidence that the shooter also suffered from a serious mental illness such as schizophrenia (Griffin 2013).

Although much of the American public perceives a strong and direct link between serious mental illness and gun violence (Barry et al. 2013), such a link is not supported by the research evidence. Some small subgroups of persons with serious mental illness are at certain times at heightened risk of committing violence toward others. However, only a very small proportion of all incidents of violence toward others (including but not limited to firearm violence) is attributable to mental illness (3%–5%) (Swanson et al. 1990, 2015). The majority of people with serious mental illness are never violent, and most instances of violence committed by this group do not involve firearms (Swanson et al. 2013, 2015). Other risk factors, such as substance abuse, are stronger predictors of future violence than is mental illness (McGinty et al. 2014a; Swanson et al. 2015). In contrast, mental illnesses such as depression significantly increase risk for suicide, which accounts for over 60% of firearm deaths in the United States each year (Nock et al. 2008; Rihmer 2007; Swanson et al. 2015).

In this chapter we focus on the relationship between mental illness and perpetration of violence toward others and summarize the current research evidence regarding this complex relationship. The evidence regarding the relationship between mental illness, firearms, and suicide, which accounts for the highest mortality rates due to gun violence, is reviewed in Chapter 2, "Firearms and Suicide in the United States."

Epidemiological Relationship Between Mental Illness and Violence Toward Others

Prevalence of Mental Illnesses

Mental illness is a significant public health problem in the United States. In a given year, about 20% of the U.S. population, including adults, adolescents, and children, experience a mental illness, and a high proportion of these individuals do not receive adequate treatment (Frank and Glied 2006). The best available data indicate that among adults, anxiety disorders are the most prevalent type of mental health condition (18.1%), followed by mood disorders such as major depressive disorder or bipolar disorder (9.5%), impulse-control disorders such as attention-deficit/hyperactivity disorder (8.9%), and substance use disorders (3.8%) (Kessler et al. 2005b). Among adolescents, 31.9% experience an anxiety disorder, 14.3% experience a mood disorder, 19.6% experience an impulse-control disorder, and 11.4% experience a substance use disorder at some point between ages 13 and 18 (Merikangas et al. 2010). About 4% of American adults experience serious mental illness, which includes conditions that cause impairment and disability, such as schizophrenia, bipolar disorder, and major depression (National Institute of Mental Health 2014).

Although the vast majority of persons with mental illness never become violent toward others, mental illness can increase the risk for perpetration of violence in some instances (Swanson et al. 2015). However, incidents of gun violence perpetrated by individuals with serious mental illness are very rare when compared to the yearly number of incidents of gun violence in the United States (Swanson et al. 2015). Therefore, the epidemiological studies of the relationship between serious mental illness and gun violence summarized in this chapter examine the role of mental illness in perpetration of all serious violence toward others, including but not limited to gun violence, rather than gun violence specifically.

Links Between Mental Illness and Violence

The earliest large-scale epidemiological studies of the prevalence of violence among the population with mental illness took place in the 1990s. In the first of these, the Epidemiologic Catchment Area (ECA) study (Swanson et al. 1990), researchers randomly selected households in five U.S. cities: New Haven, Connecticut; Baltimore, Maryland; St. Louis, Missouri; Raleigh-Durham, North Carolina; and Los Angeles, California. To measure the prevalence of mental disorders among persons living in the selected households, the ECA researchers administered structured diagnostic interviews. To measure violence, the researchers asked questions about the frequency and type of violent behaviors, such as pushing, hitting, or threatening to harm or harming someone with a weapon. Violence considered attributable to symptoms of mental illness was defined as acts that occurred as a direct result of the symptoms or manifestations of mental illness, such as hallucinations or delusions. Prevalence of substance use disorders was also assessed. In addition, ECA researchers collected survey data on demographic characteristics, socioeconomic status, and violent behavior (Swanson et al. 1990).

Using pooled data from three of the ECA sites (Baltimore, St. Louis, and Los Angeles), Swanson and colleagues examined the association between mental illness and violence toward others (Swanson et al. 1990). They found a relatively small but statistically significant positive association: approximately 12% of persons with serious mental illness (defined as schizophrenia, bipolar disorder, or major depression) had committed any minor or serious violence in the past year, compared to about 2% of persons without a mental illness or substance use disorder. The authors also used the ECA data to estimate the proportion of all violence in the United States that is attributable to mental illness, and concluded that approximately 3%–5% of all violence toward others, including but not limited to gun violence, is directly related to mental illness.

In addition, the ECA researchers found that a number of demographic factors, including youth, male gender, low socioeconomic status, and particularly substance abuse, were strong predictors of violence among ECA participants with and without mental illness (Swanson et al. 1990). Although 12% of persons with a serious mental illness had committed any minor or serious violence in the past 12 months, only 7% of persons with serious mental illness but no comorbid substance abuse had demonstrated violent behavior in the same period. Similarly, Swanson and colleagues found that the lifetime prevalence of committing violence was 15% for persons without mental illness or substance abuse, 33% for those with serious mental illness alone, and 55% for those with comorbid serious mental illness and substance abuse.

The investigation by Swanson et al. (1990) laid the groundwork for much of the epidemiological research to come and established several key points, including the following:

1. Most persons with mental illness are never violent.
2. Most violence (95%–97%), including but not limited to gun violence, is not attributable to mental illness.
3. The risk of violence toward others is heightened among a subset of persons with serious mental illness.
4. Risk factors such as substance abuse and low socioeconomic status are strong predictors of violence in populations with and without mental illness.

The ECA findings have been replicated in several subsequent studies. In the MacArthur Violence Risk Assessment Study (Steadman et al. 1998), researchers followed 1,136 persons with mental illness for 1 year following discharge from a psychiatric hospital. Data were collected from 1992 to 1995, and study participants were interviewed every 10 weeks to assess violent behavior. In addition, researchers used interviews with family and friends, hospital records, and police records to augment self-reports of violent behavior (Steadman et al. 1998). Violence among the study cohort with mental illness was compared with violence among a comparison group composed of 519 individuals living in the same neighborhoods (defined by census tracts) in which study participants resided after they were discharged from the hospital (Steadman et al. 1998). Comparison group participants were interviewed once about violent behavior in the past 10 weeks.

Using these data, Steadman et al. (1998) found that persons with mental illness alone and no comorbid substance abuse were no more likely than other members of the community to commit violence. They found, however, that substance abuse, either alone or in concert with mental illness, substantially increased the risk of violence. Importantly, both the patient and comparison groups in this study were drawn from disadvantaged neighborhoods with higher base rates of violent crime than among the ECA study participants. One interpretation of the MacArthur study's findings (Steadman et al. 2015) is that these socioeconomic and environmental influences on violence are stronger than the effects of mental illness on violence, in effect overpowering the relationship between serious mental illness and violence observed in the ECA study.

In a 2015 study, Steadman and colleagues went back to the original MacArthur study data to examine the prevalence of gun violence and of violent acts against stranger victims among the study cohort. The authors found that 2% of the study participants committed a violent act involving a firearm in the year following a psychiatric hospitalization, 6% committed a violent act involving a stranger victim, and 1% committed violence that involved both a gun and a stranger victim. The low prevalence of firearm violence directed at strangers among this population suggests that policies designed specifically to prevent persons with mental illness from having guns may have a limited effect on rates of gun violence in the United States.

Van Dorn et al. (2012) analyzed data from the National Epidemiologic Survey on Alcohol and Related Conditions, a two-wave national survey of 34,653 respondents conducted in 2001–2003 (wave 1) and 2004–2005 (wave 2). Respondents with serious mental illness, again defined as schizophrenia, bipolar disorder, and major depression, were asked the following questions to measure violence (Van Dorn et al. 2012):

Since the last interview, did you

a. use a weapon like a stick, knife, or gun in a fight?
b. hit someone so hard that you injured them or they had to see a doctor?
c. start a fire on purpose to destroy someone's property or just to see it burn?
d. force someone to have sex with you against their will?
e. get into a physical fight when or right after drinking?
f. get into a fight when under the influence of [a] drug?
g. physically hurt another person in any way on purpose?
h. get into a fight that came to swapping blows with someone like a husband, wife, boyfriend, or girlfriend?
i. get into a lot of fights you started?

Serious violence was defined as items a–d; *substance-related violence* was defined as items e and f.

Similar to Swanson et al.'s (1990) ECA study results, findings from Van Dorn et al.'s (2012) study suggested that persons with serious mental illness, with or without comorbid substance use, were at a statistically significant heightened risk of committing violence toward others. The latter researchers also found a significant gradient in prevalence of violence by type of condition. Less than 1% of respondents with no mental illness or substance use disorders committed violence, compared with 8.4% of persons with serious mental illness alone, 7.9% of persons with substance use disorders alone, and 18.1% of persons with comorbid serious mental illness and substance abuse (Van Dorn et al. 2012). Among persons with mental illnesses other than schizophrenia, bipolar disorder, or major depression, the prevalence of violence was 3.4%. Comorbid substance abuse significantly heightened risk of violence among this group as well: persons with mental illnesses other than the three conditions defined as serious mental illness and comorbid substance abuse had a prevalence of violence of 15.7%. Childhood abuse and neglect, household antisocial behavior (e.g., arrests, fighting, or substance abuse among household members), binge drinking, and stressful life events were also associated with increased risk of violence.

Risk of Violence in Subpopulations of Persons With Serious Mental Illness

The research evidence clearly shows that although the vast majority of persons with mental illness rarely commit acts of violence toward others (and of these acts only a small proportion involve firearms), small subgroups of persons with mental illness are at heightened risk of violence as a result of their condition (Consortium for Risk-Based Firearm Policy 2013; Swanson et al. 2015). The research evidence suggests that two groups of adults in particular—involuntarily committed inpatients and persons experiencing first-episode psychosis—are at elevated risk of committing violence toward others (Choe et al. 2008; Consortium for Risk-Based Firearm Policy 2013; Large and Nielssen 2011). Based on reviews and meta-analyses averaging the results of multiple studies, the prevalence of any minor or serious violence is 36% among involuntarily committed inpatients (Choe et al. 2008; Swanson et al. 2015) and 37% among persons with first-episode psychosis (Large and Nielssen 2011; Swanson et al. 2015). The definition of *violence* used to estimate these prevalence rates includes both minor acts, such as hitting and pushing, and serious acts, such as threatening to harm or harming someone with a weapon (Choe et al. 2008). Compared with the approximate 2.3% base rate of violence in the overall U.S. population, rates of violence toward others are also elevated among persons with serious mental illness seen in hospital emergency departments (23%), discharged from inpatient psychiatric care (13%), living in the community (10%), and receiving outpatient treatment (8%) (Choe et al. 2008; Swanson et al. 2015).

One feature of serious mental illness that heightens risk for perpetration of violence is psychosis (Large and Nielssen 2011). The research evidence consistently shows a modest association between psychosis and violent offending.

Psychosis is characterized by "profound disturbances in thought, perception, and behavior" (Douglas et al. 2009, p. 681). These disturbances can include delusions, hallucinations, derealization, depersonalization, disorganized thought patterns, and behavioral disturbances such as extreme agitation or lethargy. *Delusions* are defined as false beliefs, often held with conviction even in the face of acts suggesting that the beliefs cannot possibly be true. *Hallucinations* involve hearing or seeing things that are not there, and *derealization* and *depersonalization* are defined as the sense that the external world (*derealization*) and oneself as an autonomous human being (*depersonalization*) are no longer real. *Disorganized thought patterns* and *behavioral disturbances* are often characterized by extreme changes in mood, deterioration of personal hygiene, and social withdrawal (Douglas et al. 2009).

Psychotic symptoms, particularly hallucinations and delusions, can be elements of serious mental illnesses such as schizophrenia, bipolar disorder, and (less frequently) major depression. They can also be caused by substance abuse (Douglas et al. 2009). Psychosis can result in violence in several ways. First, psychotic symptoms, such as auditory hallucinations commanding an individual to hurt a family member, may directly motivate individuals to commit violence (Douglas et al. 2009). Alternatively, individuals can develop delusional beliefs that others are intending to hurt them, and might then lash out in violence in self-defense. Second, some types of psychosis can destabilize behavior and impair judgment and decision making. This can reduce the ability to effectively manage interpersonal conflicts, leading to impulsive acts of violence (Douglas et al. 2009). Third, psychosis can disinhibit violent behavior by impairing an individual's ability to experience empathy, remorse, or anxiety. In a meta-analysis of 204 studies examining the relationship between psychosis and violence, Douglas et al. (2009) concluded that psychosis is associated with a modest but consistent elevated risk of violence. Importantly, the research evidence to date does not paint a clear picture of which specific symptoms of psychosis, and in which settings and populations, the risk of violence toward others is increased. Additional research in this area is needed.

A person's first episode of psychosis is a particularly high-risk period for perpetration of violence. In a meta-analysis of nine studies examining violence among persons experiencing first-episode psychosis, Large and Nielssen (2011) concluded that about one-third of patients had exhibited some form of violence prior to entering treatment and that about 1 in 6 had committed a serious act of violence such as assaulting another person. However, fewer than 1 in 100 persons with first-episode psychosis in the studies reviewed had committed an assault resulting in serious injury to another person.

Conduct disorder, although not classified as a serious mental illness, is also associated with risk of violence. The diagnosis of conduct disorder encompasses a group of behavioral and emotional symptoms and issues in youth, including difficulty following rules and exhibiting socially unacceptable behaviors (Hodgins et al. 2008). Among children, a robust body of research evidence shows that conduct disorder increases risk of violence (Frank and McGuire 2011; Loeber et al. 2009; Mueser et al. 1999; Murray and Farrington 2010). Furthermore, persons with serious mental illness who also have a history of conduct disorder are at increased risk of aggressive behavior and violent crime (Hodgins et al. 2008).

Comorbid Risk Factors for Violence in the Population With Serious Mental Illness

The presence of comorbid risk factors in violence is a common finding in both population-level studies, such as the ECA and MacArthur Violence Risk Assessment studies (Steadman et al. 1998; Swanson et al. 1990), and studies of subgroups of persons with serious mental illness (Large and Nielssen 2011). Studies consistently show that youth, male gender, low socioeconomic status, history of childhood abuse or neglect, history of violent behavior, and substance use are risk factors for perpetration of violence (Consortium for Risk-Based Firearm Policy 2013; Swanson et al. 1990, 2015). These risk factors for violence are not specific to the population with serious mental illness but are strong predictors of violence in the U.S. population as a whole (Consortium for Risk-Based Firearm Policy 2013; Swanson et al. 1990, 2015; Van Dorn et al. 2012).

In addition, many of these risk factors are more prevalent among persons with serious mental illness (Elbogen and Johnson 2009; Swanson et al. 2015). A robust body of literature shows that childhood abuse and neglect are associated with mental illness (and substance abuse) in adulthood (Elbogen and Johnson 2009; Kendler et al. 2000; Van Dorn et al. 2012), and the prevalence of substance abuse is significantly heightened among persons with serious mental illness (Elbogen and Johnson 2009). The onset of serious mental illness typically occurs in late adolescence or young adulthood and therefore often significantly disrupts potential educational and career achievement (Frank and Glied 2006). As a result, low socioeconomic status among persons with serious mental illness, many of whom rely on Supplemental Security Income benefits, is common (Frank and Glied 2006). An estimated 46% of Americans with serious mental illness have comorbid substance abuse or dependence at some point during their lifetime (Elbogen and Johnson 2009), compared with 14.6% of the overall U.S. population (Kessler et al. 2005a).

Prediction of Future Violence Among Individuals With Serious Mental Illness

To prevent acts of violence among persons with serious mental illness before they occur requires the ability to accurately predict which individuals are likely to commit violent acts toward others. However, the usefulness of current risk assessment tools for identifying individuals who are likely to become violent is limited. Although such tools are fairly accurate at identifying persons with serious mental illness who are *unlikely* to perpetrate violence toward others, they yield far less accurate predictions of which individuals *will* become violent. This lack of accuracy is largely due to the low base rates of violence among persons with serious mental illness: rare events are inherently difficult to predict (Buchanan 2008; Fazel et al. 2012).

In a 2012 systematic review and meta-analysis, Fazel et al. (2012) studied the effectiveness of risk assessments in 73 different study populations. The authors found that existing risk assessment tools produced low to moderate positive predictive values for violent offending; the median was 41% (interquartile range: 27%–60%). This means that of all the individuals who screened positive as being likely to commit violence, 41% went on to commit a violent act within the periods studied. Negative predicted values—that is, the proportions of persons who screened negative who did not go on to commit any violence—were higher; the median was 91% (interquartile range: 81%–95%).

Although existing risk assessment tools are reasonably good at correctly identifying individuals who are unlikely to become violent, they are far less accurate at identifying which persons will become violent in the future (Swanson et al. 2015). Violence risk assessment instruments and their role in the discussion of mental illness and gun violence are discussed in Chapter 9, "Structured Violence Risk Assessment." In summary, the relatively low positive predictive value of most risk assessment instruments makes it difficult to accurately identify and intervene with those specific individuals who will go on to perpetrate violence against others (McGinty et al. 2014a).

Epidemiology of Mental Illness and Violent Victimization

Although the American public has come to associate mental illness with perpetration of gun violence, particularly mass shootings, persons with serious mental illness are more likely to be the victims rather than the perpetrators of violent crime. Teplin et al. (2005) examined victimization in an epidemiological study of persons with serious mental illness receiving treatment at one of 16 mental health treatment agencies in Chicago, Illinois. The researchers defined persons with serious mental illness as individuals taking psychiatric medications for the previous 2 years or who had been admitted to a psychiatric hospital at any point during their lifetime. The researchers randomly selected persons with serious mental illness from the waiting rooms and client lists of organizations and interviewed them using the National Crime Victimization Survey. Because this instrument is a national survey, they were able to compare prevalence of victimization among their study sample of persons with serious mental illness with national rates (Teplin et al. 2005).

The researchers found that 25% of persons with serious mental illness were victims in the past year of violent crime, defined as attempted or completed rape/sexual assault, robbery, assault, or personal theft, compared with 3% of the overall U.S. population (Teplin et al. 2005). The annual incidence rate of violent crime in the group with serious mental illness was 168.2 incidents per 1,000 persons, compared with the general population rate of 39.9 incidents per 1,000 persons. Even after the researchers controlled for demographic differences, violent crime rates were nearly 12 times higher among persons with serious mental illness than in the overall U.S. population (Teplin et al. 2005).

These findings are supported by several additional studies. In a review of 10 studies of violent victimization among persons with mental illness, Choe et al. (2008) found that in study populations comprising outpatients with mental illness, 20%–34% had been violently victimized in the past year. In studies combining inpatients and outpatients, 35% of persons with mental illness had been victims of violence in the previous year.

Several factors increase the risk of violent victimization among persons with serious mental illness. The deinstitutionalization of individuals with chronic mental illness, which began in the mid-1950s, moved individuals with serious mental illness out of public mental hospitals and into the community (Frank and Glied 2006; Teplin et al. 2005) (see Chapter 8, "Accessing Mental Health Care," for more detailed discussion of this subject). With the introduction of new antipsychotic medications, mental health treatment leaders and policy makers believed that persons with serious mental illness could be effectively treated in the community (Frank and Glied 2006). However, this vision fell short.

Many communities had insufficient outpatient treatment resources to serve the population with serious mental illness, and the community mental health centers intended to care for this group were often underfunded (Frank and Glied 2006). In addition, the broader social services needed by persons with serious mental illness, including housing, employment, and disability support services, were unavailable in many communities (Frank and Glied 2006). As a result, rates of homelessness and incarceration among persons with serious mental illness have increased considerably (Frank and Glied 2006). Homelessness, unemployment, poverty, and criminal justice involvement all increase risk of victimization by placing persons with serious mental illness in situations where they are vulnerable to assault, robbery, or other crimes.

Translating Epidemiological Research Into Policy and Practice: A Public Health Approach

The evidence summarized in the previous section, "Epidemiological Relationship Between Mental Illness and Violence Toward Others," suggests a somewhat complex path forward for gun violence prevention interventions. On the one hand, some persons with serious mental health conditions, such as schizophrenia and bipolar disorder, are at heightened risk of perpetrating violence toward others, especially during high-risk periods such as the times surrounding inpatient psychiatric hospitalizations and first-episode psychosis. On the other hand, the large majority of gun violence is not caused by mental illness, and other risk factors, especially history of violent behavior and substance abuse, have a much stronger association with perpetration of violence. Potential interventions to reduce gun violence could be narrowly focused toward high-risk individuals with serious mental illness or toward the far larger group of perpetrators whose acts are not driven by a mental health disorder. In the remainder of this chapter, we consider the research evidence surrounding both types of interventions. In both cases, we approach gun violence prevention from the standpoint of public health theory.

Mental Illness and Gun Violence

The public health approach to addressing population health and social problems, such as gun violence and mental illness, seeks to reduce morbidity and mortality through interventions at multiple levels. A common model used to guide public health interventions, the Social-Ecological Model (National Center for Injury Prevention and Control, Division of Violence Prevention 2014), asserts that public health prevention strategies should address multiple levels of the problem, including individual, immediate social network (e.g., family and close friends), community, and societal levels. For example, hospitalization and follow-up treatment for a person with mental illness showing signs of presenting a danger toward others represent an individual-level intervention. Enlisting family and friends to help that person adhere to treatment is an intervention directed toward the immediate social network. Enactment of so-called gun-free school zones is an example of a community-level intervention to reduce gun violence. At the societal level, state and federal policies to prevent access to firearms by individuals at elevated risk of perpetrating acts of violence are another gun violence prevention strategy. In the public health approach to addressing complex, multifaceted problems such as gun violence, interventions at each of these levels are needed.

At the societal level, a common public health approach is regulating the upstream causes of a given problem. For example, legal regulation of tobacco use is a key strategy in the prevention of lung cancer. Similarly, many public health experts advocate increased regulation of the sugar-sweetened beverage industry (e.g., by raising soda taxes or passing laws that forbid soda and other sweetened drinks from being sold in schools) as a way to slow and reverse steep increases in childhood obesity in the United States (Kersh and Morone 2002).

In the case of gun violence, an obvious solution with the potential to have widespread impact on rates of firearm violence is to increase legal regulation of firearms. However, such regulation is limited by the constitutional landscape surrounding this issue (Vernick et al. 2011). In 2008 and 2010, landmark Supreme Court rulings affirmed that individual firearm ownership is a constitutional right in the United States. As a result, legal firearm prohibitions must be directed toward groups at clearly heightened risk of violence, such as felons, without infringing on the rights of law-abiding gun owners (Vernick et al. 2011).

Public health theory suggests that interventions focusing on risk factors for violence, which are prevalent throughout the entire U.S. population, will have a larger impact on overall rates of gun violence than individual-level interventions focused on decreasing violent behavior among persons with serious mental illness. In this context, the epidemiological research on the relationship between mental illness and violence summarized in the first section of this chapter can play a critical role by identifying groups of individuals who are at high risk of perpetrating violence. Firearm restrictions, even if only temporary, could be directed toward these high-risk groups.

In the remainder of this chapter, we focus on two categories of interventions directly supported by the epidemiological evidence on the relationship between mental illness and gun violence: 1) interventions focused on high-risk subgroups of persons with serious mental illness and 2) interventions focused on risk for violence in the overall population, including but not limited to persons with mental illness.

Interventions to Reduce Gun Violence Among Persons With Serious Mental Illness

Mental Health Treatment

In the public policy debates surrounding recent mass shootings, many experts, advocates, and policy makers have called for improvements to the mental health treatment system in the United States (Glied and Frank 2014; McGinty et al. 2014a). These improvements are much needed: almost 40% of Americans with serious mental illness and almost 60% of Americans with any mental illness do not receive treatment in a given year (Substance Abuse and Mental Health Services Administration 2013). Unmet mental health care needs even among those who receive treatment, indicating lack of or minimally adequate services, are common. In 2012, among adults who did receive some type of mental health service in the past year, 17.8% (6.1 million) reported an unmet need for mental health care (Substance Abuse and Mental Health Services Administration 2013). Furthermore, many persons with serious mental illness do not have access to social services demonstrated by evidence to support effective mental health treatment, such as supported housing and employment (Frank and Glied 2006).

An important component of a public health approach toward both mental illness and violence is ensuring that persons with mental illness receive the treatments they need to control symptoms that can lead to violence toward others (and suicide) and improve overall health and well-being. Mental illnesses are treatable health conditions. Effective treatments exist for serious conditions such as schizophrenia and bipolar disorder, first-episode psychosis, and conduct disorder.

The best available research evidence suggests that treatment does have the potential to reduce violent behavior among some individuals with serious mental illness (Nielssen and Large 2010; Swanson et al. 2008; Van Dorn et al. 2013). Effective medications to control the symptoms of psychosis have been available for the past 60 years, since Thorazine was introduced in the United States in 1954 (Frank and Glied 2006). In addition, a robust body of research evidence suggests that first-episode psychosis, which often signals the onset of a serious, chronic condition such as schizophrenia, is amenable to intervention. Randomized treatment studies show that intervention services for psychosis can improve symptoms and restore functioning, particularly if used early (Nordentoft et al. 2014; van der Gaag et al. 2013).

The research also demonstrates that early intervention following the onset of psychosis is critical to controlling the symptoms that can lead to violent behavior. Furthermore, specialized early intervention programs for psychosis have the potential to improve long-term social outcomes, such as education and employment. These programs can include a combination of medication, cognitive and behavioral psychotherapy, family education and support, and educational and vocational rehabilitation and should ideally last 2–5 years following a first episode of psychosis (Nordentoft et al. 2014; van der Gaag et al. 2013).

A small number of studies demonstrate that continuous and effective mental health treatment can reduce involvement with the criminal justice system and rates of violent crime among persons with serious mental illness. Van Dorn et al. (2013) examined the effects of medication and outpatient mental health services on arrests among 4,056 Florida adults with schizophrenia and bipolar disorder. They found that medication possession and receipt of outpatient services reduced the likelihood of any misdemeanor or felony arrests. As in other studies of violent behavior in the population with mental illness, this study assessed likelihood of all arrests rather than arrests specifically related to gun violence.

Swanson et al. (2008) assessed the effect of antipsychotic medications on violent behavior among persons with schizophrenia. The authors found that the proportion of participants demonstrating any violent behavior declined from 16% to 9% among participants taking antipsychotic medications. Importantly, the results of this study showed that although medication adherence reduced violence in the overall sample of participants with schizophrenia, antipsychotic medications did not reduce violent behavior among the subset of persons with a history of childhood antisocial conduct (Swanson et al. 2008). This finding again highlights that history of violent behavior is a strong predictor of future violent behavior.

In another study, Nielssen and Large (2010) compared rates of homicide among persons experiencing first-episode psychosis with rates among treated individuals with psychotic illness. They found that the rate of homicides (including but not limited to firearm homicides) perpetrated during the first episode of psychosis was 15.5 times higher than the annual rate of homicide after treatment for psychosis, suggesting that early treatment of first-episode psychosis has the potential to prevent some homicides (Nielssen and Large 2010). In addition to evidence suggesting that effective treatment for serious mental illness can reduce violent behavior among some individuals, studies also show that effective treatments for conduct disorder, including cognitive-behavioral therapy (Hodgins et al. 2008) and psychosocial, psychotherapeutic, familial, and multimodal approaches (Masi et al. 2014), can reduce rates of aggressive behavior and violence among those affected (Frank and McGuire 2011; Heller et al. 2013).

Many violent offenders have contact with mental health treatment systems (Glied and Frank 2014), but mental health providers and systems administrators face significant barriers to implementing an effective, continuous system of care for persons with serious mental illnesses. Many of these individuals rotate in and out of criminal justice systems and the community, which results in disruptions in insurance coverage and treatment (Van Dorn et al. 2013). Furthermore, psychosis is often accompanied by lack of insight into the nature of the illness and the need for treatment (Tait et al. 2003). For a variety of reasons, some persons with serious mental illness refuse treatment when it is available (Tait et al. 2003). Those with serious mental illness may qualify for involuntary treatment in rare cases when they pose a significant and imminent danger to themselves or others, but the vast majority of persons with serious mental illness do not meet this criterion (for further discussion of these issues, see Chapter 7, "Mental Illness, Dangerousness, and Involuntary Commitment"; Chapter 8, "Accessing Mental Health Care"; and Chapter 11, "Treatment Engagement, Access to Services, and Civil Commitment Reform") (Craw and Compton 2006; Segal 2012).

In summary, mental health service systems present important opportunities to identify and treat the subgroups of persons with mental illness who are at heightened risk of violence. Violence and suicide risk assessments are routine elements of psychiatric evaluations and ongoing treatment (see Chapter 2, "Firearms and Suicide in the United States"; Chapter 9, "Structured Violence Risk Assessment"; and Chapter 10, "Decreasing Suicide Mortality"), and some experts have recommended widespread screening for and treatment of substance use disorder among people with serious mental illness as one important strategy to reduce the risk of violence in this population (Glied and Frank 2014). This could be achieved, for example, by training mental health providers in the routine use of evidence-based screening, brief intervention, and referral to treatment for people with serious mental illness, and using these tools as a quality metric in treatment programs (Glied and Frank 2014).

Improving access to and utilization of mental health treatment in the United States has the potential to benefit millions of Americans with mental illness, and many opportunities exist within mental health service systems to identify and treat the subgroups of persons with mental illness who are at heightened risk of violence. However, the epidemiological research evidence clearly shows that the vast majority of persons with mental illness will never be violent and that most gun violence is not caused by mental illness. Therefore, improved access to and resources in mental health treatment, although valuable, are unlikely to substantially reduce gun violence directed toward others in the United States (Glied and Frank 2014).

Mental Illness–Focused Firearm Restrictions

In the aftermath of recent mass shootings, state and federal policy makers proposed multiple policies designed to prevent persons with mental illness from having guns (McGinty et al. 2014a). Many of these policies focused on broad groups of persons with mental illness, whereas some were directed toward persons with specific diagnoses, such as schizophrenia (McGinty et al. 2014a). Neither of these approaches is supported by the research evidence, which, as reviewed earlier in the section "Epidemiological Relationship Between Mental Illness and Violence Toward Others," shows that the vast majority of persons with mental illness, regardless of specific diagnoses, are never violent (Glied and Frank 2014; Swanson et al. 2015). Instead, the epidemiological research evidence suggests that mental illness–focused policies and interventions should be designed to reduce the risk of perpetration of violence by the subgroups of persons with serious mental illness known to be at high risk of committing gun violence (Consortium for Risk-Based Firearm Policy 2013; Glied and Frank 2014).

One important subgroup at significantly heightened risk of violence consists of persons involuntarily committed to inpatient psychiatric care (Choe et al. 2008). Federal law disqualifies anyone who has been involuntarily committed (as well as persons found incompetent to stand trial and persons placed under conservatorship because of serious mental illness) from purchasing or possessing a firearm (Gun Control Act of 1968, 18 U.S.C. § 922[d][4]). One promising study (Swanson et al. 2013) suggests that reducing access to firearms in this population does have the potential to reduce the small proportion of gun violence perpetrated by persons with serious mental illness who have been involuntarily committed, at least under conditions in which records for disqualifying conditions are made available for background checks and a comprehensive background check system is in place.

In 2007, Connecticut began reporting persons prohibited by federal law from purchasing or possessing firearms due to serious mental illness to the National

Instant Criminal Background Check System, the federal background check system for firearm sales (see Chapter 6, "Mental Illness and the National Instant Criminal Background Check System," for discussion). To test the effects of implementation of the federal law in Connecticut on violent crime, Swanson and colleagues assembled two cohorts of people with serious mental illness using administrative records from Connecticut's public mental health and criminal justice agencies for the period 2002–2009. The first cohort included persons with serious mental illnesses, including schizophrenia, bipolar disorder, and major depression, who were prohibited from buying a gun under federal law due to involuntary commitment or adjudication of mental incompetence. The second cohort included individuals with the same diagnoses who had a voluntary psychiatric hospitalization during the study period but were not prohibited by federal law from buying a gun for any reason.

Implementation of the federal gun restriction policy for individuals with serious mental illness was associated with reduced likelihood of arrest for violent crime in the cohort of persons prohibited from having a gun due to involuntarily commitment or adjudication of mental incompetence (Swanson et al. 2013). In contrast, implementation of the law had no effect on arrest for violent crime in the second cohort of persons with serious mental illnesses who had been voluntarily hospitalized but who were legally allowed to buy a gun. The authors also found that the majority of violent crime in the study population with serious mental illness was committed by individuals who did not meet federal criteria (involuntary commitment or adjudication of mental incompetence) for gun prohibition as a result of serious mental illness. This important finding suggests that other risk factors, such as history of violent behavior, alcohol abuse, and drug abuse, were important contributors to violent crime in the cohort of persons with serious mental illness. These are also important risk factors for gun violence and other violent crime in the overall U.S. population, suggesting that interventions specifically directed toward such risk factors may have a larger impact on overall rates of violence in the United States than interventions that apply broadly to persons with serious mental illness as a category.

This finding by Swanson et al. (2013) suggests that current federal law prohibiting persons who have been involuntarily committed, found incompetent to stand trial, or placed under legal conservatorship because of serious mental illness can reduce some violent offending among persons with serious mental illness. Nevertheless, because of the small proportion of all violence (including but not limited to gun violence) that is attributable to serious mental illness (3%–5%), implementation of federal mental illness–focused firearm restrictions alone will not significantly reduce overall rates of gun violence in the United States. However, the results of the study by Swanson and colleagues suggest that this implementation can meaningfully reduce perpetration of violence among persons with serious mental illness. The benefits of this reduction are tangible and not insignificant to the potential victims as well as to the perpetrators with serious mental illness, who as a result of effective limitation of access to firearms may avoid criminal justice involvement.

Swanson et al. (2013) also found that the majority of violent crimes in the study population with serious mental illness were committed by individuals who did not meet federal criteria (involuntary commitment or adjudication of mental incompetence) for gun prohibition as a result of serious mental illness. This means that most individuals with serious mental illness had never been legally deemed a danger to self or others (and involuntarily committed as a result) and suggests that risk factors such as a history of violent behavior, a history of alcohol abuse, and a history of drug abuse were important contributors to violent crime in the cohort of persons with serious mental illness. These are also important risk factors for gun violence and other violent crime in the overall U.S. population, suggesting that interventions directed toward these risk factors may have a larger impact on overall rates of violence in the United States than interventions focused specifically on persons with serious mental illness.

Interventions for Individuals Meeting Evidence-Based Criteria for Risk of Future Violence

A consistent finding across epidemiological studies of the relationship between mental illness and violence (including but not limited to firearm violence) concerns the role of comorbid risk factors (Steadman et al. 1998; Swanson et al. 1990; Van Dorn et al. 2012). These risk factors, such as substance abuse, heighten the risk of other-directed violence among the overall population and are not specific to the population with serious mental illness (Van Dorn et al. 2012). However, many risk factors, including substance abuse and socioeconomic risk factors such as poverty and unemployment, are overrepresented among persons with mental illness (Frank and Glied 2006; Swanson et al. 2015). Given that these risk factors affect wide segments of the U.S. population, focusing gun violence prevention policies and interventions on these risk factors for violence has the potential to meaningfully reduce perpetration of gun violence by persons with and without mental illness.

In the aftermath of the Sandy Hook Elementary School shooting in December 2012, the public dialogue surrounding mental illness and gun violence reached a peak. In March 2013, the Consortium for Risk-Based Firearm Policy, a group of national experts in mental health and gun violence prevention, convened at the Johns Hopkins School of Public Health in Baltimore, Maryland, to discuss the research evidence surrounding mental illness and gun violence. The goals of the group were to 1) reach a consensus on the epidemiological research evidence regarding the relationship between mental illness and violence and 2) make evidence-based policy recommendations.

On the basis of the research evidence, the consortium came to a consensus around a guiding principle for development of policy recommendations: restricting firearm access based on certain dangerous behaviors is supported by the research evidence, whereas restricting access based on a diagnosis of mental illness is not (Consortium for Risk-Based Firearm Policy 2013). The consortium then developed a set of policy recommendations utilizing available research and public health principles to create new prohibitions on individuals' ability to purchase and possess firearms based on the presence of evidence-based risk factors for violence. The consortium's recommendations addressed specific risk factors that had been demonstrated by research evidence to significantly increase the risk of violence, whether mental illness is present or not. These recommendations included the following (Consortium for Risk-Based Firearm Policy 2013):

1. *Individuals convicted of a violent misdemeanor should be prohibited from purchasing or possessing firearms for 10 years. Misdemeanor convictions involving the use of a deadly weapon, use of force, threat of force, or stalking are included in this prohibition.* The research evidence demonstrates that individuals convicted of violent misdemeanors are at increased risk of future violent crimes (Cook et al. 2005; Vittes et al. 2013; Wintemute et al. 2001), and laws to prevent firearm access among this group have been shown to reduce gun violence. For example, California's law prohibiting firearm ownership among violent misdemeanants resulted in reduced arrest rates for violent crime (Wintemute et al. 2001).
2. *Individuals subject to temporary domestic violence restraining orders should be prohibited from purchasing and possessing firearms for the duration of the temporary order.* Most victims of intimate partner homicide are killed with a gun (Fox and Zawitz 2009; Moracco et al. 1998), and the research clearly shows an increased risk of homicide when an abuser has a firearm (Bailey et al. 1997; Campbell et al. 2003; Kellermann et al. 1993). Laws in this area can be very effective: one study found that cities in states with laws prohibiting respondents to domestic violence restraining orders from purchasing or possessing guns had 25% fewer firearm-related intimate partner homicides (Zeoli and Webster 2010). In most states, temporary orders are the first step in the domestic violence restraining order process. The period encompassed by the temporary order is often the period immediately following initiation of separation in violent relationships and can be particularly dangerous.
3. *Individuals convicted of two or more offenses of driving while intoxicated (DWI) or driving under the influence (DUI) in a period of 5 years should be prohibited from purchasing or possessing firearms for at least 5 years.* Alcohol abuse is consistently associated with violence toward others (Afifi et al. 2012; Friedman 1998; Kelleher et al. 1994; Rivara et al. 1997), and individuals with mul-

tiple DUI arrests are at significantly higher risk of committing future violent crimes (Freeman et al. 2011; Lucker et al. 1991; McMillen et al. 1992).

4. *Individuals convicted of two or more misdemeanor crimes involving controlled substances in a 5-year period should be prohibited from purchasing or possessing firearms for at least 5 years.* Illegal use of controlled substances is also consistently associated with heighted risk of violence toward others (Afifi et al. 2012; Boles and Miotto 2003; Friedman 1998). The physical and psychological effects of controlled substances, including agitation, reduced impulse control, disinhibition, and cognitive impairment, can heighten the risk for violent behavior (Friedman 1998; Miller et al. 1991). In addition, involvement in illicit drug markets is strongly associated with violence (Goldstein et al. 1989).

Although these recommendations do not specifically address mental illness, they are examples of policies addressing risk factors that the research evidence shows strongly predict future violence among both persons with mental illness and persons in the overall population without mental illness. Addressing these risk factors may significantly reduce morbidity and mortality of gun violence associated with mental illness without focusing firearm restrictions directly on individuals with mental illness. For example, substance abuse in particular is more prevalent among persons with serious mental illness than in the overall population, suggesting that such policies could be effective at preventing violence by these persons. Future research to study the effects of these policies among persons with mental illness and the overall U.S. population is needed.

Suggested Directions for Future Research

The research evidence summarized in this chapter suggests several important directions for future research.

1. *Evaluation of innovative policies and interventions to prevent violence by persons with serious mental illness.* Additional research is needed to inform the design of effective interventions to decrease morbidity and mortality of gun violence associated with mental illness. To date, only one study conducted in a single state (Connecticut) has assessed the effects of the federal law prohibiting firearm purchase and possession by certain categories of persons with serious mental illness on violent crime (Swanson et al. 2013). Additional research is needed to assess how implementation of the federal law affects violence in states with different policy, political, and demographic contexts.

   Several states have additional serious mental illness firearm restrictions. For example, although federal law only prohibits firearm purchase and possession following a full involuntary civil commitment, California has a firearm prohibition for 5 years following a short-term involuntary hospitalization.

Evaluation of this and other policies designed to decrease perpetration of violence overall and gun violence specifically by subgroups of individuals with serious mental illness at heightened risk of violence is needed.

In addition to considering the effects of such policies on gun violence and violent crime overall, future research should assess the potential unintended consequences of these policies. The mental health treatment and advocacy communities have expressed considerable concern that policies to prevent persons with mental illness from having guns exacerbate the stigma surrounding mental illness (Gostin and Record 2011; McGinty et al. 2013). Although one study has shown that messages promoting policies to prevent "dangerous people" with serious mental illness from having guns do not heighten already widespread public stigma (McGinty et al. 2013), little is known about how such policies influence self-stigma, which research has shown can prevent persons with mental illness from seeking treatment (Eisenberg et al. 2009).

2. *Evaluation of gun violence prevention policies and programs specifically addressing risk factors for violence identified by research evidence, such as substance abuse.* Research evidence has identified persons convicted of misdemeanor crimes (Wintemute et al. 2001) and respondents to domestic violence restraining orders (Zeoli and Webster 2010) as two groups at high risk of committing future violence. Studies have also demonstrated that policies prohibiting access to firearms among these two groups are effective at reducing violence. To date, however, there is a lack of rigorous studies evaluating how gun violence prevention policies addressing alcohol and drug abuse, which are two of the primary risk factors for violence among persons with and without serious mental illness, influence gun violence. Studies of policies focused on early identification and treatment of comorbid substance abuse among persons with serious mental illness are also needed.
3. *Evaluation of strategies to improve widespread implementation of evidence-based treatments and services shown by prior research to prevent violence among persons with serious mental illness.* Although prior research suggests that effective health care and social services can reduce violence among persons with mental illness, few of these services are widely implemented. Effective services for the early treatment of psychosis (Nordentoft et al. 2014), comorbid substance use (Fischer et al. 1999; Glasner-Edwards and Rawson 2010), and conduct disorder (Frank and McGuire 2011; Heller et al. 2013)—all shown to heighten risk of future violence in this population—do exist. Similarly, evidence-based social services such as supported housing and employment (Burt 2012), which have the potential to address socioeconomic risk factors for violence perpetration and victimization among persons with serious mental illness, have also been created and evaluated in some communities (Drake et al. 2009).

However, most persons with serious mental illness do not have access to or do not receive these services (Frank and Glied 2006). Future studies should assess innovative strategies to improve the uptake and sustained delivery of these services in multiple service settings, including but not limited to health care settings, accessed by persons with serious mental illness. In addition, future studies should evaluate strategies to better coordinate health care and social services for the subgroup of persons with serious mental illness who are at heightened risk of violence.

Conclusion

Epidemiological research evidence on the relationship between mental illness and violence clearly demonstrates four key points: 1) most persons with mental illness are never violent, 2) a very small fraction of gun violence is attributable to mental illness, 3) risk of violence toward others is heightened among a subset of persons with serious mental illness, and 4) risk factors such as low socioeconomic status and substance abuse are strong predictors of violence in populations with and without mental illness. This evidence suggests that gun violence prevention initiatives intended to specifically address persons with mental illness should focus on the small subgroups of people with serious mental illness who are at heightened risk of committing violence, such as those who have been involuntarily committed to inpatient psychiatric care or those experiencing first-episode psychosis. Improving mental health treatment resources and access to these resources would benefit millions of Americans with mental illness. Nevertheless, the evidence clearly suggests that even the most effective mental health interventions will not significantly decrease the morbidity and mortality of gun violence directed toward others, because individuals with mental illness account for only a small fraction of the overall public health problem of gun violence.

Most importantly, the research reviewed in this chapter also suggests that rather than focusing primarily on individuals with mental illness, future public health–based gun violence prevention policies and interventions should focus on groups meeting other evidence-based risk criteria for violence, such as substance abuse and history of violent behavior. At the population level, these factors have a stronger association with risk of future violence than does mental illness and they affect large segments of Americans with and without mental health disorders.

Suggested Interventions

- Firearm prohibitions should be expanded to include:
  - More individuals with a history of violent behavior, which greatly increases the risk for perpetration of future violence toward others. Specifically, individuals convicted of violent misdemeanor crimes and those subject to *ex parte* domestic violence restraining orders should be temporarily prohibited from purchasing or possessing firearms.
  - Individuals with a history of risky substance use, which heightens risk of violence toward others. Specifically, individuals convicted of multiple DWIs or DUIs and multiple misdemeanor crimes involving controlled substances should be temporarily prohibited from purchasing or possessing firearms.
- Effective services for the early treatment of psychosis, which include a combination of medication, cognitive-behavioral therapy, family education and support, and educational and vocational rehabilitation, should be widely implemented.
- Persons at high risk of substance abuse, including but not limited to those with serious mental illness, should be screened for substance abuse and provided evidence-based treatment when abuse or addiction is identified. Substance abuse is an important risk factor for perpetration of violence toward others.

References

Afifi TO, Henriksen CA, Asmundson GJ, et al: Victimization and perpetration of intimate partner violence and substance use disorders in a nationally representative sample. J Nerv Ment Dis 200(8):684–691, 2012 22850303

Bailey JE, Kellermann AL, Somes GW, et al: Risk factors for violent death of women in the home. Arch Intern Med 157(7):777–782, 1997 9125010

Barry CL, McGinty EE, Vernick JS, et al: After Newtown—public opinion on gun policy and mental illness. N Engl J Med 368(12):1077–1081, 2013 23356490

Boles SM, Miotto K: Substance abuse and violence: a review of the literature. Aggress Violent Behav 8(2):155–174, 2003

Buchanan A: Risk of violence by psychiatric patients: beyond the "actuarial versus clinical" assessment debate. Psychiatr Serv 59(2):184–190, 2008 18245161

Burt MR: Impact of housing and work supports on outcomes for chronically homeless adults with mental illness: LA's HOPE. Psychiatr Serv 63(3):209–215, 2012 22307878

Campbell JC, Webster D, Koziol-McLain J, et al: Risk factors for femicide in abusive relationships: results from a multisite case control study. Am J Public Health 93(7):1089–1097, 2003 12835191

Choe JY, Teplin LA, Abram KM: Perpetration of violence, violent victimization, and severe mental illness: balancing public health concerns. Psychiatr Serv 59(2):153–164, 2008 18245157

Consortium for Risk-Based Firearm Policy: Guns, Public Health, and Mental Illness: An Evidence-Based Approach for State Policy. Baltimore, MD, Johns Hopkins University, December 2, 2013. Available at: http://www.jhsph.edu/research/centers-and-institutes/johns-hopkins-center-for-gun-policy-and-research/publications/GPHMI-State.pdf. Accessed July 5, 2014.

Cook PJ, Ludwig J, Braga AA: Criminal records of homicide offenders. JAMA 294(5):598–601, 2005 16077054

Craw J, Compton MT: Characteristics associated with involuntary versus voluntary legal status at admission and discharge among psychiatric inpatients. Soc Psychiatry Psychiatr Epidemiol 41(12):981–988, 2006 17041737

Department of Health and Mental Hygiene and the Judiciary: Forensic Populations and the Department of Health and Mental Hygiene: Report to the General Assembly as Required by the Joint Chairmen's Report, April 2007, p 101. Baltimore, MD, Department of Health and Mental Hygiene and the Judiciary, February 19, 2008

Douglas KS, Guy LS, Hart SD: Psychosis as a risk factor for violence to others: a meta-analysis. Psychol Bull 135(5):679–706, 2009 19702378

Drake RE, Skinner JS, Bond GR, et al: Social Security and mental illness: reducing disability with supported employment. Health Aff (Millwood) 28(3):761–770, 2009 19414885

Eisenberg D, Downs MF, Golberstein E, et al: Stigma and help seeking for mental health among college students. Med Care Res Rev 66(5):522–541, 2009 19454625

Elbogen EB, Johnson SC: The intricate link between violence and mental disorder: results from the National Epidemiologic Survey on Alcohol and Related Conditions. Arch Gen Psychiatry 66(2):152–161, 2009 19188537

Fazel S, Singh JP, Doll H, et al: Use of risk assessment instruments to predict violence and antisocial behaviour in 73 samples involving 24,827 people: systematic review and meta-analysis. BMJ 345:e4692, 2012 22833604

Fischer G, Gombas W, Eder H, et al: Buprenorphine versus methadone maintenance for the treatment of opioid dependence. Addiction 94(9):1337–1347, 1999 10615719

Fox JA, Zawitz MW: Homicide Trends in the United States. Crime Data Brief. NCJ 173956. Washington, DC, Bureau of Justice Statistics, January 1999. Available at: http://bjs.gov/content/pub/pdf/htiuscdb.pdf. Accessed July 5, 2014.

Frank RG, Glied SA: Better but Not Well: Mental Health Policy in the United States Since 1950. Baltimore, MD, Johns Hopkins University Press, 2006

Frank R, McGuire TG: Mental health treatment and criminal justice outcomes, in Controlling Crime: Strategies and Tradeoffs. Edited by Cook P, Ludwig J, McCrary J. Chicago, IL, University of Chicago Press, 2011, pp 167–215

Freeman J, Maxwell JC, Davey J: Unraveling the complexity of driving while intoxicated: a study into the prevalence of psychiatric and substance abuse comorbidity. Accid Anal Prev 43(1):34–39, 2011 21094294

Friedman AS: Substance use/abuse as a predictor to illegal and violent behavior: a review of the relevant literature. Aggress Violent Behav 3(4):339–355, 1998

Friedman E: Va. Tech shooter Seung-Hui Cho's mental health records released. ABC News, August 19, 2009. Available at: http://abcnews.go.com/US/seung-hui-chos-mental-health-records-released/story?id=8278195#.UKUxeWd418c. Accessed November 15, 2012.

Glasner-Edwards S, Rawson R: Evidence-based practices in addiction treatment: review and recommendations for public policy. Health Policy 97(2–3):93–104, 2010 20557970

Glied S, Frank RG: Mental illness and violence: lessons from the evidence. Am J Public Health 104(2):e5–e6, 2014 24328636

Goldstein PJ, Brownstein HH, Ryan PJ, et al: Crack and homicide in New York City, 1988: a conceptually based event analysis. Contemp Drug Probl 16(4):651–687, 1989

Gostin LO, Record KL: Dangerous people or dangerous weapons: access to firearms for persons with mental illness. JAMA 305(20):2108–2109, 2011 21610243

Griffin A: Lanza's psychiatric treatment revealed in documents. Hartford Courant, December 28, 2013. Available at: http://articles.courant.com/2013-12-28/news/hc-lanza-sandy-hook-report1228-20131227_1_peter-lanza-adam-lanza-nancy-lanza. Accessed June 27, 2014.

Heller S, Pollack HA, Ander R, et al: Preventing Youth Violence and Dropout: A Randomized Field Experiment. Cambridge, MA, National Bureau of Economic Research, 2013

Hodgins S, Cree A, Alderton J, et al: From conduct disorder to severe mental illness: associations with aggressive behaviour, crime and victimization. Psychol Med 38(7):975–987, 2008 17988416

Kelleher K, Chaffin M, Hollenberg J, et al: Alcohol and drug disorders among physically abusive and neglectful parents in a community-based sample. Am J Public Health 84(10):1586–1590, 1994 7943475

Kellermann AL, Rivara FP, Rushforth NB, et al: Gun ownership as a risk factor for homicide in the home. N Engl J Med 329(15):1084–1091, 1993 8371731

Kendler KS, Bulik CM, Silberg J, et al: Childhood sexual abuse and adult psychiatric and substance use disorders in women: an epidemiological and cotwin control analysis. Arch Gen Psychiatry 57(10):953–959, 2000 11015813

Kersh R, Morone J: The politics of obesity: seven steps to government action. Health Aff (Millwood) 21(6):142–153, 2002 12442849

Kessler RC, Berglund P, Demler O, et al: Lifetime prevalence and age-of-onset distributions of DSM-IV disorders in the National Comorbidity Survey Replication. Arch Gen Psychiatry 62(6):593–602, 2005a 15939837

Kessler RC, Chiu WT, Demler O, et al: Prevalence, severity, and comorbidity of 12-month DSM-IV disorders in the National Comorbidity Survey Replication. Arch Gen Psychiatry 62(6):617–627, 2005b 15939839

Large MM, Nielssen O: Violence in first-episode psychosis: a systematic review and meta-analysis. Schizophr Res 125(2–3):209–220, 2011 21208783

Loeber R, Burke J, Pardini DA: Perspectives on oppositional defiant disorder, conduct disorder, and psychopathic features. J Child Psychol Psychiatry 50(1–2):133–142, 2009 19220596

Lucker GW, Kruzich DJ, Holt MT, et al: The prevalence of antisocial behavior among U.S. Army DWI offenders. J Stud Alcohol 52(4):318–320, 1991 1875703

Masi G, Milone A, Paciello M, et al: Efficacy of a multimodal treatment for disruptive behavior disorders in children and adolescents: focus on internalizing problems. Psychiatry Res 219(3):617–624, 2014 25060833

McGinty EE, Webster DW, Barry CL: Effects of news media messages about mass shootings on attitudes toward persons with serious mental illness and public support for gun control policies. Am J Psychiatry 170(5):494–501, 2013 23511486

McGinty EE, Webster DW, Barry CL: Gun policy and serious mental illness: priorities for future research and policy. Psychiatr Serv 65(1):50–58, 2014a 23852317

McGinty EE, Webster DW, Jarlenski M, et al: News media framing of serious mental illness and gun violence in the United States, 1997–2012. Am J Public Health 104(3):406–413, 2014b 24432874

McMillen DL, Adams MS, Wells-Parker E, et al: Personality traits and behaviors of alcohol-impaired drivers: a comparison of first and multiple offenders. Addict Behav 17(5):407–414, 1992 1442235

Merikangas KR, He JP, Burstein M, et al: Lifetime prevalence of mental disorders in U.S. adolescents: results from the National Comorbidity Survey Replication—Adolescent Supplement (NCS-A). J Am Acad Child Adolesc Psychiatry 49(10):980–989, 2010 20855043

Miller NS, Gold MS, Mahler JC: Violent behaviors associated with cocaine use: possible pharmacological mechanisms. Int J Addict 26(10):1077–1088, 1991 1683859

Moracco KE, Runyan CW, Butts JD: Femicide in North Carolina, 1991–1993: a statewide study of patterns and precursors. Homicide Stud 2(4):422–446, 1998

Mueser KT, Rosenberg SD, Drake RE, et al: Conduct disorder, antisocial personality disorder and substance use disorders in schizophrenia and major affective disorders. J Stud Alcohol 60(2):278–284, 1999 10091967

Murray J, Farrington DP: Risk factors for conduct disorder and delinquency: key findings from longitudinal studies. Can J Psychiatry 55(10):633–642, 2010 20964942

National Center for Injury Prevention and Control: Data From Web-based Injury Statistics Query and Reporting System (WISQARS). Atlanta, GA, Centers for Disease Control and Prevention, 2010

National Center for Injury Prevention and Control: WISQARS Nonfatal Injury Reports, 2011–2012. Atlanta, GA, Centers for Disease Control and Prevention, 2012. Available at: http://webappa.cdc.gov/sasweb/ncipc/nfirates2001.html. Accessed May 28, 2014.

National Center for Injury Prevention and Control: Ten Leading Causes of Death and Injury. Atlanta, GA, Centers for Disease Control and Prevention, 2014. Available at: http://www.cdc.gov/injury/wisqars/leadingcauses.html. Accessed May 15, 2014.

National Center for Injury Prevention and Control, Division of Violence Prevention: The Social-Ecological Model: A Framework for Prevention. Atlanta, GA, Centers for Disease Control and Prevention, 2014. Available at: http://www.cdc.gov/violenceprevention/overview/social-ecologicalmodel.html. Accessed July 30, 2014.

National Institute of Mental Health: Serious Mental Illness (SMI) Among Adults. Bethesda, MD, National Institutes of Mental Health, 2014. Available at: http://www.nimh.nih.gov/health/statistics/prevalence/serious-mental-illness-smi-among-us-adults.shtml. Accessed April 1, 2014.

Nielssen O, Large M: Rates of homicide during the first episode of psychosis and after treatment: a systematic review and meta-analysis. Schizophr Bull 36(4):702–712, 2010 18990713

Nock MK, Borges G, Bromet EJ, et al: Suicide and suicidal behavior. Epidemiol Rev 30(1):133–154, 2008 18653727

Nordentoft M, Rasmussen JO, Melau M, et al: How successful are first episode programs? A review of the evidence for specialized assertive early intervention. Curr Opin Psychiatry 27(3):167–172, 2014 24662959

Rihmer Z: Suicide risk in mood disorders. Curr Opin Psychiatry 20(1):17–22, 2007 17143077

Rivara FP, Mueller BA, Somes G, et al: Alcohol and illicit drug abuse and the risk of violent death in the home. JAMA 278(7):569–575, 1997 9268278

Sallinger R: James Holmes saw three mental health professionals before shooting. CBS News, August 21, 2012. Available at: http://www.cbsnews.com/news/james-holmes-saw-three-mental-health-professionals-before-shooting/. Accessed November 15, 2012.

Sanchez R, Brumfield B: Fort Hood shooter was Iraq vet being treated for mental health issues. CNN.com, April 4, 2014. Available at: http://www.cnn.com/2014/04/02/us/fort-hood-shooter-profile/. Accessed May 15, 2014.

Santos F: Life term for gunman after guilty plea in Tucson killings. New York Times, August 7, 2012. Available at: http://www.nytimes.com/2012/08/08/us/loughner-pleads-guilty-in-2011-tucson-shootings.html?ref=jaredleeloughner. Accessed November 15, 2012.

Segal SP: Civil commitment law, mental health services, and U.S. homicide rates. Soc Psychiatry Psychiatr Epidemiol 47(9):1449–1458, 2012 22072224

Steadman HJ, Mulvey EP, Monahan J, et al: Violence by people discharged from acute psychiatric inpatient facilities and by others in the same neighborhoods. Arch Gen Psychiatry 55(5):393–401, 1998 9596041

Steadman HJ, Monahan J, Pinals DA, et al: Gun violence and victimization of strangers by persons with a mental illness: data from the MacArthur Violence Risk Assessment Study. Psychiatr Serv Jun 15, 2015 26073414 [Epub ahead of print]

Substance Abuse and Mental Health Services Administration: Results from the 2012 National Survey on Drug Use and Health: Mental Health Findings (NSDUH Series H-47, HHS Publ No SMA 13-4805). Rockville, MD, Substance Abuse and Mental Health Services Administration, 2013

Swanson JW, Holzer CE III, Ganju VK, et al: Violence and psychiatric disorder in the community: evidence from the Epidemiologic Catchment Area surveys. Hosp Community Psychiatry 41(7):761–770, 1990 2142118

Swanson JW, Swartz MS, Van Dorn RA, et al: Comparison of antipsychotic medication effects on reducing violence in people with schizophrenia. Br J Psychiatry 193(1):37–43, 2008 18700216

Swanson J, Robertson AG, Frisman LK, et al: Preventing gun violence involving people with serious mental illness, in Reducing Gun Violence in America: Informing Policy with Evidence and Analysis. Edited by Webster DW, Vernick JS. Baltimore, MD, Johns Hopkins University Press, 2013, pp 33–51

Swanson JW, McGinty EE, Fazel S, Mays VM: Mental illness and reduction of gun violence and suicide: bringing epidemiologic research to policy. Ann Epidemiol 25(5):366–376, 2015 24861430

Tait L, Birchwood M, Trower P: Predicting engagement with services for psychosis: insight, symptoms and recovery style. Br J Psychiatry 182(2):123–128, 2003 12562739

Teplin LA, McClelland GM, Abram KM, et al: Crime victimization in adults with severe mental illness: comparison with the National Crime Victimization Survey. Arch Gen Psychiatry 62(8):911–921, 2005 16061769

van der Gaag M, Smit F, Bechdolf A, et al: Preventing a first episode of psychosis: meta-analysis of randomized controlled prevention trials of 12 month and longer-term follow-ups. Schizophr Res 149(1–3):56–62, 2013 23870806

Van Dorn R, Volavka J, Johnson N: Mental disorder and violence: is there a relationship beyond substance use? Soc Psychiatry Psychiatr Epidemiol 47(3):487–503, 2012 21359532

Van Dorn RA, Desmarais SL, Petrila J, et al: Effects of outpatient treatment on risk of arrest of adults with serious mental illness and associated costs. Psychiatr Serv 64(9):856–862, 2013 23677480

Vernick JS, Rutkow L, Webster DW, et al: Changing the constitutional landscape for firearms: the U.S. Supreme Court's recent Second Amendment decisions. Am J Public Health 101(11):2021–2026, 2011 21940936

Vittes KA, Vernick JS, Webster DW: Legal status and source of offenders' firearms in states with the least stringent criteria for gun ownership. Inj Prev 19(1):26–31, 2013 22729164

Wintemute GJ, Wright MA, Drake CM, et al: Subsequent criminal activity among violent misdemeanants who seek to purchase handguns: risk factors and effectiveness of denying handgun purchase. JAMA 285(8):1019–1026, 2001 11209172

Zeoli AM, Webster DW: Effects of domestic violence policies, alcohol taxes and police staffing levels on intimate partner homicide in large U.S. cities. Inj Prev 16(2):90–95, 2010 20363814

2

Firearms and Suicide in the United States

Matthew Miller, M.D., M.P.H., Sc.D.
Catherine Barber, M.P.A.
Deborah Azrael, Ph.D.

Common Misperceptions

☒ People who are serious enough about suicide to use firearms will find another equally lethal way to end their lives if firearms are made less readily available.

☒ In the United States, places where suicide rates are highest are places where rates of mental illness are higher, where more people think about suicide, and where more people attempt suicide.

☒ Physicians who screen patients for risk of suicide generally ask about firearms and firearm safety.

Evidence-Based Facts

☑ Access to firearms increases suicide risk by increasing the likelihood that suicidal acts will involve guns—and therefore, on average, prove fatal.

This chapter draws in part from previous reviews that the authors have written; support has been provided by the Joyce Foundation. We thank our research assistant Steven Rausher for his indefatigable efforts and Harper Favreau for her valuable assistance.

☑ In the United States, places where suicide rates are highest are not places where rates of mental illness are higher. Neither are they places where more people think about suicide, plan suicide, or attempt suicide. Instead, they are places where more Americans live in homes with firearms.

☑ Physicians who screen patients for suicide often do not ask about access to firearms or discuss firearm safety.

Our main purpose in this chapter is to review the empirical literature on the association between firearm availability and suicide in the United States. We provide background on the measure of firearm exposure most often used in population-level studies (household firearm ownership), explain why access to highly lethal means of suicide increases suicide risk, and conclude with implications for suicide prevention.

Suicide in the United States

On an average day in the United States, more than 100 Americans die by suicide; over half of these suicides involve the use of firearms (Centers for Disease Control and Prevention, National Center for Health Statistics 2013). In 2013, a reported total of 41,149 people died by suicide in the United States; of these, 21,175 used firearms. More people died by suicide in 2013 than by unintentional overdoses (38,851) or in motor vehicle crashes (33,804), falls (30,208), or homicides (16,121). For Americans 35 and younger, suicide is the second leading cause of death (Centers for Disease Control and Prevention, National Center for Health Statistics 2013).

Over the past several decades, suicide rates have been more stable than homicide rates (Miller et al. 2012). Nevertheless, suicide rates have varied by as much as 30% over the past 25 years. For example, suicide rates declined from a peak rate of 12.9/100,000 in 1986 to 10.4/100,000 in 2000, driven largely by a decline in the rate of firearm suicide. Since 2000, suicide rates have risen, reaching 13.0/100,000 in 2013, with increases apparent across all major methods, particularly hanging (Centers for Disease Control and Prevention, National Center for Health Statistics 2013). In contrast to homicide rates, suicide rates are higher in rural than in urban areas, mostly because of higher rates of firearm suicide in rural areas (Branas et al. 2004).

Age, sex, race, and other demographic characteristics—including marital status, income, educational attainment, and employment status—all influence suicide mortality (Nock et al. 2008). Suicide rates are higher, for example, among people who are white or Native American than among people who are black, Hispanic, or Asian American and are higher for middle-aged and older males than for teens and young adults (Centers for Disease Control and Prevention, National Center for Health Statistics 2013). A consistent finding across numerous studies is that the strongest individual-level risk factor for a fatal suicidal act is a previous suicide attempt; other strong risk factors include psychiatric and substance use disorders (Shaffer et al. 1996).

Firearm Ownership in the United States

In 2001, 2002, and 2004, but not since, the Centers for Disease Control and Prevention included an item in its Behavioral Risk Factor Surveillance System (BRFSS) to assess the prevalence of household firearm ownership in the United States (Okoro et al. 2005). The BRFSS survey, conducted in all 50 states, is of a sufficient size (more than 200,000 respondents annually) that in the years the BRFSS was conducted, household gun ownership could be determined at the state level for all 50 states, as well as for some Metropolitan Statistical Areas and other substate areas. Results indicated that in 2000, 2001, and 2004, about one-third of adults lived in a home with a firearm—the same proportion reported by smaller surveys designed to provide estimates of gun ownership (Hepburn et al. 2007; Ilgen et al. 2008; Morin 2014; National Opinion Research Center 2010).

For periods before and since the BRFSS surveys, gun ownership trend data have been supplied by the General Social Survey (National Opinion Research Center 2010). These data indicate that the percentage of households with firearms has fallen from approximately half of all households in the early 1990s to just over one-third by 1999, a percentage that has remained relatively stable since that time. Notably, the percentage of *individuals* owning firearms has remained relatively constant over the past several decades. Changing household demographics, chiefly a fall in the number of households with an adult male, have been proposed to explain the decline in the household ownership rate in the 1990s (Smith 2000). Compared with other Americans, gun owners are disproportionately male, married, older than 40, and more likely to live in nonurban areas. Their long guns (rifles, shotguns) are owned mainly for sport (hunting and target shooting), whereas their handguns are typically for protection against crime (Cook and Ludwig 1997; Hepburn et al. 2007).

Prior to the three iterations of the BRFSS, researchers generally used proxies to measure firearm ownership rates at state and substate levels. A validation study by Azrael et al. (2004) found that among all proxies, the percentage of suicides that are committed with firearms correlates most strongly and consistently with cross-sectional, survey-based measures of household firearm ownership at county, state, and regional levels. Household firearm ownership is a good measure of the accessibility of guns used in U.S. suicides for a number of reasons: over 75% of firearm suicides among adults and nearly all suicides among children occur in the home (Karch et al. 2012; Kellermann et al. 1992); few suicide decedents who lived in homes without guns used firearms to kill themselves (Kellermann et al. 1992); and the vast majority of firearms used in firearm suicides involve a firearm owned by a member of the household (Kellermann et al. 1992).

Why Ready Availability of Firearms Might Impose Suicide Risk

The argument that restricting access to a highly lethal method of suicide can save lives rests on three well-established observations. First, many suicidal crises are fleeting (Deisenhammer et al. 2009; de Moore et al. 1994; Drum et al. 2009; Eddleston et al. 2006; Hawton et al. 1995; Li et al. 2002; Simon et al. 2001). Data in support of this contention come from surveys of people who have seriously considered suicide and those who have engaged in suicidal acts. For example, among college students in the United States who had seriously considered suicide in the previous year, approximately 30% reported that their suicidal period lasted under 1 hour (Drum et al. 2009). In a study that assessed characteristics of people taking large paracetamol (acetaminophen) overdoses in the United Kingdom, 75% of whom said they wanted to die, over 50% took the overdose within 1 hour of first thinking of it (Hawton et al. 1995).

Other surveys of people who have survived suicide attempts have found that the interval between deciding on suicide and actually attempting was 10 minutes or less for 24%–74% of attempters (with shorter times reported by patients who nearly died in their attempts) (Deisenhammer et al. 2009; Hawton et al. 1995; Simon et al. 2001; Williams et al. 1980). Eddleston et al. (2006) interviewed patients who had attempted suicide by ingesting pesticides, a suicide method for which the time from ingestion to death can be quite long. These patients reported, on average, that they took the poison after less than 30 minutes of thought, often following an argument; this interval did not differ significantly between those who survived and those who died.

Second, the method people use in suicidal acts depends, to a large extent, on a method's ready availability, over and above—and perhaps even independent of—the attempters' assessment of a method's intrinsic lethality (which indeed may not be correlated with its actual lethality) (de Moore et al. 1994; Eddleston et al. 2006; Hawton et al. 1995; Li et al. 2002). For example, in the few near-lethal suicide attempt studies involving firearms (de Moore et al. 1994; Peterson et al. 1985), firearms were readily available in the home in all cases, and this ready availability was usually the reason given for using firearms rather than another method. The case fatality ratio (the percentage of attempts by a given method that result in death) for commonly used methods varies by nearly an order of magnitude, and firearms are far more likely to prove lethal than are most other commonly used methods (Table 2–1) (Vyrostek et al. 2004). This observation suggests that when access to suicide methods with particularly high intrinsic lethality is reduced, on average less lethal means, if any, will be chosen.

TABLE 2–1. Case fatality ratio for select suicide methods used in the United States

Suicide method	Case fatality ratio (range)	Reference(s)
Firearm	83%–91%	Miller et al. 2004 Spicer and Miller 2000 Vyrostek et al. 2004
Drowning	66%–84%	Miller et al. 2004 Spicer and Miller 2000
Suffocation/hanging	61%–83%	Elnour and Harrison 2008 Miller et al. 2004 Spicer and Miller 2000 Vyrostek et al. 2004
Charcoal burning	50%	Lee et al. 2014
Poison, gas	42%–64%	Elnour and Harrison 2008 Miller et al. 2004 Spicer and Miller 2000
Jumping	31%–79%	Elnour and Harrison 2008 Miller et al. 2004 Spicer and Miller 2000 Vyrostek et al. 2004
Cutting/piercing	1%–3%	Elnour and Harrison 2008 Miller et al. 2004 Spicer and Miller 2000 Vyrostek et al. 2004
Poison, drug	2%	Elnour and Harrison 2008 Miller et al. 2004 Spicer and Miller 2000

Third, the prognosis if one survives a suicide attempt is relatively good. In a review of more than 90 studies of suicide attempt survivors, Owens et al. (2002) found that fewer than 10% of those people who survived a suicide attempt went on to die by suicide. This observation holds true even for suicide attempters who have made medically serious attempts, such as those involving jumping in front of a train (O'Donnell et al. 1994), and for those whose attempts were aborted or otherwise averted (Seiden 1978). The implication of this favorable prognosis with respect to dying by suicide is that saving someone's life in the short run is very likely to save his or her life in the long run.

Empirical Studies

Inclusion and Exclusion Criteria for Studies in This Review

From a suicide prevention perspective, the central question about the relationship between firearm availability and suicide risk is whether reducing access to firearms saves lives. This question guided our systematic literature search inasmuch as we sought to identify empirical studies that examined whether exposure to firearms was associated with increased risk of suicide, not merely an increased risk of firearm suicide, in the United States. To locate English-language, peer-reviewed articles regarding reducing access to firearms (or means restriction), we used an iterative process that included 1) searches of multiple electronic databases, including PubMed, Google Scholar, PsycINFO, EBSCOhost, and ERIC, using the term *suicide* in combination with the terms *availability, access, means, means restriction,* and *restriction* and variants of the term *firearm* (e.g., *firearm**, *gun**); and 2) review of abstracts, full articles, reference lists from unidentified articles, and so forth.

Our literature search included only manuscripts that analyzed empirical data and excluded letters to editors, commentaries, and news articles. We included U.S. studies only if they used actual measures of firearm exposure (e.g., self-reported household firearm ownership, roster of handgun purchasers) or validated proxies of firearm ownership. We excluded studies of firearm legislation, because these generally have not measured whether actual exposure to guns—the principal question at issue here—changed as a result of the legislation. Studies that assessed only the association between firearm availability and firearm suicide (rather than overall suicide) were not included, with the exception of studies that measured the impact of firearm storage practices on firearm suicide rates.

A total of 25 empirical studies met our inclusion criteria. These studies include cross-sectional ecological (i.e., population-level) studies that compared suicide rates across U.S. subpopulations that have differing levels of firearm ownership; ecological time-series studies that compared suicide rates at the population level over a time period in which firearm exposure at the population level changed appreciably; individual-level case-control studies; and cohort studies that measured firearm exposure in a defined population at baseline and observed suicide risk over time. Most of the ecological studies used measures of household gun ownership as an indicator of the accessibility of firearms.

Ecological Studies (Firearm Prevalence and Suicide)

Firearm suicide rates and overall suicide rates in the United States are higher where gun ownership is more prevalent. By contrast, rates of suicide by methods other than firearms are not significantly correlated with rates of household firearm ownership. This pattern has been reported in ecological studies that have adjusted for several potential confounders, including measures of psychological distress, alcohol and illicit drug use and abuse, poverty, education, and unemployment (Miller et al. 2004, 2007, 2012, 2015), as well as for underlying suicide attempt rates (Miller et al. 2013a). Earlier studies that relied on validated cross-sectional proxies of firearm ownership showed similar relationships (Miller et al. 2002a, 2002b, 2002c).

One time-series ecological study exploited the decline in U.S. household firearm ownership rates that occurred between 1981 and 2002 to examine the relationship between household firearm prevalence, measured at the regional level using data from the General Social Survey, and suicide rates. Over the study period, household firearm ownership fell substantially—from approximately one in two households to one in three households (Miller et al. 2006). A strong and significant relationship was found between declines in household firearm ownership and declines in rates of firearm suicide and overall suicide, but no significant relationship was found between declines in firearm ownership and rates of nonfirearm suicide. The authors noted that the declines in household firearm ownership and suicide rates occurred over a period when other investigators, using individual-level data from national surveys, found no changes in the prevalence of underlying mental illness, suicidal ideation, and suicide attempts (Kessler et al. 2005; Youth Risk Behavior Surveillance System 2012).

The magnitude of the differences in lethal self-directed violence in states with high versus low firearm prevalence can be seen in Table 2–2 (Miller et al. 2013a). Although the aggregate number of people residing in the 16 states with the highest gun ownership rates and the 6 states with the lowest gun ownership rates is approximately equal, and suicide attempt rates are similar, almost twice as many adults (11,428) completed suicide in the highest gun ownership states than in the lowest gun ownership states (6,038). The difference in total suicides over a 2-year period is almost entirely attributable to differences in firearm suicides (7,275 vs. 1,697), with virtually no difference in the number of nonfirearm suicides (4,153 vs. 4,341).

Individual-Level Studies

Household firearm ownership has also consistently been found to be a strong predictor of suicide risk in studies that examined individual-level data. Every U.S. case-control study that has examined the issue has found that the presence of a gun in the home or the purchase of a gun from a licensed dealer is a strong risk factor for suicide in the U.S. population overall (Cummings et al. 1997; Dahlberg et al. 2004; Grassel et al. 2003; Kellermann et al. 1992; Wiebe 2003) and, separately, for adolescents (Brent et al. 1988, 1991, 1993a, 1994, 1999),

TABLE 2–2. Suicides and suicide attempts in U.S. states with the highest and lowest gun ownership levels, 2008–2009

Population group by state gun ownership level	Person-years	No. of firearm suicides	No. of nonfirearm suicides	Total no. of suicides	Suicidal acts (%)
Highest gun ownership states[a,b]					
All adults	62,383,037	7,275	4,153	11,428	0.41
Adult men	30,273,657	6,263	2,905	9,168	0.38
Adult women	32,109,380	1,012	1,248	2,260	0.44
Adults ages 18–29 years	13,829,694	1,303	960	2,263	1.04
Adults age ≥30 years	48,553,343	5,972	3,193	9,165	0.24
Lowest gun ownership states[c,d]					
All adults	62,447,876	1,697	4,341	6,038	0.49
Adult men	29,810,942	1,572	3,207	4,779	0.38
Adult women	32,636,934	125	1,134	1,259	0.60
Adults ages 18–29 years	13,335,648	219	778	997	0.97
Adults age ≥30 years	49,112,228	1,478	3,563	5,041	0.26

[a]Highest gun ownership states are Alabama, Alaska, Arkansas, Idaho, Iowa, Kentucky, Louisiana, Mississippi, Montana, Nebraska, North Dakota, Oklahoma, South Dakota, Tennessee, West Virginia, and Wyoming.

[b]In highest gun ownership states, 51% of adults live in households with firearms.

[c]Lowest gun ownership states are Connecticut, Hawaii, Massachusetts, New Jersey, New York, and Rhode Island.

[d]In lowest gun ownership states, 15% of adults live in households with firearms.

adults and seniors (Conwell et al. 2002), males and females (Bailey et al. 1997; Kung et al. 2003), and Caucasians and African Americans (Kung et al. 2005).

The relative risk associated with firearms in the home is large, varying from two- to tenfold depending on the age group and the manner in which firearms are stored in the home (Brent et al. 1991; Conwell et al. 2002; Grossman et al. 2005; Miller and Hemenway 1999; Shenassa et al. 2004). A meta-analysis of individual-level studies (Anglemyer et al. 2014) pooled data from 12 U.S. and two international studies and reported that household firearm access increased the odds of suicide more than threefold. Brent's (2001) review of the early literature points out that the odds of suicide among persons in gun-owning (vs. non-gun-owning) households are increased four- to fivefold after adjustment for psychiatric disorders, but the odds are increased further among those persons without apparent psychopathology (although baseline suicide risk is much lower in this group). In addition, there appears to be an analogue of a dose-response relationship in the firearm-suicide literature: the presence of a gun matters, but so too does the manner in which it is stored (Conwell et al. 2002; Grossman et al. 2005; Kellermann et al. 1992; Shenassa et al. 2004), with less safely stored guns conferring greater risk.

The only large U.S. cohort study to examine the firearm-suicide connection found that California residents who purchased handguns from licensed dealers were over twice as likely to die by suicide as were age- and sex-matched members of the general population (Wintemute et al. 1999). In this study, too, the increase in suicide risk was attributable entirely to an excess risk of suicide with a firearm. Risk of suicide was elevated not only immediately after the purchase but throughout the 6-year study period. This finding is consistent with results from a case-control study by Cummings et al. (1997) in which the relative risk for suicide by persons with a history of family handgun purchase was greatest within the first year after purchase but remained elevated throughout the 5-year study period.

As in ecological studies, individual-level studies that examine method-specific suicide risk have found that the relationship between firearm availability and overall suicide is driven by the relationship between firearm availability and firearm suicide (Cummings et al. 1997; Grassel et al. 2003; Wiebe 2003; Wintemute et al. 1999).

Inferential Considerations

Drawing causal inferences about the relationship between firearm availability and the risk of suicide from existing case-control and ecological studies has been questioned on the grounds that these studies may not have adequately controlled for the possibility that members of households with firearms are inherently more suicidal than members of households without firearms (National Research Council 2005). Although this critique is theoretically grounded, in fact a number of studies have addressed this question directly. First, several individual-level case-control studies that found higher suicide risk among people in homes with guns controlled for measures of psychopathology (Bailey et al. 1997; Brent et al. 1988, 1993b, 1994; Conwell et al. 2002; Cummings et al. 1997; Kellermann et al. 1992; Wiebe 2003), and the findings suggested that the suicide risk associated with access to firearms was independent of underlying psychopathology.

Second, studies that have examined whether people who live in homes with guns have higher rates of psychiatric illness, substance abuse, or other known suicide risk factors generally have failed to find any indication that rates of these risk factors are higher in gun-owning than in non-gun-owning homes (Kolla et al. 2011; Oslin et al. 2004). For example, four case-control studies found comparable rates of psychiatric illness, psychosocial distress, and suicidal ideation among adult members of households with versus without firearms (Betz et al. 2011; Ilgen et al. 2008; Miller et al. 2009; Sorenson and Vittes 2008). Several studies have been done among adolescents who have attempted suicide; the most recent found that living in a home with a gun was not related to the probability of a suicide attempt (Simonetti et al. 2015). In contrast, in an earlier paper using data from the National Longitudinal Study on Adolescent Health, Resnick et al. (1997) found that living in a home with a gun was associated with increased risk of a suicide attempt among some, but not all, adolescents (see also Borowsky et al. 2001). Consistent with most individual-level analyses, ecological analyses have found that rates of suicide attempts (Miller et al. 2013a) and of suicidal ideation (Miller et al. 2015) are not significantly related to rates of household gun ownership at the population level.

Third, the risk of suicide associated with a household firearm pertains not only to gun owners, who, it could be argued, may have bought a gun with suicide in mind, but to *all* household members (Cummings et al. 1997; Kellermann et al. 1992; Wintemute et al. 1999). Additional observations also strongly suggest that the risk of suicide imposed by firearms is distinct from gun owners' underlying suicidality: the relative risk of suicide is larger for adolescents than for the gun owner, the risk persists for years after firearms are purchased, and less than 10% of firearms used in suicides are purchased close to the time of suicide (Kellermann et al. 1992; Vriniotis et al. 2015; Wintemute et al. 1999).

Data From Other Countries

Studies from countries other than the United States have helped build the evidence base in support of the conclusion that reducing access to a highly lethal and commonly used suicide method can save lives. Several carefully evaluated international studies have found that changes in suicide rates have paralleled changes in the availability of highly lethal, commonly used methods of suicide.

One of the most convincing and carefully studied examples comes from Sri Lanka, where, in the early 1990s, suicide rates were among the highest in the world (Gunnell et al. 2007). In subsequent years the suicide rate in Sri Lanka declined dramatically, by 50% over a 10-year period, from 47/100,000 in 1995 to 24/100,000 in 2005, coincident with a series of bans on several of the most commonly used and highly human-toxic agents.

The decline in suicide during this period in Sri Lanka was driven by a decline in poisoning suicides. Nonpoisoning suicides did not change appreciably over the period, although an increase in the number of hanging deaths first apparent in the 1980s continued but did not come close to offsetting the much steeper decline in pesticide poisoning suicides. Investigators carefully assessed secular trends in other suicide risk factors, including unemployment, alcohol misuse, divorce, and Sri Lanka's civil war (1983–2009) (Gunnell et al. 2007), as well as birth-cohort effects (Knipe et al. 2014), and found that they did not explain observed declines in pesticide and overall suicide over the time period. Moreover, as pointed out by Eddleston and Bateman (2011), the profound fall in suicides in Sri Lanka occurred without any psychosocial intervention aimed at reducing suicidality. A similarly dramatic drop in suicides was observed in Western Samoa when the pesticide paraquat became less available (Bowles 1995).

Other compelling evidence comes from the United Kingdom, where Kreitman (1976) analyzed data from England and Wales and separately from Scotland, for the years 1960–1971. He found that over the study period, aggregate-level reductions in the carbon monoxide concentration in domestic gas were associated with steep declines in suicide by domestic gas, accompanied by a 30% drop in overall suicide in England and Wales (and a smaller drop in Scotland). The magnitude of the decline in overall suicide rates varied by age and gender (greatest among older males, least among young women) but was of sufficient size to reduce overall suicide in all age and sex subgroups. In other non-U.S. studies where no significant correlation has been found between overall suicide rates and reduced access to a particular suicide method, the method under study typically represented too small a proportion of overall suicides or was of such low lethality that expectations of a statistically significant effect on overall suicide rates would be unreasonable (e.g., paracetamol in the United Kingdom [Hawton et al. 2013]).

Ongoing Challenges

How best to achieve reductions in ready access to firearms for those who are at risk of suicide is perhaps the most vital suicide prevention challenge currently facing the United States. From a global perspective, reducing access to highly toxic pesticides can save more lives than any other approach to suicide prevention, principally because 1) the capacity to reduce access and save lives from pesticide poisoning resides in a centralized mechanism, 2) the stock of highly human-toxic pesticides can be exhausted, and 3) equally effective but less human-toxic compounds are available for eradicating pests.

In contrast, firearms in the United States are both widely distributed and durable, and any changes in firearm access at the individual or household level will occur largely, but not exclusively, as the result of household-level decision making about guns. Current efforts to address the risk of access to firearms have by and large been developed and tested in the clinical context. It is encouraging in this regard that the most developed literature—on parents of youth with psychiatric problems—finds that families counseled by clinicians to reduce access to firearms and/or medications at home are more likely to do so than those not counseled (Brent et al. 2000; Kruesi et al. 1999; McManus et al. 1997).

More limited evidence suggests that such counseling might be more broadly effective. For example, studies that speak to the acceptability of *lethal means counseling* generally find that patients are open to providers speaking with them about firearm safety (Walters et al. 2012). Little is yet known, however, about how clinicians can most effectively communicate risk and motivate behavioral change around firearm access for people potentially at risk for suicide, including those with established psychiatric risk factors such as major depression, substance abuse, and posttraumatic stress disorder, and for others struggling with existential crises stemming from issues such as job loss, divorce, financial strain, and legal problems.

The limited evidence about how to optimally engage patients most effectively and the fact that few clinicians have been trained in lethal means counseling may help explain why, despite endorsement by several professional medical societies, counseling patients about limiting access to firearms during high-risk periods is not a widespread practice (Giggie et al. 2007; Grossman et al. 2000; McManus et al. 1997). For example, in a national random sample of the members of the American College of Emergency Physicians (Price et al. 2013), the majority of respondents had never been formally trained regarding firearm safety counseling, did not believe patients would see them as credible sources, and did not believe that anticipatory guidance on firearm safety would have any impact on suicide risk.

As effective messages are developed and clinicians are trained, rigorous studies will be needed to test the impact of lethal means counseling (Barber and Miller 2014) in a variety of populations and settings. Ideally, large enough populations (e.g., Veterans Affairs, military, large health maintenance organizations) will be studied to detect changes not only in firearm storage but also in suicide.

Opportunities to influence firearm-related behavior also exist outside the clinical context. For example, many gun organizations promote a culture of safety aimed at preventing unintentional firearm injuries, and extending the culture of safety to include suicide prevention may be a natural fit for these groups.

Efforts to this end are already under way in some locations. For example, members of the New Hampshire Firearm Safety Coalition, a coalition of gun advocates, firearm retailers, and public health professionals, have collaborated to design suicide prevention materials aimed at gun shop personnel and their customers (Vriniotis et al. 2015). Materials promote what has been called the "eleventh commandment" of firearm safety: be alert to signs of suicide in loved ones and keep firearms from them until they have recovered.

Similar campaigns aimed at gun shows, gun shops, and firearm instructors are under way or in the works in Tennessee, Missouri, Colorado, California, New York, Utah, and elsewhere, some initiated by suicide prevention groups and others by gun retailers themselves. The Maryland Licensed Firearm Dealers Association, for example, voted unanimously to adapt the New Hampshire campaign for their membership (Maryland Licensed Firearm Dealers Association 2015). As with efforts in the clinical context, interventions in the context of gun shops and other places will require rigorous evaluation. Other opportunities for suicide prevention outside the clinical context include personalizing firearms so that only the gun owner can fire them. This technology, a reality today, would provide a measure of suicide protection for other members of the household, although it would not likely reduce suicide risk for the gun owner.

Conclusion

In the United States, places where suicide rates are highest are not places where rates of mental illness are higher. Neither are they places where more people think about suicide, plan suicide, or attempt suicide. Instead, they are places where more Americans live in homes with firearms. Access to firearms increases suicide risk by making it more likely that suicidal acts will involve guns—and therefore, on average, prove fatal. No credible evidence suggests otherwise.

Taken as a whole, the literature reviewed in this chapter confirms that ready access to firearms imposes a suicide risk above and beyond the risk that would otherwise pertain were access to firearms made more difficult. The consistency of findings across different populations, using different study designs, and by different researchers is striking. The conclusion that reducing access to firearms can reduce suicide rates is made even more persuasive in light of the literature's conformity with studies from other countries that demonstrate the lifesaving effects of reducing access to other commonly used, physically and cognitively accessible methods of suicide, such as pesticides and domestic gas.

The challenge today is to develop, implement, and evaluate interventions to reduce access to firearms for individuals at risk of suicide. As interventions prove effective, they should be used to promote social norms that support their widespread adoption not only as the standard of care among medical and behavioral health providers, but also as the right thing to do for other professionals and concerned citizens who come in contact with people potentially at risk for suicide.

Suggested Interventions

- Research to evaluate the effectiveness of lethal means counseling in preventing suicide and to improve lethal means counseling should be undertaken with federal or foundation support.
- Providers who counsel people in crisis (e.g., substance abuse counselors, mental health clinicians, medical providers, social workers, clergy, first responders) should be trained in lethal means counseling to help reduce a suicidal person's access to firearms.
- Providers' home institutions and professional organizations should include steps to reduce a suicidal person's access to firearms in their protocols for assessing and managing suicidal risk.
- Medical, mental health, and public health organizations should partner with gun owner organizations to promote suicide prevention as a basic tenet of firearm safety and to expand voluntary off-site storage options for households that opt to store their guns elsewhere because family members are at risk of causing harm to themselves or others.

References

Anglemyer A, Horvath T, Rutherford G: The accessibility of firearms and risk for suicide and homicide victimization among household members: a systematic review and meta-analysis. Ann Intern Med 160(2):101–110, 2014 24592495

Azrael D, Cook PJ, Miller MJ: State and local prevalence of firearms ownership: measurement, structure, and trends. J Quant Criminol 20(1):43–62, 2004

Bailey JE, Kellermann AL, Somes GW, et al: Risk factors for violent death of women in the home. Arch Intern Med 157(7):777–782, 1997 9125010

Barber CW, Miller MJ: Reducing a suicidal person's access to lethal means of suicide: a research agenda. Am J Prev Med 47(3 suppl 2):S264–S272, 2014 25145749

Betz ME, Barber C, Miller M: Suicidal behavior and firearm access: results from the Second Injury Control and Risk Survey. Suicide Life Threat Behav 41(4):384–391, 2011 21535097

Borowsky IW, Ireland M, Resnick MD: Adolescent suicide attempts: risks and protectors. Pediatrics 107(3):485–493, 2001 11230587

Bowles J: Suicide in Western Samoa: an example of a suicide prevention program in a developing country, in Preventive Strategies on Suicide (Advances in Suicidology Vol 2). Edited by Diekstra RFW, Gulbinat W, Kienhorst I, et al. Leiden, The Netherlands, Brill Academic Publishers, 1995, pp 173–206

Branas CC, Nance ML, Elliott MR, et al: Urban-rural shifts in intentional firearm death: different causes, same results. Am J Public Health 94(10):1750–1755, 2004 15451745

Brent DA: Firearms and suicide. Ann NY Acad Sci 932:225–239, discussion 239–240, 2001

Brent DA, Perper JA, Goldstein CE, et al: Risk factors for adolescent suicide: a comparison of adolescent suicide victims with suicidal inpatients. Arch Gen Psychiatry 45(6):581–588, 1988 3377645

Brent DA, Perper JA, Allman CJ, et al: The presence and accessibility of firearms in the homes of adolescent suicides: a case-control study. JAMA 266(21):2989–2995, 1991 1820470

Brent DA, Perper JA, Moritz G, et al: Firearms and adolescent suicide: a community case-control study. Am J Dis Child 147(10):1066–1071, 1993a 8213677

Brent DA, Perper JA, Moritz G, et al: Psychiatric risk factors for adolescent suicide: a case-control study. J Am Acad Child Adolesc Psychiatry 32(3):521–529, 1993b 8496115

Brent DA, Perper JA, Moritz G, et al: Suicide in affectively ill adolescents: a case-control study. J Affect Disord 31(3):193–202, 1994 7963072

Brent DA, Baugher M, Bridge J, et al: Age- and sex-related risk factors for adolescent suicide. J Am Acad Child Adolesc Psychiatry 38(12):1497–1505, 1999 10596249

Brent DA, Baugher M, Birmaher B, et al: Compliance with recommendations to remove firearms in families participating in a clinical trial for adolescent depression. J Am Acad Child Adolesc Psychiatry 39(10):1220–1226, 2000 11026174

Centers for Disease Control and Prevention, National Center for Health Statistics: Compressed Mortality File 1999–2013. CDC WONDER Online Database, compiled from Compressed Mortality File 1999–2013. 2013. Available at: http://wonder.cdc.gov/mortsql.html. Accessed January 23, 2015.

Conwell Y, Duberstein PR, Connor K, et al: Access to firearms and risk for suicide in middle-aged and older adults. Am J Geriatr Psychiatry 10(4):407–416, 2002 12095900

Cook PJ, Ludwig J: Guns in America: National Survey on Private Ownership and Use of Firearms (NCJ 1654476). Washington, DC, U.S. Department of Justice, 1997

Cummings P, Koepsell TD, Grossman DC, et al: The association between the purchase of a handgun and homicide or suicide. Am J Public Health 87(6):974–978, 1997 9224179

Dahlberg LL, Ikeda RM, Kresnow M-J: Guns in the home and risk of a violent death in the home: findings from a national study. Am J Epidemiol 160(10):929–936, 2004 15522849

Deisenhammer EA, Ing CM, Strauss R, et al: The duration of the suicidal process: how much time is left for intervention between consideration and accomplishment of a suicide attempt? J Clin Psychiatry 70(1):19–24, 2009 19026258

de Moore GM, Plew JD, Bray KM, Snars JN: Survivors of self-inflicted firearm injury: a liaison psychiatry perspective. Med J Aust 160(7):421–425, 1994 8007865

Drum DJ, Brownson C, Denmark AB, et al: New data on the nature of suicidal crises in college students: shifting the paradigm. Prof Psychol Res Pr 40(3):213–222, 2009

Eddleston M, Bateman DN: Major reductions in global suicide numbers can be made rapidly through pesticide regulation without the need for psychosocial interventions. Soc Sci Med 72(1):1–2, discussion 3–5, 2011 21106286

Eddleston M, Karunaratne A, Weerakoon M, et al: Choice of poison for intentional self-poisoning in rural Sri Lanka. Clin Toxicol (Phila) 44(3):283–286, 2006 16749546

Elnour AA, Harrison J: Lethality of suicide methods. Inj Prev 14(1):39–45, 2008 18245314

Giggie MA, Olvera RL, Joshi MN: Screening for risk factors associated with violence in pediatric patients presenting to a psychiatric emergency department. J Psychiatr Pract 13(4):246–252, 2007 17667737

Grassel KM, Wintemute GJ, Wright MA, et al: Association between handgun purchase and mortality from firearm injury. Inj Prev 9(1):48–52, 2003 12642559

Grossman DC, Cummings P, Koepsell TD, et al: Firearm safety counseling in primary care pediatrics: a randomized, controlled trial. Pediatrics 106(1 Pt 1):22–26, 2000 10878144

Grossman DC, Mueller BA, Riedy C, et al: Gun storage practices and risk of youth suicide and unintentional firearm injuries. JAMA 293(6):707–714, 2005 15701912

Gunnell D, Fernando R, Hewagama M, et al: The impact of pesticide regulations on suicide in Sri Lanka. Int J Epidemiol 36(6):1235–1242, 2007 17726039

Hawton K, Ware C, Mistry H, et al: Why patients choose paracetamol for self poisoning and their knowledge of its dangers. BMJ 310(6973):164, 1995 7833757

Hawton K, Bergen H, Simkin S, et al: Long term effect of reduced pack sizes of paracetamol on poisoning deaths and liver transplant activity in England and Wales: interrupted time series analyses. BMJ 346:f403, 2013 23393081

Hepburn L, Miller M, Azrael D, et al: The U.S. gun stock: results from the 2004 National Firearms Survey. Inj Prev 13(1):15–19, 2007 17296683

Ilgen MA, Zivin K, McCammon RJ, et al: Mental illness, previous suicidality, and access to guns in the United States. Psychiatr Serv 59(2):198–200, 2008 18245165

Karch DL, Logan J, McDaniel D, et al: Surveillance for violent deaths—National Violent Death Reporting System, 16 states, 2009. MMWR Surveill Summ 61(6):1–43, 2012 22971797

Kellermann AL, Rivara FP, Somes G, et al: Suicide in the home in relation to gun ownership. N Engl J Med 327(7):467–472, 1992 1308093

Kessler RC, Berglund P, Borges G, et al: Trends in suicide ideation, plans, gestures, and attempts in the United States, 1990–1992 to 2001–2003. JAMA 293(20):2487–2495, 2005 15914749

Knipe DW, Metcalfe C, Fernando R, et al: Suicide in Sri Lanka 1975–2012: age, period and cohort analysis of police and hospital data. BMC Public Health 14:839, 2014 25118074

Kolla BP, O'Connor SS, Lineberry TW: The base rates and factors associated with reported access to firearms in psychiatric inpatients. Gen Hosp Psychiatry 33(2):191–196, 2011 21596213

Kreitman N: The coal gas story: United Kingdom suicide rates, 1960–71. Br J Prev Soc Med 30(2):86–93, 1976 953381

Kruesi MJ, Grossman J, Pennington JM, et al: Suicide and violence prevention: parent education in the emergency department. J Am Acad Child Adolesc Psychiatry 38(3):250–255, 1999 10087685

Kung HC, Pearson JL, Liu X: Risk factors for male and female suicide decedents ages 15–64 in the United States: results from the 1993 National Mortality Followback Survey. Soc Psychiatry Psychiatr Epidemiol 38(8):419–426, 2003 12910337

Kung HC, Pearson JL, Wei R: Substance use, firearm availability, depressive symptoms, and mental health service utilization among white and African American suicide decedents aged 15 to 64 years. Ann Epidemiol 15(8):614–621, 2005 16118006

Lee AR, Ahn MH, Lee TY, et al: Rapid spread of suicide by charcoal burning from 2007 to 2011 in Korea. Psychiatry Res 219(3):518–524, 2014 25048757

Li XY, Yu YC, Wang YP, et al: Characteristics of serious suicide attempts treated in general hospitals. Chinese Journal of Mental Health 16:681–684, 2002

Maryland Licensed Firearm Dealers Association. Suicide Prevention. MLFDA.org, 2015. Available at: http://mlfda.org/suicide/suicideletter2/suicideletter2.html. Accessed January 23, 2015.

McManus BL, Kruesi MJ, Dontes AE, et al: Child and adolescent suicide attempts: an opportunity for emergency departments to provide injury prevention education. Am J Emerg Med 15(4):357–360, 1997 9217524

Miller M, Hemenway D: The relationship between firearms and suicide: a review of the literature. Aggress Violent Behav 4(1):59–75, 1999

Miller M, Azrael D, Hemenway D: Firearm availability and suicide, homicide, and unintentional firearm deaths among women. J Urban Health 79(1):26–38, 2002a 11937613

Miller M, Azrael D, Hemenway D: Firearm availability and unintentional firearm deaths, suicide, and homicide among 5–14 year olds. J Trauma 52(2):267–274, discussion 274–275, 2002b 11834986

Miller M, Azrael D, Hemenway D: Household firearm ownership and suicide rates in the United States. Epidemiology 13(5):517–524, 2002c 12192220

Miller M, Hemenway D, Azrael D: Firearms and suicide in the northeast. J Trauma 57(3):626–632, 2004 15454813

Miller M, Azrael D, Hepburn L, et al: The association between changes in household firearm ownership and rates of suicide in the United States, 1981–2002. Inj Prev 12(3):178–182, 2006 16751449

Miller M, Lippmann SJ, Azrael D, Hemenway D: Household firearm ownership and rates of suicide across the 50 United States. J Trauma 62(4):1029–1034, discussion 1034–1035, 2007 17426563

Miller M, Barber C, Azrael D, et al: Recent psychopathology, suicidal thoughts and suicide attempts in households with and without firearms: findings from the National Comorbidity Study Replication. Inj Prev 15(3):183–187, 2009 19494098

Miller M, Azrael D, Barber C: Suicide mortality in the United States: the importance of attending to method in understanding population-level disparities in the burden of suicide. Annu Rev Public Health 33:393–408, 2012 22224886

Miller M, Barber C, White RA, et al: Firearms and suicide in the United States: is risk independent of underlying suicidal behavior? Am J Epidemiol 178(6):946–955, 2013a 23975641

Miller M, Warren M, Hemenway D, et al: Firearms and suicide in U.S. cities. Inj Prev 21(e1):e116–e119, 2015 24302479

Morin R: The demographics and politics of gun-owning households. FacTank: News in the Numbers. Washington, DC, Pew Research Center, July 15, 2014. Available at: http://www.pewresearch.org/fact-tank/2014/07/15/the-demographics-and-politics-of-gun-owning-households/. Accessed January 23, 2015.

National Opinion Research Center: General Social Survey. Chicago, IL, University of Chicago, 2010

National Research Council: Firearms and Violence: A Critical Review. Washington, DC, National Academies Press, 2005

Nock MK, Borges G, Bromet EJ, et al: Suicide and suicidal behavior. Epidemiol Rev 30:133–154, 2008 18653727

O'Donnell I, Arthur AJ, Farmer RD: A follow-up study of attempted railway suicides. Soc Sci Med 38(3):437–442, 1994 8153748

Okoro CA, Nelson DE, Mercy JA, et al: Prevalence of household firearms and firearm-storage practices in the 50 states and the District of Columbia: findings from the Behavioral Risk Factor Surveillance System, 2002. Pediatrics 116(3):e370–e376, 2005 16140680

Oslin DW, Zubritsky C, Brown G, et al: Managing suicide risk in late life: access to firearms as a public health risk. Am J Geriatr Psychiatry 12(1):30–36, 2004 14729556

Owens D, Horrocks J, House A: Fatal and non-fatal repetition of self-harm: systematic review. Br J Psychiatry 181:193–199, 2002 12204922

Peterson LG, Peterson M, O'Shanick GJ, et al: Self-inflicted gunshot wounds: lethality of method versus intent. Am J Psychiatry 142(2):228–231, 1985 3970248

Price JH, Thompson A, Khubchandani J, et al: Perceived roles of emergency department physicians regarding anticipatory guidance on firearm safety. J Emerg Med 44(5):1007–1016, 2013 23352862

Resnick MD, Bearman PS, Blum RW, et al: Protecting adolescents from harm: findings from the National Longitudinal Study on Adolescent Health. JAMA 278(10):823–832, 1997 9293990

Seiden RH: Where are they now? A follow-up study of suicide attempters from the Golden Gate Bridge. Suicide Life Threat Behav 8(4):203–216, 1978 217131

Shaffer D, Gould MS, Fisher P, et al: Psychiatric diagnosis in child and adolescent suicide. Arch Gen Psychiatry 53(4):339–348, 1996 8634012

Shenassa ED, Rogers ML, Spalding KL, et al: Safer storage of firearms at home and risk of suicide: a study of protective factors in a nationally representative sample. J Epidemiol Community Health 58(10):841–848, 2004 15365110

Simon OR, Swann AC, Powell KE, et al: Characteristics of impulsive suicide attempts and attempters. Suicide Life Threat Behav 32(1 suppl):49–59, 2001 11924695

Simonetti JA, Mackelprang JL, Rowhani-Rahbar A, et al: Psychiatric comorbidity, suicidality, and in-home firearm access among a nationally representative sample of adolescents. JAMA Psychiatry 72(2):152–159, 2015 25548879

Smith TW: 1999 National Gun Policy Survey of the National Opinion Research Center: Research Findings. Chicago, IL, National Opinion Research Center, University of Chicago, 2000

Sorenson SB, Vittes KA: Mental health and firearms in community-based surveys: implications for suicide prevention. Eval Rev 32(3):239–256, 2008 18456876

Spicer RS, Miller TR: Suicide acts in 8 states: incidence and case fatality rates by demographics and method. Am J Public Health 90(12):1885–1891, 2000 11111261

Vriniotis M, Barber C, Frank E, et al: A suicide prevention campaign for firearm dealers in New Hampshire. Suicide Life Threat Behav 45(2):157–163, 2015 25348506

Vyrostek SB, Annest JL, Ryan GW: Surveillance for fatal and nonfatal injuries—United States, 2001. MMWR Surveill Summ 53(7):1–57, 2004 15343143

Walters H, Kulkarni M, Forman J, et al: Feasibility and acceptability of interventions to delay gun access in VA mental health settings. Gen Hosp Psychiatry 34(6):692–698, 2012 22959420

Wiebe DJ: Homicide and suicide risks associated with firearms in the home: a national case-control study. Ann Emerg Med 41(6):771–782, 2003 12764330

Williams CL, Davidson JA, Montgomery I: Impulsive suicidal behavior. J Clin Psychol 36(1):90–94, 1980 7391258

Wintemute GJ, Parham CA, Beaumont JJ, et al: Mortality among recent purchasers of handguns. N Engl J Med 341(21):1583–1589, 1999 10564689

Youth Risk Behavior Surveillance System: Trends in the prevalence of suicidal behaviors: National YRBS: 1991–2011. Atlanta, GA, Centers for Disease Control and Prevention, 2012. Available at: http://www.cdc.gov/healthyyouth/yrbs/pdf/us_suicide_trend_yrbs.pdf. Accessed January 24, 2015.

3

Gun Violence, Urban Youth, and Mental Illness

Carl C. Bell, M.D., DLFAPA

Common Misperceptions

☒ Urban youth homicide rates due to gun violence are dramatically increasing.

☒ Urban youth gun violence is a socioeconomic problem and does not involve mental health issues.

☒ Urban youth gun violence cannot be effectively prevented.

Evidence-Based Findings

☑ From 1994 to 2010, homicide rates among youth ages 10–24 years decreased by 50%.

☑ Urban youth gun violence is a complex behavioral problem involving many different biological, psychological, and sociological facets.

☑ Programs directed toward decreasing violence among urban youth have been shown to be effective for more than 100 years.

Unfortunately, long-held misperceptions about youth violence and more specifically urban youth gun violence persist. In his comprehensive youth violence report, Dr. David Satcher, the U.S. Surgeon General from 1998 to 2002, outlined several prevalent myths regarding youth violence that endure to this day (U.S. Department of Health and Human Services 2001). His list included the following:

- Future juvenile offenders can be identified in childhood.
- Child abuse and neglect is a strong predictor of violence in later life.
- African American and Hispanic youth are far more likely to be violent than any other ethnic/racial group.
- The United States is threatened by superpredators, a term later defined by Howell (2009) as amoral, feral subhumans bent on maiming, raping, and murdering Americans for little or no reason.
- Trying juvenile offenders in adult criminal court is a wiser course of action than trying them in juvenile courts.
- Most violent offenders get caught.
- Programs intended to decrease violence among urban youth are ineffective.

These myths and assumptions have hampered the public's and policy makers' political will to address the issue of urban youth gun violence and have contributed to the misdirected solution of increasing incarceration (National Research Council 2014). The most common result of these myths is a paralyzing public fear of the country's children.

Addressing the issue of urban youth gun violence has been hindered even further by the reality that most studies of youth violence prior to 1992 did not measure variables regarding guns or gun use (Wilkinson and Fagan 2002). In addition, because of political maneuvering, research on guns has been effectively blocked since 1996 (Marshall 2013). When President Obama removed the block by executive order in January 2013 (The White House 2013), the Centers for Disease Control and Prevention (CDC) and the CDC Foundation requested that the Institute of Medicine and National Research Council convene a committee to develop a research agenda on causes and prevention of firearm-related violence. This group developed a "full range of high-priority topics that could be explored with significant progress made in 3–5 years" (Institute of Medicine and National Research Council 2013, p. 2). One of the goals was to identify "factors associated with youth having access to, possessing, and carrying guns" (p. 5).

Despite the dearth of research data, it has become clear that firearms have been increasingly used in homicides. For example, firearms were used in nearly 8 of 10 homicides in 1991, compared with 6 of 10 in 1976 (U.S. Department of Justice, Office of Justice Programs, Office of Juvenile Justice and Delinquency Prevention 1996). The increase in the 1980s and 1990s in the numbers of homicides committed by juveniles in which juveniles were also victims was directly due to the use of firearms. Between 1980 and 1997, three-quarters of homicide victims ages 12–17 were killed with firearms (Butts et al. 2002). For the purposes of this chapter, *youth homicide* refers to homicide perpetrated with a gun.

Historical Context

To fully understand urban youth violence and its relationship to firearms, one benefits from an examination of this phenomenon in its historical context. With the formation of the Black Psychiatrists of America in 1969, there was a call for the National Institute of Mental Health (NIMH) to develop a center to study minority problems (Black Psychiatrists of America 1969). In 1971, Dr. James Ralph, an African American psychiatrist, was appointed as the chief of NIMH's Center for Minority Group Mental Health Programs. He began to advocate for a greater focus on the problem of homicide in the African American community. In 1972, Dr. Alvin Poussaint published *Why Blacks Kill Blacks,* a psychodynamic explanation of African American youth homicide rates (Poussaint 1972).

These efforts resulted in research on homicides among young African Americans, and patterns based on this research began to emerge relatively quickly (Black Psychiatrists of America 1980; Dennis 1980; Dennis et al. 1981; Gorwitz and Dennis 1976). In the late 1970s, homicides (typically measured as the rate of incidents per 100,000 people), most of which involved firearms, ranked as the fifth highest cause of death among African American males and the ninth highest cause of death among African American females (National Center for Health Statistics 1977). In 1985, homicide was the leading cause of death for African American males and females ages 15–34 (Koop 1985; U.S. Department of Health and Human Services 1985), and the vast majority of these homicides involved firearms.

Measurements of youth violence with or without firearms are derived from two primary sources: official law enforcement reports and confidential youth surveys. Official law enforcement reports provide a reliable way to obtain relevant epidemiological data, especially those relating to homicide. Youth surveys often contain information about youth violence that goes unreported and undetected by more formal studies. The official law enforcement reports have always suggested that African Americans are generally more violent with or without firearms than are European Americans. For example, ever since the Federal Bureau of Investigation (FBI) began collecting homicide statistics in 1929 (Bell and Jenkins 1990), the agency's statistics have consistently indicated that African American homicide rates are 6–12 times higher than European American homicide rates. However, confidential youth surveys suggest that African American and European American males have equal rates of self-reported violence (U.S. Department of Health and Human Services 2001). Other studies suggest that when socioeconomic status is held constant, the racial differences in homicide rates decrease substantially (Griffith and Bell 1989).

In 1985, U.S. Surgeon General C. Everett Koop issued a major call to action that focused on violence as a public health problem (Koop 1985). The seminal work of Dr. Carolyn Block began to uncover the complex dynamics of youth violence (Block 1985). In 1986, African American homicide rates rose, with the homicides typically involving guns. African American males were found to be six times more likely than European American males to be victims of homicide, and African American females were found to be four times more likely than European American females to be victims of homicide (Block 1985). At that time, most of the African American homicides took place in the context of interpersonal altercations between family and friends, and were not associated with predatory violence, such as robbery homicide.

By 1990, it had become clear that youth homicide was a complex phenomenon (Bell and Jenkins 1990). For example, prior to 1981, gang-related homicides accounted for about 1% of the nation's homicide deaths. However, in Chicago, gang-related homicides accounted for 5% of the total homicides but 25% of youth homicides overall and 50% of Hispanic youth homicides (Block 1985). In addition, in the late 1980s, drug-related homicides were estimated to account for less than 10% of all homicides in Chicago. This rate was thought to be characteristic of most cities, with the notable exception of Washington, D.C., where drug-related homicides were estimated to represent 80% of total homicide deaths (Bell and Jenkins 1990).

Thus, the emerging data and patterns demonstrated that the stereotypical assumptions about African American homicides—that they are related to gangs, drugs, and robberies—were in error. Americans were starting to realize that most homicides, with or without firearms, involved someone the victim knew. Thus, the public health focus for homicide prevention took root (Bell 1987; Bell et al. 1986). In a development that turned out to be critical concerning urban youth violence, in 1995, President Clinton tasked his White House cabinet to address the issue of violence against women, and from 1995 to 2000, Attorney General Janet Reno and Secretary of Health and Human Services Donna Shalala chaired the Advisory Council on Violence Against Women.

By 2000, it became clear that many identifiable categories of violence could result in homicide. At that time, most public health data collectors considered homicides as indicators of violence. Nonlethal types of violence were not closely surveilled or well measured. Thus, an early review identifying over 15 types of violence (Table 3–1) did not specify relative frequency of homicides in each category or weapons utilized, but was in fact conceptualized based on types of homicide. Homicides related to any of these categories were due primarily to firearms.

TABLE 3–1. Types of violence

Group or mob violence
Individual violence
Systemic violence, such as war, racism, and sexism
Institutional violence, such as preventing inmates from getting the benefit of prophylactic medications to prevent hepatitis
Hate-crime violence, such as terrorism
Multicide (e.g., mass murder, murder sprees, and serial killing)
Psychopathic violence
Predatory violence, also known as instrumental or secondary violence
Interpersonal altercation violence, also known as expressive or primary violence (e.g., domestic violence, child abuse, elder abuse, and peer violence)
Drug-related violence, such as systemic drug-related violence (whereby drug dealers kill to sell drugs), pharmacological drug-related violence (whereby an individual perpetrates violence because of drug intoxication), economic-compulsive drug-related violence (whereby a drug addict uses violence to obtain drugs), and negligent drug-related violence (such as a drunk driver who kills a pedestrian)
Gang-related violence
Violence by mentally ill individuals
Lethal violence directed toward self (suicide)
Lethal violence directed toward others (homicide)
Lethal violence directed toward others and self (suicide preceded by homicide)
Violence by organically brain damaged individuals
Legitimate/illegitimate violence
Nonlethal violence

Source. Reprinted from Bell CC: "Violence Prevention 101: Implications for Policy Development," in *Perspectives on Crime and Justice: 2000–2001 Lecture Series,* Vol 5. Washington, D.C., National Institute of Justice, March 2002, p. 67. Available at: http://www.ncjrs.gov/pdffiles1/nij/187100.pdf. Accessed May 23, 2014.

At the time this review was published, public health homicide prevention efforts were developing throughout the United States. Although these efforts were helpful, many unfortunately lacked the specificity and coordination that would have maximized their positive results. For example, each type of defined gun-related homicide as delineated in Table 3–1 calls for different prevention, intervention, and postvention strategies, which often conflict with one another (Bell 1997). These differences have to be taken into account when designing programs so as to achieve maximum success.

Early Approaches to Urban Youth Violence and Firearms

Despite the increasing understanding of the complex phenomenon of violence with firearms, a rational, coherent public policy approach to this problem based on facts has eluded implementation. In part, the lack of lucid violence prevention public policy has been due to the complicated, multidetermined nature of human behavior. However, another dynamic involves the effect of public media, which often drive public policy. Many people, including policy makers, often derive their understanding of the epidemiology of violence from headlines and lead stories. However, the media tend to report unusual or attention-grabbing events, such as mass shootings at a mall or a college campus. Thus, the public and policy makers have come to believe that these types of incidents are representative of the problem with gun violence, when in fact the instances of interpersonal gun-related violence are much more common and deadly.

For example, media coverage contributed to the many years of public attention focused on the problem of drug-related and gang-related violence. Preventive interventions directed specifically toward these forms of violence, based on and designed by criminal justice and police strategies or representing community efforts, such as the CeaseFire program (Kotlowitz 2008), were viewed as appropriate interventions. In 1985, homicide, usually by means of a gun, was deemed a public health problem and gained national attention. As a result of the misconception that drug offenders were primarily responsible for most homicides, the punishment for drug-related offenses became much more strict. The percentage of sentenced drug offenders went from about 13% in 1985 to more than 30% in 2005 (Bell 2005). During this period, the myth of the superpredator was promulgated (Howell 2009); however, as discussed in the previous section, "Historical Context," the great majority of homicides at that time were the result of interpersonal altercations.

Between 1983 and 1993, the official crime statistics demonstrate an increase in arrest rates for youth violence (U.S. Department of Health and Human Services 2001). The response to these findings was the promulgation of policies to get tough on crime (National Research Council 2014). Gun control laws were passed, boot camps were started, and youth were sent from juvenile justice systems to adult criminal courts. However, Satcher's Youth Violence Report found that although most youth who perpetrated violent crimes were not arrested, youth of color were disproportionally arrested for such crimes (U.S. Department of Health and Human Services 2001). Furthermore, although arrests for youth violent crimes decreased in the mid-1990s, the surveys that measured self-reports of violence did not show a similar decrease in self-reports of violent behavior (U.S. Department of Health and Human Services 2001). Accordingly, the evidence did not support the popular belief that increased arrest rates were resulting in decreasing violence. Unfortunately, the strict criminal justice approach to delinquent youth behavior did not change commensurately, even though the data did not support its efficacy (Bonnie et al. 2013; National Research Council 2014; U.S. Department of Health and Human Services 2001). Criminal justice or law enforcement approaches, while addressing one facet of gun-related youth violence, were overall not effective in decreasing juvenile firearm-related homicide. For example, research revealed that gun buyback programs do not work. Similarly, trying to identify urban youth who are predisposed to gun violence also did not work (U.S. Department of Health and Human Services 2001).

Douglas and Bell (2011) asserted that these law enforcement and criminal justice–driven policies and approaches to youth violence were momentous errors for two important reasons. First, these policies and approaches did not consider age-related neurodevelopmental issues that play a role in youth violence. Second, these policies represented a narrow criminal justice approach to the problem of youth violence instead of wider, evidence-based public health approaches. The National Academy of Sciences' report *Reforming Juvenile Justice* (Bonnie et al. 2013) supported taking a developmental approach to urban youth who were delinquent and violent, and emphasized the need for public health–based interventions.

In addition, the available science indicating that urban youth violence might be more effectively addressed by designing interventions for decreasing interpersonal violence was not considered in the development or implementation of the law enforcement or community initiatives. In fact, the high rates of African American interpersonal altercation homicides have driven the overall homicide rates for all categories of people since 1927, when the FBI first started gathering homicide data (Bell and Jenkins 1990).

As Figure 3–1 demonstrates, in the mid-1990s, the interpersonal altercation homicide rates began to decline (Greenfield et al. 1998). The growth in the availability of domestic violence shelters in the United States between 1970 and 1990, due in large part to the increasing influence of the women's movement (Rosen 2001), was highly successful in decreasing rates of homicide due to intimate violence. The National Advisory Council on Violence Against Women found that these shelters were directly responsible for the drastically decreased rates of violence by intimates, which fell from 16.5 per 100,000 in 1976 to 3.5 per 100,000 in 1996 (see Figure 3–1; Greenfield et al. 1998). For years prior to 1995, about 50,000 gun-related deaths occurred each year (30,000 suicides and 20,000 homicides) (Bell and Jenkins 1990). However, in 2010, there were 31,672 gun-related deaths, of which about 20,000 were suicides and about 11,000 were homicides (Murphy et al. 2013). Similarly, the gradual decrease in homicide rates from 1976 to 1996 was primarily due to the decrease in domestic homicides among blacks (Bureau of Justice Statistics 2007).

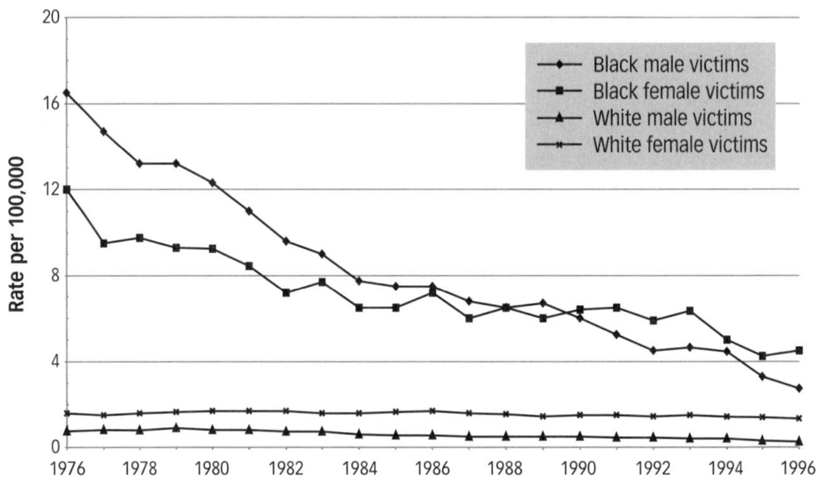

FIGURE 3–1. Rates of murder by intimates (per 100,000 persons ages 20–44) from 1976 to 1996.

Source. Greenfield LA, Rand MR, Craven D, et al.: *Violence by Intimates* (NCJ-167237). Washington, D.C., U.S. Department of Justice, Office of Justice Programs, Bureau of Justice Statistics, March 1998, p. 7.

Urban Youth Violence

The drop in interpersonal altercation homicides resulted in lower youth homicide rates, many of which were gang related. Suicide, homicide, and firearm-related death rates among youth ages 15–19 years were between 6 and 15 per 100,000 in the 1970s. These rates increased slightly in the 1980s, but by 1995, they had doubled. In 1995, firearm-related deaths numbered in the low 20s per 100,000, homicides in the upper teens per 100,000, and suicides numbered 10 or 11 per 100,000 (Figure 3–2) (Child Trends Data Bank 2012). After 1995, the rates of firearm-related homicide and suicide deaths began to decrease significantly. By 2010, these rates had halved, decreasing nearly to 1968 levels (see Figure 3–2) (Child Trends Data Bank 2012).

Similarly, national rates of homicide for youth ages 10–24 declined from 15.2 per 100,000 in 1994 to 7.5 per 100,000 in 2010 (Figure 3–3) (Centers for Disease Control and Prevention 2013). Data from the Child Trends Data Bank (2012), which were collected from multiple sources, demonstrate similar findings. By 2010, firearm-related deaths for youths ages 15–19 were down to 10.6 per 100,000 from a high of 24.5 per 100,000 in 1995; homicides were down to 8.3 per 100,000 from their highest rate of 18.1 per 100,000 in 1995; and suicides were down from 10.5 per 100,000 in 1995 to 7.5 per 100,000 in 1995.

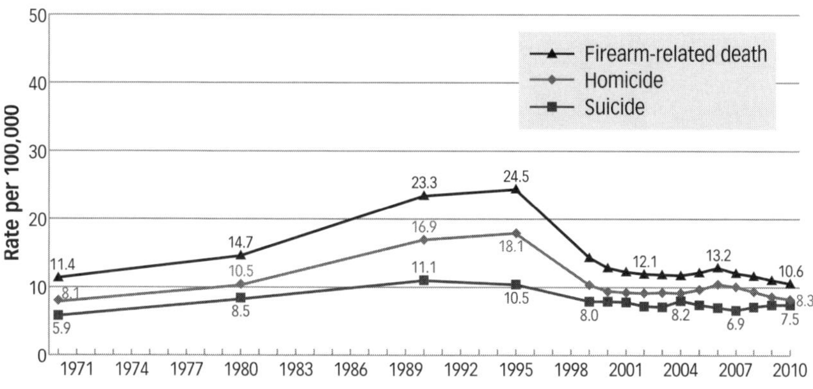

FIGURE 3–2. Rates (per 100,000) of homicide, suicide, and firearm-related deaths among youth ages 15–19, selected years 1970–2010.

Data for 1970–1980: National Center for Health Statistics. (2002) Health United States, 2002 With Chartbook on Trends in the Health of Americans. National Center for Health Statistics. Tables 46, 47, and 48. Data for 1995–2013: Centers for Disease Control and Prevention. Web-based Injury Statistics Query and Reporting System (WISQARS) [Online], 2015. National Center for Injury Prevention and Control, Centers for Disease Control and Prevention (producer). Available at: www.cdc.gov/injury/wisqars/fatal.html.

Source. Child Trends Data Bank: "Teen Homicide, Suicide and Firearm Deaths." Bethesda, M.D., Child Trends, March 2012. Available at: http://www.childtrends.org/wp-content/uploads/2014/10/70_Homicide_Suicide_Firearms.pdf. Accessed May 23, 2014.

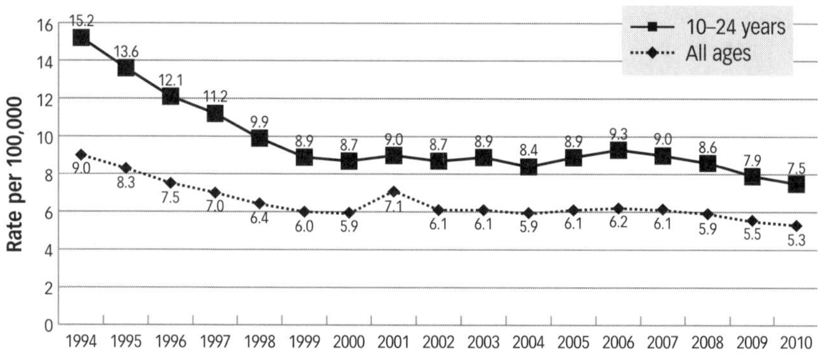

FIGURE 3–3. National youth homicide rates (per 100,000).

Rates for all ages are age-adjusted to the standard 2000 population; rates for the 10- to 24-year age group are age-specific.

Source. Centers for Disease Control and Prevention, National Center for Injury Prevention and Control, Division of Violence Prevention. Available at: http://www.cdc.gov/ViolencePrevention/youthviolence/stats_at-a_glance/. Accessed May 23, 2014.

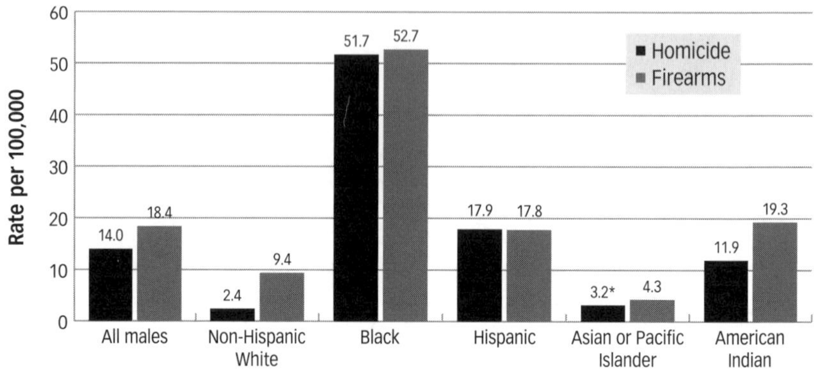

FIGURE 3–4. Rates of homicide (per 100,000) and firearm deaths among males ages 15–19, by race and Hispanic origin, 2010.

*Should be interpreted with caution because it is based on 20 or fewer deaths and may be unstable. Centers for Disease Control and Prevention. Web-based Injury Statistics Query and Reporting System (WISQARS) [Online], 2015. National Center for Injury Prevention and Control, Centers for Disease Control and Prevention (producer). Available at: www.cdc.gov/injury/wisqars/fatal.html.
Source. Child Trends Data Bank: "Teen Homicide, Suicide and Firearm Deaths." Bethesda, MD, Child Trends, March 2012. Available at: http://www.childtrends.org/wp-content/uploads/2014/10/70_Homicide_Suicide_Firearms.pdf. Accessed May 23, 2014.

Of course, these rates vary by culture, race, ethnicity, and gender. In 2010, the firearm-related death rates and homicide rates for black youth ages 15–19 were in the low 50s per 100,000; for the other groups, the rates were below 19.5 per 100,000 (see Figure 3–4; Child Trends Data Bank 2012). Data regarding youth violence and firearms among individuals ages 10–24 collected for the year 2005 also demonstrate significant variability based on race and ethnicity. These data indicate that homicide rates among all persons ages 10–24 decreased from 15.6 deaths per 100,000 persons in 1991 to 9.0 deaths per 100,000 in 2005 (Douglas and Bell 2011). Homicide rates for non-Hispanic blacks in this age range dropped from 62.6 per 100,000 in 1991 to 32.8 per 100,000 in 2005 (Douglas and Bell 2011). During these years, the firearm homicide rate among males ages 10–24 was highest for non-Hispanic blacks, with 51.4 deaths per 100,000, and was lowest for non-Hispanic whites, with 2.4 deaths per 100,000. Naturally, rates of firearm-related deaths, homicides, and suicides are higher for older youth (ages 20–24 years) than younger youth (ages 15–19 years). Among older youth, the overall homicide rate in 2010 for all persons was 13.2 per 100,000; for blacks, it was 28.8 per 100,000 (Centers for Disease Control and Prevention 2013).

Gang-Related Homicide

Gang membership is a major determinant for carrying a firearm (Bjerregaard and Lizotte 1995; Lizotte et al. 2000). Accordingly, an understanding of gang-related homicide is necessary for an understanding of the relationship between gun violence and urban youth. Early examinations of gang-related homicides indicated that about half of gang-related homicides are committed to benefit the gang; the other half represent interpersonal altercations between gang members of the same gang (Bell 2002). Thus, from a public health perspective, identifying specific patterns of homicide for which specific intervention strategies can be crafted and implemented is a complex challenge.

Although the numbers of youth gangs and youth gang members have increased, the numbers of youth gang–related homicides have paradoxically decreased (Egley and Howell 2013). In the 33 U.S. cities included in the National Violent Death Reporting System and/or the National Youth Gang Survey, gang–related mortalities or homicides between 2003 to 2008 were below 7 per 100,000 (Figure 3–5) (Centers for Disease Control and Prevention 2012a).

In addition, the estimates for gang-related homicides in large cities differ significantly from those in small cities and suburbs. For example, the U.S. Department of Justice's National Gang Center, using FBI data (Federal Bureau of Investigation 2010), suggested that the two gang "capitals" of the United States—Chicago and Los Angeles—account for 20% of all gang-related homicides in the United States (National Gang Center 2014b). In contrast, across the United States, the National Gang Center estimated that gang-related homicides account for around 12% of all homicides annually (National Gang Center 2014a). Highly populated areas accounted for the vast majority of gang homicides: nearly 70% occurred in cities with populations over 100,000 and 19% occurred in suburban counties in 2011 (National Gang Center 2014b). The National Gang Center (2014b) estimates that about half of Chicago's homicides are gang related. The National Gang Center estimates that half of Chicago's homicides are gang related. As noted above, gang-related mortalities or homicides between 2003 and 2008 were below 7 per 100,000 (Figure 3–5) (Centers for Disease Control and Prevention 2012a). This estimate is consistent with the estimate of the current superintendent of the Chicago Police Department that puts Chicago's overall homicide rate at 14 per 100,000 Chicago citizens (McCarthy 2014). These findings confirm that homicides in general are relatively rare, and gang-related homicides in specific are even less frequent.

A major problem confounding the gathering of homicide statistics, especially those related to gun violence and gang-related homicides, is the lack of clarity with which gang-related homicides are classified. The definition of *gang-related homicide* can be broad, referring to any homicide in which the victim or perpetrator is a gang member; for example, if a man who is a known member of

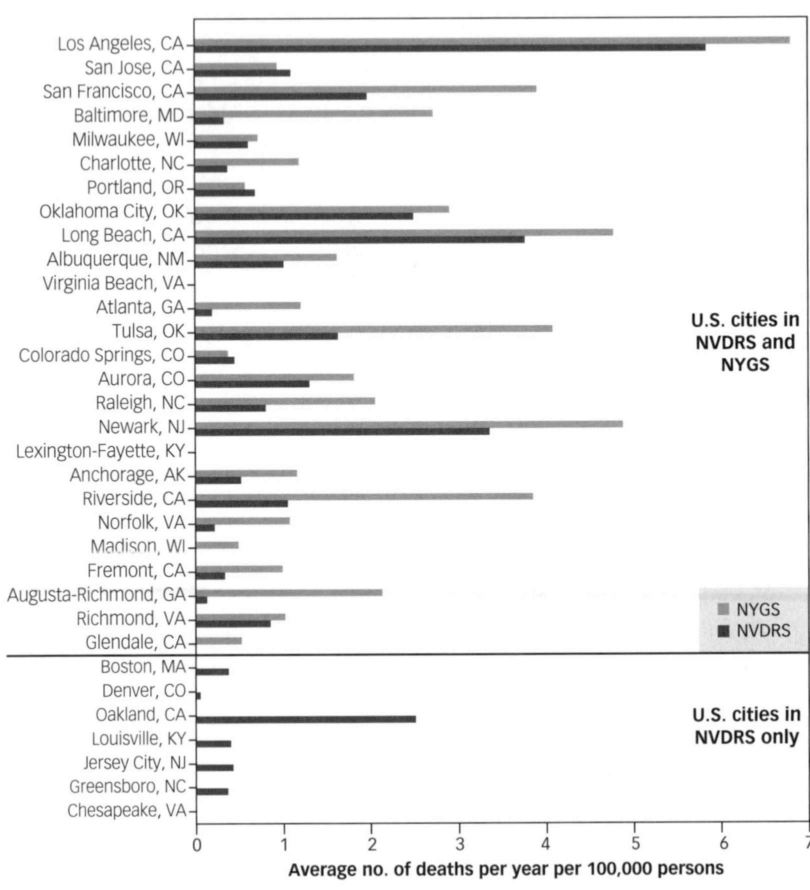

FIGURE 3–5. Estimated gang-related mortality rates among 33 U.S. cities included in the National Violent Death Reporting System (NVDRS) and/or the National Youth Gang Survey (NYGS), 2003–2008.

Cities are listed in descending order by population size. City population estimates were determined by 2000 U.S. Census levels. Cities were in the 17 states participating in NVDRS during 2003–2008 and ranked among the 100 largest cities in the United States based on U.S. Census Bureau statistics. Surveillance years for participating cities vary.

Source. Centers for Disease Control and Prevention: "Gang Homicides—Five U.S. Cities, 2003–2008." *MMWR Morbidity and Mortality Weekly Report* 61(3):46–51, 2012.

a gang kills his wife, that homicide may be classified as gang related. A more narrow definition limits the designation of a gang-related homicide to a homicide in which the motive of the perpetrator(s) furthers the interest and activities of the gang. In addition, the term *gang-related homicide* often subsumes lethal outcomes from a variety of circumstances, such as gang rivalries, drug market participation, solitary crimes involving individual gang members, or arguments between gang acquaintances. Therefore, there is no single characteristic type of gang-related homicide problem, but rather many gang-related homicide problems (National Gang Center 2014a).

Another reason that gathering statistics concerning gang-related homicide is complicated involves decreasing rates of clearance (Isackson 2013). A homicide is described as cleared when the police are able to determine the circumstances around the homicide. In Chicago, which has had the best homicide surveillance for decades, one source reported that clearance rates fell from 48% in 2008 to 26% in 2012 (Isackson 2013). Homicides that occur as a result of interpersonal altercations are typically easy to solve or clear; more complicated homicides, such as those related to gang activity, are harder to clear. The decreasing numbers of interpersonal homicides have resulted in fewer homicides being cleared, changing the statistical calculations of percentages of causes of homicides.

As the more statistically frequent types of homicide (e.g., interpersonal altercation homicides) have decreased, homicides with more opaque causes (e.g., gang-related homicides) represent an increasingly larger percentage of total homicides but not an absolute in rates of gang-related homicides. For example, prior to 1995 in Aurora, Illinois, city police cleared 80% of the homicides as family, friend, and acquaintance homicides. After a large influx of Latinos into the city in 1995, gang-related activity increased, and concomitantly the police department's homicide clearance rate went down to only 20% (personal consultation with the Aurora police department, 1995). In cities with populations over 100,000, such as Aurora, the percentage of gang-related homicides increased approximately 10% from 2009 to 2010 (National Gang Center 2014b), although there was little change in the absolute rates of such homicides.

Similarly, statistics for Chicago demonstrate that an apparent increase in gang-related homicide rates is mostly due to the decrease in domestic homicides. For example, in 1990, street gang–related homicides accounted for 12% of all Chicago homicides (Jenkins and Bell 1992). As noted, the gang-related homicide rates for Chicago between 2007 and 2011 have been estimated to account for 50% of all the homicides in Chicago (National Gang Center 2014b). Again, this change represents only a relative, not an absolute, increase of urban youth homicides, many of which are gang related. In other words, as non-gang-related homicide rates fall and gang homicide rates remain stable, a greater proportion of all homicides in the city involve members of street gangs.

Moreover, for most large cities, the rates of homicide can vary depending on which neighborhood is examined. For example, the overall Chicago homicide rate is 14.5 per 100,000 (McCarthy 2014). However, in the neighborhood of West Lawndale, the homicide rate is 44.5 per 100,000, and the homicide rate for gang members in West Lawndale is 1,685 per 100,000 (McCarthy 2014). Los Angeles and other major cities that have gang problems show similar cluster effects for both their overall homicide and gang homicide rates. Most residents of any major city in the United States can list the "bad neighborhoods" where 75%–80% of the homicides in the city occur. These neighborhoods with high homicide rates also tend to have more than their share of social problems, including substance use, teen pregnancy, inadequate schools and access to education, low employment rates, limited job opportunities, and poor housing.

Dr. Satcher's Youth Violence Report

Although not specifically focused on gun violence, Satcher's 2001 report did an exemplary job of outlining the trends in, the pathways to, and the risk and protective factors for youth violence (U.S. Department of Health and Human Services 2001). Reviewing the lessons from this seminal report is important and relevant because an ultimate form of youth violence is homicide and firearms have been increasingly used in homicides (Butts et al. 2002; U.S. Department of Justice, Office of Justice Programs, Office of Juvenile Justice and Delinquency Prevention 1996). Satcher's report emphasizes that popular assertions that "nothing works" to prevent youth violence, which are often used to justify inaction or failing to attempt initiatives, are false according to the available science (U.S. Department of Health and Human Services 2001).

As the report points out, the assumptions regarding the major risk factors associated with youth violence are not as powerful as expected. Only three variables traditionally associated with youth violence had large effect sizes ($r>0.30$): weak social ties ($r=0.39$); having antisocial, delinquent peers ($r=0.37$); and gang membership ($r=0.31$) (U.S. Department of Health and Human Services 2001). The variables commonly suspected to "predict" future violence had strikingly and surprisingly small effect sizes ($r<0.20$) (U.S. Department of Health and Human Services 2001). These included psychological conditions; hyperactivity; poor parent-child relations; harsh, lax, or inconsistent discipline; weak social ties; problem (antisocial) behavior; antisocial attitudes and beliefs; having antisocial peers; exposure to TV violence; poor attitude toward performance in school; medical or physical problems; low IQ; other problematic family conditions such as coming from a broken home or being separated from parents; dishonesty (males only); and parental abuse and/or neglect.

Satcher's report also highlighted and admirably underscored protective factors that prevented risk factors from becoming predictive factors (U.S. Department of Health and Human Services 2001). These included individual factors (intolerant attitude toward deviance, high IQ, being female, positive social orientation, perceived sanctions for transgressions); factors relating to family (warm, supportive relationships with parents or other adults; parents' positive evaluation of peers; parental monitoring); factors relating to school (commitment to school, recognition for involvement in conventional activities); and factors relating to peer group (friends who engage in conventional behavior) (U.S. Department of Health and Human Services 2001).

Finally, the report highlighted various youth violence intervention and prevention programs that have demonstrated efficacy in decreasing rates of youth homicide (U.S. Department of Health and Human Services 2001). The most highly effective programs combine components that address both individual and environmental conditions. Principles suggested in the design of programs to prevent and intervene in youth violence included assisting in building individual skills and competencies, providing parent effectiveness training, improving the social climate of the school, and changing the type and level of involvement in peer groups. Furthermore, in schools, interventions directed at creating changes in the social context appear to be more effective, on average, than those that attempt to change individual attitudes, skills, and risk behaviors.

The Statistical Problem of Measuring Urban Youth's Gun Violence

To determine whether youth violence prevention and intervention strategies are actually working, we need ways to accurately measure the rates of youth violence and to assess whether morbidity and mortality rates due to firearms are changing and, if so, whether the changes are directly or indirectly attributable to the interventions. Unfortunately, measuring whether rates of gun violence among urban youth are actually increasing or decreasing presents a thorny statistical problem. Addressing public policy implementation issues, which relies in large part on the public's perceptions of whether these rates are increasing or decreasing, is even trickier.

Considering all of the various types of youth violence (Table 3–1), the easiest rates to measure are those of lethal violence. Fortunately, such events are extraordinarily rare in society. However, the rarity of these events is often obfuscated by media reports that declare homicide is one of the leading causes of death in adolescents, or in certain neighborhoods, or in populations such as youth in a gang. For example, the media may report that the statistical homicide rate of youth in gangs in the Chicago neighborhood of West Lawndale is 1,685 per 100,000 (McCarthy 2014). Although accurate in an absolute sense, these reports fail to contextualize the data. *When the incidence of low-base-rate events is being measured, the leading cause of such events is still a statistically small number.*

Clearly, from a public health and policy perspective, putting systems in place to stop events that occur at such low frequency is challenging. Similarly, measuring relative increases or decreases in rates of such small numbers is statistically challenging. For example, in 2009, the national age-adjusted homicide rate was 5.5 per 100,000 population (Centers for Disease Control and Prevention 2012b), a very low base rate of incidence. Even in Chicago, dubbed by the media as the homicide capital of the United States in 2013 (Stableford 2013), the homicide rate was 14.5 per 100,000 people, still a low base rate number. Even in specific neighborhoods with significantly higher relative rates of gang-related homicides, such as West Lawndale (44.5 per 100,000), Roseland (35 per 100,000), or South Chicago (71 per 100,000) (McCarthy 2014), the absolute base rate was still low.

Finding a scientifically valid and reliable method to determine whether rates of youth violence involving firearms are increasing or decreasing is difficult due to the relatively low frequency of the event. The fact that homicide rates are so low, even in areas in which relative frequency of homicide rates is high, makes it difficult to obtain any statistical power to lend scientific credence in the determination of whether or not the homicide rates actually are going up or down. Work from the suicide prevention field indicates that large sample sizes are necessary to provide the statistical power needed for studies of events with low base rates (Institute of Medicine 2002). Accordingly, a scientific study that might be able to prove or disprove the ability of a program or intervention to decrease or prevent urban youth gun violence resulting in a homicide would need an experimental and control population of several hundred thousand people in each condition (Institute of Medicine 2002).

Nevertheless, the existing evidence regarding the incidence of urban youth gun homicide flies in the face of conventional media analysis and public beliefs, which tend to focus attention on the sensational. After every new tragedy, the media declare we are having an epidemic of mass homicides or suicide preceded by homicides by people with mental illness (rarely is the suicide seen as the driving factor for the mass murder) (Bell 2013b). One result of relying on the media to provide accurate information about the public health issues of mental illness and gun violence is that the less sensational but more prevalent and common problems associated with mental illness and gun violence go unnoticed and unaddressed.

Although less newsworthy, data have consistently demonstrated that statistically the most common homicides have been those that occur in the context of interpersonal altercations. In other words, arguments between family and friends or acquaintances that escalate to murder are more common than gang-related homicide, drug-related homicide, mass murder, serial killing, hate crime, police shootings, homicide by individuals with mental illness, or even predatory homicide. In their efforts to provide the public with some perspective on and critical analysis of sensational media reporting, some policy makers try to remind the public that there are more gun-related deaths from suicides than homicides (Centers for Disease Control and Prevention 2012b). Efforts are made to highlight the fact that mass shootings by individuals with or without mental illness (Gold 2013) or "suicides preceded by mass murder" (Bell 2013b) are statistically rare events that account for only a tiny fraction of all firearm homicides.

The notion of trying to use accurate surveillance to size a problem and then design evidence-based methodologies to prevent, intervene in, and provide services to ameliorate the damage from youth violence with a solid public health approach will probably not be newsworthy, despite its utility in providing information to decrease morbidity and mortality of gun violence in populations of youth. Although gang-based violence and drug-based violence should continue to be addressed, programs aimed at these phenomena will not significantly decrease morbidity and mortality from gun violence. Advocacy of legal or regulatory interventions such as requiring psychiatrists to report to the state the names of all their patients who might be dangerous and have guns is also likely to be futile (Law Center to Prevent Gun Violence 2014).

The overarching societal dynamics associated with gun violence and media reporting make it difficult for science to drive public policy and political will. Emotional reactivity to high-profile events involving firearms may fuel "political will" to take action. However, complex problems cannot be solved by interventions based on emotional responses. If the actions taken are not grounded in an appreciation of the best available evidence and its complexity, proposed solutions are likely to be faulty, shortsighted, and ultimately ineffective.

Mental Illness, Urban Youth, Gang Membership, and Violence

Because of the dearth of research on people of color (Parekh 2014; U.S. Public Health Service 2001), there is almost no solid research that directly addresses the issue of the prevalence of mental illness in gangs/urban youth and violence. There is some evidence indicating that a disproportionate number of youth in the criminal justice system have mental illness (Bell 2012b, 2014; Teplin et al. 2002); however, considering the prevalence of mental illness in the United States, using mental illness as a marker for urban youth gun violence is preposterous (Gold 2013).

Nevertheless, recent data indicate that a large proportion of urban children of color in special education, juvenile justice, foster care, and mental health clinics have histories of neurodevelopmental disorders (most likely due to fetal alcohol exposure) (Bell 2012a, 2014; Bell and Chimata 2015), and some of these youth have issues with perpetrating violence. Clinical experience with this population suggests that many of these patients have a history of incarceration due to gun violence behavior that stems from their poor affect regulation (Bell and McBride 2010). Despite the probable increased prevalence of mental illness in youth in juvenile detention centers, it would be a travesty to stereotype and assume that all youth in correctional settings are violent. In 2008, over 2 million youth under age 18 were arrested, and of these about 95% had not been accused of violent crimes such as murder, rape, or aggravated assault (Gottesman and Schwarz 2011).

In addition to the difficulty of disentangling the issue of the prevalence of mental illness of youth in gangs or in juvenile justice detention facilities who perpetrate gun violence, there is also the complexity of understanding the differing degrees or depths of youth involvement in gangs. The vast majority of youth in gangs are marginal (Young and Gonzalez 2013)—that is, they only join a gang for protection or because they live in a certain neighborhood, but they do not fully endorse gang lifestyles and values. In fact, the vast majority of gang members could be classified by the DSM-II (American Psychiatric Association 1968) designation of being dyssocial (i.e., they follow the rules and regulations of the gang, such as being loyal or displaying honor toward each other, but they engage in antisocial behavior toward outsiders). Gang members who are dyssocial readily recognize gang members who are antisocial. Antisocial gang members have no loyalty toward fellow gang members and are a threat to people both inside and outside the gang.

What little research is available on the subject of youth, violence, and psychiatric disorders has suggested a high rate of psychiatric disorders (other than substance use disorders) among gang members (Coid et al. 2013) and among adolescents detained in the justice system (e.g., Colins et al. 2009). However, the most striking finding regarding research on youth, firearm violence, and psychiatric disorders is the absence of psychiatric disorders. Coid et al. (2013) noted that to their knowledge, "no previous research has investigated whether gang violence is related to psychiatric morbidity (other than substance misuse)" (p. 985). As the Institute of Medicine and National Research Council (2013) indicated, more research on the issue of the nature of the association between mental illness, youth, and firearms is clearly needed.

Decreasing Morbidity and Mortality Due to Gun Violence in Urban Youth Populations

Gun violence in the United States has been decreasing over recent decades (Institute of Medicine and National Research Council 2013). This is due, in part, to the decrease in domestic homicides, which as discussed above (see "Early Approaches to Urban Youth Violence and Firearms") has also resulted in a statistically relative increase in gang-related homicides. However, evidence also indicates that the youth homicide rates are also decreasing (see Figure 3–3). The nation and Chicago are doing something right, as indicated by the scientifically documented decreases in urban youth firearm-related death rates. It is worthwhile to examine what kinds of interventions are driving down the rates of gun-related violence or homicide.

The lessons learned from the Institute of Medicine's (2002) *Reducing Suicide* report, Satcher's youth violence report (U.S. Department of Health and Human Services 2001), and the Institute of Medicine's 2009 prevention report (O'Connell et al. 2009) are slowly but surely helping the nation shift gears in addressing youth violence and firearm-related deaths. One of the most important of these lessons represents a basic principle of public health: instead of trying to catalogue risk factors to which the most vulnerable individuals are subject, public health is trying to understand protective factors and promote changes in behavior to keep youth from engaging in risky, unhealthy behaviors.

Satcher advised a focus on three youth populations that would lead to improving the nation's public health: those in protective services, in special education, and in the juvenile justice system (U.S. Department of Health and Human Services et al. 2000). These three systems are where the most vulnerable youth wind up if their families and communities fail them (Bell 2013a). The usual Western approach to problem solving—being deficit focused and trying to ameliorate risk factors for urban youth gun violence—has not proven effective when dealing with these social and systems issues. However, public health interventions, which routinely focus on systems and on multidisciplinary initiatives, provide a different direction: focusing on the protective factors that prevent the risk factors from becoming predictive factors.

Violence Prevention 100 Years Ago

The power of this public health model to make changes in lives of youth has already been demonstrated. A little more than 100 years ago, after the 1891 Chicago fire, the city of Chicago grew as a result of the influx of European immigrants. Within decades, over 70% of Chicago's residents were either immigrants or first-generation Americans. Parents were working overtime to scrape out a living, and children had to work to contribute to the family's livelihood. Children were described as "ill fed, ill housed, ill clothed, illiterate, and wholly untrained and unfitted for any occupation" (Kelley and Stevens 1895, p. 55); families were described as "disrupted by poverty and unfamiliar community circumstances" (Beuttler and Bell 2010, p. 4). These descriptions could also be applied to many modern urban contexts.

From 1875 to 1920, these conditions caused rates of domestic violence among the European immigrant population in Chicago to be extraordinarily high (Adler 2003), and juvenile delinquency and violence were rampant. Fortunately, Jane Addams and colleagues founded Hull House as a social settlement house "to aid in the solution of the social and industrial problems which are engendered by the modern conditions of life in a great city" (Beuttler and Bell 2010, p. 5). This group of industrious women also developed the first juvenile court and the Institute for Juvenile Research (the birthplace of child psychiatry) to strengthen families and to understand the causes of delinquency. Their methods, supported by the science of the day, proved successful for families disrupted by poverty and for disconnected communities, and significantly reduced the problem of violence committed by European American ethnic groups in Chicago more than 100 years ago.

Insights From Chicago

Although the science was less precise, Jane Addams and her colleagues utilized methods and interventions that were similar to current programs providing successful interventions to reduce violence and delinquency in Chicago Public Schools. From 1992 to 1999, Aban Aya Youth Project researchers, led by Brian Flay, conducted violence, drug use, and early sexual activity prevention research in 12 Chicago Public Schools (Flay et al. 2004). This program focused on youth in grades 5–8 and their parents and teachers.

The Aban Aya Youth Project conducted a cluster-randomized trial in which groups of students were assigned to a social development curriculum (SDC), a social development curriculum with school-wide climate and parental and community components (a school-community intervention; SCI), or a control condition. The SDC and SCI groups received 16–21 lessons per year focusing on social competence skills necessary to manage high-risk situations that fostered violence, drug use, and sexual behaviors. The control group received an attention-placebo health enhancement curriculum (HEC) of equal intensity focusing on nutrition, physical activity, and general health care.

The study found that boys in the SDC and SCI conditions demonstrated significant reductions in the rate of increased violent behavior (by 35% and 47%, respectively, compared with the HEC) (Flay et al. 2004). The experimental universal preventive SDC and SCI interventions, respectively, also resulted in significant reductions in the rates of increase in provoking behavior (41% and 59%), school delinquency (31% and 66%), drug use (32% and 34%), and recent sexual intercourse (44% and 65%) for boys (Flay et al. 2004). There was also improvement in the rate of increased condom use (95% and 165%). Additionally, the SCI was significantly more effective than the SDC alone for a combined behavioral measure (79% improvement vs. 51%) (Flay et al. 2004).

In 2007, an independent team of national researchers examined 53 universal school-based programs to prevent violent and aggressive behavior (Hahn et al. 2007) and affirmed Aban Aya as one of seven programs that had greatest design suitability and good execution (Centers for Disease Control and Prevention 2007). Based on its solid research methodology and positive outcomes, the Aban Aya program's core theory was crafted into seven field principles (described later in this section). Government and community partners could use these seven principles to cultivate resiliency (Bell 2001) and reduce the likelihood that risk factors (e.g., poverty, neighborhood disruption, exposure to violence) would lead to violence and other negative behaviors in youth (Bell et al. 2002).

Use of the seven field principles in the Chicago Public Schools (Flay et al. 2004) helped to reduce violence in the schools by about 50% (Bell et al. 2001) and to decrease child abuse in Illinois (Griffin et al. 2011; Redd et al. 2005). The seven field principles have also been effective in several other public health contexts, including HIV prevention (Bell et al. 2008), suicide prevention (Kaslow et al. 2010), and engaging and treating depressed African American youth (Breland-Noble et al. 2006, 2011, 2012). They have also formed the basis for an internationally utilized intervention to reduce the immediate and midterm psychological effects of trauma (Hobfoll et al. 2007). The seven field principles are as follows (Bell 2001):

1. *Rebuilding the village/constructing social fabric (technically known as building "collective efficacy").* The social disorganization theory of delinquency, of which urban youth gun violence is an extreme form, suggests that poverty, single-headed households, isolation from neighbors to help raise youth, and weakened community relationships and networks lead to reduced formal and informal social controls (Shaw and McKay 1942). Sampson et al. (1997) demonstrated that of the 49 equally poor urban neighborhoods in Chicago, only 6 had high rates of violence, whereas the other 43 had homicide rates comparable to those in the rest of the city. This difference was attributed to collective efficacy—that is, the outcome of the effect of social fabric within the various communities. Accordingly, in communities whose social fabric has been shredded by city neighborhoods being torn up (Fullilove 2005), the concept of rebuilding the village has utility as a guiding principle to restore protective communities.

   The principle of rebuilding the village suggests that government institutions, organizations, businesses, families, and citizens in a community can come together and create synergy from working in concert with one another so the whole community is a safer, healthier place (Bell et al. 2001). Technically, government officials who are elected by the populace are supposed to be responsible for facilitating this task; however, any individual or body can commence a process of collaboration within a community. An example of rebuilding the village is a church or police district helping to organize block clubs to encourage neighbors to monitor the behavior of each other's children (Bell et al. 2001).
2. *Providing access to biotechnical and psychosocial technology.* A disproportionate number of youth in the criminal justice system have mental illness (Bell 2012b, 2014; Teplin et al. 2002). One hypothesis is that the provision of mental health treatment or preventive interventions to this population (Beardslee et al. 2011; Bonnie et al. 2013; O'Connell et al. 2009) could prevent subsequent acts of urban youth gun violence. This theory implies that increased provision of mental health care, social services, and educational

and employment opportunities to an identifiable at-risk population may decrease this population's risk of committing legal infractions, including future gun violence.

In addition, as noted earlier, recent data indicate that a large proportion of urban children of color receiving special education services, or those in the juvenile justice system, in foster care, and in mental health clinics, have histories of neurodevelopmental disorders (most likely due to fetal alcohol exposure) (Bell 2012a, 2014; Bell and Chimata 2015). Clinical experience with this population suggests that many of these individuals have a history of incarceration due to behavior involving gun violence stemming from their poor affect regulation (Bell and McBride 2010).

Early research indicates that prenatal administration of choline mitigates the effects of fetal alcohol exposure on the developing fetus. In addition, providing choline to young children with fetal alcohol syndrome has reduced the severity of overactivity and of learning and memory deficits, and has improved attention, fine motor skills, and cognitive functioning (Chicago Department of Public Health 2013). Because most studies on fetal alcohol exposure have found that damage done to fetuses by the mothers' drinking occurs when women do not know they are pregnant, these strategies could prevent the common problem of neurodevelopmental disorder associated with prenatal alcohol exposure (American Psychiatric Association 2013).

3. *Improving bonding, attachment, and connectedness dynamics.* In an effort to improve urban youth affect regulation and thereby decrease impulsive youth gun violence, Chicago Public Schools implemented the Cradles to Classroom intervention (Bell et al. 2001), based on attachment theory (Bowlby 1973), and the Nurse-Family Partnership (Olds et al. 2007; Sweet and Appelbaum 2004). This collaborative initiative helped teens understand child development and illustrated how the development of parenting skills and accessing community resources could result in better childhood outcomes. The results from 2002 revealed that significantly fewer girls in Chicago Public Schools who participated in this program became pregnant and dropped out of high school. Of the 495 seniors who had babies in Chicago Public Schools, all graduated and 78% were enrolled in a 2- or 4-year college; only 5 of 2,000 high school mothers had a repeat pregnancy while still in school (Lamberg 2003). The dynamics of bonding, attachment, and connectedness can be improved through multiple interventions such as these.
4. *Providing opportunities to improve self-esteem.* Low self-esteem has been associated with violent behavior, such as bullying and domestic abuse (Bell et al. 2001; Flay et al. 2004). Many sources of conflict that result in urban male gun violence derive from issues of low self-esteem (Wilkinson and Fagan 2002). Accordingly, the Aban Aya researchers hypothesized that improving self-esteem—operationally defined as 1) a sense of power, 2) a sense of uniqueness,

3) a sense of models, and 4) a sense of connectedness (Bean 1992)—might provide protection from engaging in risky behaviors that stem from low self-esteem (Flay et al. 2004). For example, students who did not expect to attend college reported a threefold greater prevalence of handgun ownership than did students expecting to attend college (Callahan and Rivara 1992). Activities to improve self-esteem are protective against engaging in risky behaviors such as weapon carrying.

5. *Increasing opportunities to learn social and emotional skills.* Social and emotional "people skills" are essential requirements for success in life and can be helpful in navigating social communication and interactions, such as reading social cues or understanding social consequences. In regard to urban youth gun violence, such skills can often de-escalate conflicts and prevent them from ending in gun violence. In addition, having the social and emotional skill of affect regulation is helpful in preventing or intervening in potentially violent situations involving firearms (Bell and McBride 2010).

   Extracurricular social and emotional skill activities were used in the Aban Aya research intervention and in the "naturalistic, large-scale public health" research done in Chicago Public Schools (O'Connell et al. 2009). Urban youth were taught and practiced social and emotional skills of mediation, conflict resolution, and anger management and were taught how to resolve disputes peacefully without harming relationships. Students were given opportunities to develop leadership skills so they could join in the effort of reducing youth gun violence within their communities (Bell et al. 2001; Flay et al. 2004).

6. *Providing a sense of safety, reestablishing the adult protective shield, and monitoring risky behaviors.* In one study, students who reported hearing gunfire in their neighborhoods at least one or two times a week also reported a fourfold higher rate of handgun ownership compared with students from neighborhoods where gunfire was never heard (Callahan and Rivara 1992). Young people need protection in their communities, schools, and homes. Communities must provide a sense of safety for their youth; otherwise, the youth will feel the need to protect themselves.

   In recognition of this need, Chicago Public Schools instituted an outside and an inside school safety initiative. The 2006 Walking School Bus (which in 2009 became known as the Safe Passage program) was a conscious effort to increase the sense of security in the public schools and during the passage to and from school. This program involved parents and other responsible adults who supervised the students' travel to and from school (Bell et al. 2001). The Safe Passage program "has led to a 20% decline in criminal incidents around Safe Passage schools, a 27% drop in incidents among students, and a 7% increase in attendance over the past two years in high schools that currently have the Safe Passage program" (Chicago Public Schools 2014, p. 1).

The inside school safety initiative involved enhanced training and expansion of both security personnel and rapid response teams. Chicago Public Schools instituted random weapon searches. In the baseline 1997–1998 school year, 107 cutting weapons were found and confiscated; in the 1998–1999 school year, 96 cutting weapons were confiscated; and in the 1999–2000 school year, 54 cutting weapons were found and confiscated. Only one gun was confiscated in the 1999–2000 school year, compared with none seized in previous years. This yield was so small that no real conclusions could be made regarding youth carrying guns to school. However, the number of random sweeps per school went from 56 in the 1997–1998 school year to 65 in the 1998–1999 school year and to 89 in the 1999–2000 school year. Considering the increasing frequency of random weapon searches over these 3 years, if weapon-carrying behavior had not changed, one would expect more rather than fewer weapons to be found (Bell et al. 2001).

7. *Minimizing the residual effects of trauma.* One study highlighting the issue of trauma in urban youth found that of teens carrying concealed firearms, more than 90% had been victimized, more than 90% had witnessed violence, and 73% had a family member who had been shot (Molnar et al. 2004). In contrast, neighborhood poverty did not predict concealed gun carrying any more than neighborhood poverty predicted high homicide rates. This study also pointed out that the vast majority of teens who had witnessed violence, been victimized, or had a family member shot did not carry concealed weapons, also indicating the influence of protective factors for this population.

   In another study highlighting how experiencing potentially traumatizing events affects gun-carrying behavior, 14% of adolescents reported carrying a handgun in the past 30 days, and 4% reported taking a handgun to school during the year. Of these, 39% personally knew someone who had been either killed or injured from gunfire, and 22% reported that carrying a handgun could make them feel safer if they were going to be in a physical fight (Wilkinson and Fagan 2002).

   As an intervention to try to decrease the effects of exposure to trauma, Chicago Public Schools developed service-learning requirements for graduation from high school. These efforts sought to augment the ability of youth to transform their helplessness into helpful community activities (Bell et al. 2001). In another large system effort to prevent violence, the Illinois Department of Children and Family Services (IDCFS) attempted to minimize the effects of exposure to trauma by providing protective factors that had been identified as shielding urban youth. These interventions utilized strategies to turn learned helplessness into learned helpfulness—that is, fostering mastery and thus generating hope. Accordingly, 50 IDCFS psychological first aid trainers provided training for more than 4,600 IDCFS staff in psychological first aid techniques (Griffin et al. 2011).

Many different activities and interventions can work toward the outcomes that the seven field principles are striving to achieve (Bell 2014). For example, organizing a community soccer program can establish relationships between neighbors and facilitate raising one another's children; starting a Little League baseball program can teach youth social and emotional skills as they learn how to play baseball with respect and emotional regulation; math clubs can provide a source for self-esteem; and religious activities or a church-sponsored garden can change the helplessness of hunger into the helpfulness of growing one's own food.

One of the advantages of using these principles as models for interventional programs to decrease the incidence of urban youth gun violence and mental illness lies in their flexibility and creativity. The principles are focused enough to be "directionally correct" but flexible enough to accommodate differing neighborhoods, cultures, and resources within a community. These are strength-based approaches that not only reduce violence but also reduce risky sexual behaviors, lower the likelihood of drug use, decrease teen pregnancy, and encourage successful school performance. These strategies have worked before and they can work again.

Conclusion

The causes of urban youth gun violence are multidetermined and extraordinarily complex. Accordingly, no single "magic bullet" criminal justice or public health approach will correct the problem; rather, a multipronged strategy is likely to get the best results. Nevertheless, scientific evidence does suggest that interventions designed to decrease the morbidity and mortality associated with urban youth gun violence can be successfully implemented. Efforts to increase urban youth's community social fabric, connectedness, social and emotional skills, self-esteem, adult protective shield, and ability to adapt to various types of stress have shown success in reducing not only urban youth gun violence but other risky behaviors as well. Until society provides all of its youth with access to the protective factors that have been demonstrated to decrease the incidence of urban youth gun violence, society will suffer the consequences.

Suggested Interventions

- Most cities in the United States have public health, criminal justice, and community initiatives that are working to solve the problem of gun violence by urban youth. Because local efforts scaffold public well-being, these efforts can always use support. Accordingly, as simple as it sounds, one major suggested intervention is to become involved with local gun violence programs for urban youth.

- Urban natural support systems (e.g., large, well-organized community churches or youth organizations such as the Boys and Girls Clubs of America) should be encouraged to take more responsibility for improving social fabric in at-risk neighborhoods. A great example of the value of this intervention can be found at http://saintsabina.org.
- Local schools should be encouraged to implement evidence-based school violence prevention programs as outlined by Hahn et al. (2007).
- An important intervention is to improve access to psychological first aid skills in adults who are in frequent contact with urban youth so that these skills are as ubiquitous as physical first aid.

References

Adler JS: "We've got a right to fight: we're married": domestic homicide in Chicago, 1875–1920. J Interdiscip Hist 34(1):27–48, 2003

American Psychiatric Association: Diagnostic and Statistical Manual of Mental Disorders, 2nd Edition. Washington, DC, American Psychiatric Association, 1968

American Psychiatric Association: Diagnostic and Statistical Manual of Mental Disorders, 5th Edition. Arlington, VA, American Psychiatric Association, 2013

Bean R: The Four Conditions of Self-Esteem: A New Approach for Elementary and Middle Schools, 2nd Edition. Santa Cruz, CA, ETR Associates, 1992

Beardslee WR, Chien PL, Bell CC: Prevention of mental disorders, substance abuse, and problem behaviors: a developmental perspective. Psychiatr Serv 62(3):247–254, 2011 21363895

Bell CC: Preventive strategies for dealing with violence among blacks. Community Ment Health J 23(3):217–228, 1987 3677590

Bell CC: Community violence: causes, prevention, and intervention. J Natl Med Assoc 89(10):657–662, 1997 9347679

Bell CC: Cultivating resiliency in youth. J Adolesc Health 29(5):375–381, 2001 11691598

Bell CC: Violence Prevention 101: implications for policy development," in Perspectives on Crime and Justice: 2000–2001 Lecture Series, Vol V. Washington, DC, National Institute of Justice, March 2002, p 67. Available at: http://www.ncjrs.gov/pdffiles1/nij/187100.pdf. Accessed May 23, 2014.

Bell CC: Correctional psychiatry, in Comprehensive Textbook of Psychiatry, 8th Edition. Edited by Sadock BJ, Sadock VA. Baltimore, MD, Lippincott Williams & Wilkins, 2005, pp 4002–4012

Bell CC: Preventing fetal alcohol syndrome. Clinical Psychiatry News 40(5):8, 2012a

Bell CC: Violence: contagion, group marginalization, and resilience or protective factors. Proceedings of the Contagion of Violence: A Workshop of the Forum on Global Violence Prevention Sponsored by the Board on Global Health, Board on Children, Youth, and Families of the Institute of Medicine of the National Academies. Washington, DC, National Academy of Sciences, 2012b, pp II.1–II.5

Bell CC: Culture: a key touchstone for treatment. Clinical Psychiatry News 41(2):10, 2013a

Bell CC: Preventing suicide preceded by mass murder. Clinical Psychiatry News 41(1):4, 2013b

Bell CC: Prevention continues to gain traction. Clinical Psychiatry News 41(3):12, 2013c

Bell CC: Fetal alcohol exposure among African Americans. Psychiatr Serv 65(5):569, 2014 24788732

Bell CC, Chimata R: Prevalence of neurodevelopmental disorders among low-income African Americans at a clinic on Chicago's South Side. Psychiatr Serv 66(5):539–542, 2015 25726976

Bell CC, Jenkins E: Prevention of black homicide, in The State of Black America—1990. Edited by Dewart J. New York, National Urban League, 1990, pp 143–155

Bell CC, McBride DF: Affect regulation and prevention of risky behaviors. JAMA 304(5):565–566, 2010 20682937

Bell CC, Prothrow-Stith D, Smallwood-Murchison C: Black-on-black homicide: the National Medical Association's responsibilities. J Natl Med Assoc 78(12):1139–1141, 1986 3806686

Bell CC, Gamm S, Vallas P, et al: Strategies for the prevention of youth violence in Chicago Public Schools, in School Violence: Contributing Factors, Management, and Prevention. Edited by Shafii M, Shafii S. Washington, DC, American Psychiatric Publishing, 2001, pp 251–272

Bell CC, Flay B, Paikoff R: Strategies for health behavior change, in The Health Behavioral Change Imperatives: Theory, Education, and Practice in Diverse Populations. Edited by Chunn J. New York, Kluwer Academic/Plenum Publishers, 2002, pp 17–40. Available at: http://people.oregonstate.edu/~flayb/MY%20PUBLICATIONS/Multiple%20behaviors/Bell,Flay,Paikoff.pdf. Accessed May 23, 2014.

Bell CC, Bhana A, Petersen I, et al: Building protective factors to offset sexually risky behaviors among black youths: a randomized control trial. J Natl Med Assoc 100(8):936–944, 2008 18717144

Beuttler FW, Bell CC: For the Welfare of Every Child—A Brief History of the Institute for Juvenile Research, 1909–2010. Chicago, University of Illinois, 2010

Bjerregaard B, Lizotte AJ: Gun ownership and gang membership. J Crim Law Criminol 86(1):37–58, 1995

Black Psychiatrists of America: New center proposed. Black Psychiatrists of America 1(1):3, 1969

Black Psychiatrists of America: Homicide in young black males. The Bottom Line 10(2):3, 1980

Block CR: Lethal Violence in Chicago Over Seventeen Years: Homicide Known to the Police, 1965–81. Chicago, Illinois Criminal Justice Information Authority, 1985

Bonnie RJ, Johnson RL, Chemers BM, et al (eds): Reforming Juvenile Justice: A Developmental Approach. Washington, DC, National Academies Press, 2013. Available at: http://www.nap.edu/catalog.php?record_id=14685. Accessed May 23, 2014.

Bowlby J: Attachment and Loss, Vol 2: Separation. New York, Basic Books, 1973

Breland-Noble AM, Bell C, Nicolas G: Family first: the development of an evidence-based family intervention for increasing participation in psychiatric clinical care and research in depressed African American adolescents. Fam Process 45(2):153–169, 2006 16768016

Breland-Noble AM, Bell CC, Burriss A, et al: "Mama just won't accept this": adult perspectives on engaging depressed African American teens in clinical research and treatment. J Clin Psychol Med Settings 18(3):225–234, 2011 21512751

Breland-Noble AM, Bell CC, Burriss A, et al: The significance of strategic community engagement in recruiting African American youth and families for clinical research. J Child Fam Stud 21(2):273–280, 2012 22984337

Bureau of Justice Statistics: Homicide Trends in the U.S.: Intimate Homicide. Washington, DC, Bureau of Justice Statistics, 2007. Available at: http://www.lb7.uscourts.gov/documents/08–37701.pdf. Accessed May 23, 2014.

Butts J, Coffeshall M, Gouvis C, et al: Youth, Guns, and the Juvenile Justice System. Washington, DC, Urban Institute, 2002

Callahan CM, Rivara FP: Urban high school youth and handguns: a school-based survey. JAMA 267(22):3038–3042, 1992 1588717

Centers for Disease Control and Prevention: The effectiveness of universal school-based programs to prevent violent and aggressive behavior—a report on recommendations of the Task Force on Community Preventive Services. MMWR Morb Mortal Wkly Rep 56(RR-7):1–16, 2007

Centers for Disease Control and Prevention: Gang homicides—five U.S. cities, 2003–2008. MMWR Morb Mortal Wkly Rep 61(3):46–51, 2012a

Centers for Disease Control and Prevention: QuickStats: suicide and homicide rates, by age group—United States, 2009. MMWR Morb Mortal Wkly Rep 61(28):543, 2012b

Centers for Disease Control and Prevention: Homicide rates among persons aged 10–24 years—United States, 1981–2010. MMWR Morb Mortal Wkly Rep 62(27):545–548, 2013 23842443

Chicago Department of Public Health: Public Health Brief: Fetal Alcohol Spectrum Disorders. Chicago, IL, Chicago Department of Public Health, 2013

Chicago Public Schools: Safe Passage Routes. Chicago, IL, Chicago Public Schools. 2014. Available at: http://www.cps.edu/Pages/safepassage.aspx. Accessed July 1, 2014.

Child Trends Data Bank: Teen Homicide, Suicide, and Firearm Deaths. Bethesda, MD, Child Trends, 2012. Available at: http://www.childtrends.org/?indicators=teen-homicide-suicide-and-firearm-deaths. Accessed May 23, 2014.

Coid JW, Ullrich S, Keers R, et al: Gang membership, violence, and psychiatric morbidity. Am J Psychiatry 170(9):985–993, 2013 23846827

Colins O, Vermeiren R, Schuyten G, et al: Psychiatric disorders in property, violent, and versatile offending detained male adolescents. Am J Orthopsychiatry 79(1):31–38, 2009 19290723

Dennis RE: Homicide among black males: social costs to families and communities. Public Health Rep 95(6):556–557, 1980 7433607

Dennis RE, Kirk A, Knuckles BN: Black Males at Risk to Low Life Expectancy: A Study of Homicide Victims and Perpetrators. Bethesda, MD, National Institute of Mental Health, Center for Studies of Minority Group Mental Health, 1981

Douglas K, Bell CC: Youth homicide prevention. Psychiatr Clin North Am 34(3):205–216, 2011 21333848

Egley A, Howell JC: Highlights of the 2011 National Youth Gang Survey (NCJ 242884). Washington, DC, U.S. Department of Justice, Office of Justice Programs, Office of Juvenile Justice and Delinquency Prevention, 2013

Federal Bureau of Investigation: Table: Crime in the United States by Volume and Rate per 100,000 Inhabitants, 1991–2010. Washington, DC, Federal Bureau of Investigation, 2010. Available at: www.fbi.gov/about-us/cjis/ucr/crime-in-the-u.s/2010/crime-in-the-u.s.-2010/tables/10tbl01.xls. Accessed May 23, 2014.

Flay BR, Graumlich S, Segawa E, et al: Effects of 2 prevention programs on high-risk behaviors among African American youth: a randomized trial. Arch Pediatr Adolesc Med 158(4):377–384, 2004 15066879

Flay BR, Snyder F, Petraitis J: Biopsychosocial causes of behavior: the theory of triadic influence, in Emerging Theories in Health Promotion Practice and Research, 2nd Edition. Edited by DiClemente RJ, Kegler MC, Crosby RA. New York, Jossey-Bass, 2009, pp 451–510

Fullilove MT: Root Shock: How Tearing Up City Neighborhoods Hurts America, and What We Can Do About It. New York, One World–Ballantine Books, 2005

Gibbons RD, Hur K, Bhaumik DK, et al: Profiling of county-level foster care placements using random-effects Poisson regression models. Health Serv Outcomes Res Methodol 7(3–4):97–108, 2007

Gold LH: Gun violence: psychiatry, risk assessment, and social policy. J Am Acad Psychiatry Law 41(3):337–343, 2013 24051585

Gorwitz K, Dennis R: On the decrease in the life expectancy of black males in Michigan. Public Health Rep 91(2):141–145, 1976 822463

Gottesman D, Schwarz SW: Juvenile Justice in the U.S.: Facts for Policymakers. Washington, DC, National Center for Children in Poverty, 2011

Greenfield LA, Rand MR, Craven D, et al: Violence by Intimates (NCJ-167237). Washington, DC, U.S. Department of Justice, Office of Justice Programs, Bureau of Justice Statistics, March 1998

Griffin G, McEwen E, Samuels BH, et al: Infusing protective factors for children in foster care. Psychiatr Clin North Am 34(3):185–203, 2011 21333847

Griffith EE, Bell CC: Recent trends in suicide and homicide among blacks. JAMA 262(16):2265–2269, 1989 2677427

Hahn R, Fuqua-Whitley D, Wethington H, et al: Effectiveness of universal school-based programs to prevent violent and aggressive behavior: a systematic review. Am J Prev Med 33(2 suppl):S114–S129, 2007 17675013

Hobfoll SE, Watson P, Bell CC, et al: Five essential elements of immediate and mid-term mass trauma intervention: empirical evidence. Psychiatry 70(4):283–315, discussion 316–369, 2007 18181708

Howell JC: Preventing and Reducing Juvenile Delinquency. Thousand Oaks, CA, Sage, 2009

Institute of Medicine: Reducing Suicide: A National Imperative. Edited by Goldsmith SK, Pellmar TC, Kleinman AM, et al. Washington, DC, National Academies Press, 2002

Institute of Medicine, National Research Council: Priorities for Research to Reduce the Threat of Firearm-Related Violence. Washington, DC, National Academies Press, 2013

Isackson I: Chicago's criminals are getting away with murder. Chicago Magazine, May 2013. Available at: http://www.chicagomag.com/Chicago-Magazine/May-2013/Getting-Away-with-Murder/index.php?cparticle=2andsiarticle=1#artanc. Accessed May 23, 2014.

Jenkins EJ, Bell CC: Adolescent violence: can it be curbed? Adolesc Med 3(1):71–86, 1992 10356167

Kaslow NJ, Leiner AS, Reviere S, et al: Suicidal, abused African American women's response to a culturally informed intervention. J Consult Clin Psychol 78(4):449–458, 2010 20658802

Kelley F, Stevens AP: Wage-earning children, in Hull House Maps and Papers. Edited by Addams J. New York, Thomas Y. Crowell & Co, 1895, pp 49–76. Available at: http://media.pfeiffer.edu/lridener/DSS/Addams/hh3.html. Accessed May 23, 2014.

Koop CE: Surgeon General's Workshop on Violence and Public Health: Source Book. Washington, DC, National Center on Child Abuse and Neglect, 1985

Kotlowitz A: If gang shootings and revenge killing were an infectious disease, how would you stop it? Chicago epidemiologist thinks he has the answer. New York Times Magazine, May 4, 2008, pp 52–59, 100–102

Lamberg L: Programs target youth violence prevention. JAMA 290(5):585–586, 2003 12902355

Law Center to Prevent Gun Violence: Mental Health Reporting in Illinois. Smartgunlaws.org, March 2, 2014. Available at: http://smartgunlaws.org/mental-health-reporting-in-illinois. Accessed August 4, 2015.

Lizotte AJ, Krohn MD, Howell JC, et al: Factors influencing gun carrying among young urban males over the adolescent–young adult life course. Criminology 38(3):811–834, 2000

Marshall E: Obama lifts ban on funding gun violence research. Science Insider, January 16, 2013. Available at: http://news.sciencemag.org/2013/01/obama-lifts-ban-funding-gun-violence-research. Accessed May 23, 2014.

McCarthy G: Leadership Breakfast: Addressing Gun and Community Violence in Chicago. March 13, 2014

Molnar BE, Miller MJ, Azrael D, et al: Neighborhood predictors of concealed firearm carrying among children and adolescents: results from the Project on Human Development in Chicago Neighborhoods. Arch Pediatr Adolesc Med 158(7):657–664, 2004 15237065

Murphy SL, Xu J, Kochanek KD: Deaths: final data for 2010. Natl Vital Stat Rep 61(4):1–117, 2013 24979972

National Center for Health Statistics: Final Mortality Statistics. Hyattsville, MD, Division of Vital Statistics, 1977

National Gang Center: Frequently Asked Questions About Gangs. Tallahassee, FL, National Gang Center, 2014a. Available at: http://www.nationalgangcenter.gov/About/FAQ#RefEgley2003. Accessed May 23, 2014.

National Gang Center: National Youth Gang Survey Analysis. Tallahassee, FL, National Gang Center, 2014b. Available at: http://www.nationalgangcenter.gov/Survey-Analysis. Accessed May 23, 2014.

National Research Council: The Growth of Incarceration in the United States: Exploring Causes and Consequences. Committee on Causes and Consequences of High Rates of Incarceration. Edited by Travis J, Western B, Redburn S, et al. Washington, DC, National Academies Press, 2014

O'Connell ME, Boat T, Warner KE (eds): Preventing Mental, Emotional, and Behavioral Disorders Among Young People: Progress and Possibilities. Washington, DC, National Academies Press, 2009

Olds DL, Sadler L, Kitzman H: Programs for parents of infants and toddlers: recent evidence from randomized trials. J Child Psychol Psychiatry 48(3–4):355–391, 2007 17355402

Parekh R (ed): The Massachusetts General Hospital Textbook on Diversity and Cultural Sensitivity in Mental Health (Current Clinical Psychiatry). New York, Springer, 2014

Poussaint A: Why Blacks Kill Blacks. New York, Emerson Hall Publishers, 1972

Redd J, Suggs H, Gibbons R, et al: A plan to strengthen systems and reduce the number of African-American children in child welfare. Illinois Child Welfare 2(1 and 2):34–46, 2005. Available at: http://www.illinoischildwelfare.org/archives/spr2007/A%20Plan%20To%20Strengthen%20Systems%20And%20Reduce%20The%20Number%20Of.pdf. Accessed May 23, 2014.

Rosen R: The World Split Open: How the Modern Women's Movement Changed America, Revised Edition. New York, Penguin Books, 2001

Sampson RJ, Raudenbush SW, Earls F: Neighborhoods and violent crime: a multilevel study of collective efficacy. Science 277(5328):918–924, 1997 9252316

Shaw CR, McKay H: Juvenile Delinquency and Urban Areas. Chicago, IL, University of Chicago Press, 1942

Stableford D: Chicago now murder capital of U.S., FBI says. Yahoo News, September 19, 2013. Available at: http://news.yahoo.com/chicago-murder-capital-of-america-fbi-142122290.html;_ylt=A0LEV7.36Y1T6XkA_u8PxQt.;_ylu=X3oDMTByZDBpbXI5BHNlYwNzcgRwb3MDNQRjb2xvA2JmMQR2dGlkAw—. Accessed August 4, 2015.

Sweet MA, Appelbaum MI: Is home visiting an effective strategy? A meta-analytic review of home visiting programs for families with young children. Child Dev 75(5):1435–1456, 2004 15369524

Teplin LA, Abram KM, McClelland GM, et al: Psychiatric disorders in youth in juvenile detention. Arch Gen Psychiatry 59(12):1133–1143, 2002 12470130

U.S. Department of Health and Human Services: Report of the Secretary's Task Force on Black and Minority Health, Vol 1: Executive Summary. DHHS Publ No PHS 0-487-637. Rockville, MD, U.S. Department of Health and Human Services, 1985

U.S. Department of Health and Human Services: Youth Violence: A Report of the Surgeon General. Rockville, MD, U.S. Department of Health and Human Services, 2001

U.S. Department of Health and Human Services, U.S. Department of Education, U.S. Department of Justice: Report of the Surgeon General's Conference on Children's Mental Health. Washington, DC, U.S. Department of Health and Human Services, 2000

U.S. Department of Justice, Office of Justice Programs, Office of Juvenile Justice and Delinquency Prevention: Combating Violence and Delinquency: The National Juvenile Justice Action Plan (NCJ 157106). Washington, DC, U.S. Department of Justice, 1996

U.S. Public Health Service: Mental Health: Culture, Race and Ethnicity. A Supplement to Mental Health: A Report of the Surgeon General. Rockville, MD, U.S. Public Health Service, 2001

The White House: Presidential memorandum: engaging in public health research on the causes and prevention of gun violence. Washington, DC, The White House, January 16, 2013. Available at: https://www.whitehouse.gov/the-press-office/2013/01/16/presidential-memorandum-engaging-public-health-research-causes-and-preve. Accessed August 4, 2015.

Wilkinson D, Fagan J: What Do We Know About Gun Use Among Adolescents? Boulder, CO, Center for the Study and Prevention of Violence, 2002

Young MA, Gonzalez V: Getting out of gangs, staying out of gangs: gang intervention and desistence strategies. National Gang Center Bulletin, No 8, January 2013

4

Mass Shootings and Mental Illness

James L. Knoll IV, M.D.
George D. Annas, M.D., M.P.H.

Common Misperceptions

- ☒ Mass shootings by people with serious mental illness represent the most significant relationship between gun violence and mental illness.
- ☒ People with serious mental illness should be considered dangerous.
- ☒ Gun laws focusing on people with mental illness or with a psychiatric diagnosis can effectively prevent mass shootings.
- ☒ Gun laws focusing on people with mental illness or a psychiatric diagnosis are reasonable, even if they add to the stigma already associated with mental illness.

Evidence-Based Facts

- ☑ Mass shootings by people with serious mental illness represent less than 1% of all yearly gun-related homicides. In contrast, deaths by suicide using firearms account for the majority of yearly gun-related deaths.
- ☑ The overall contribution of people with serious mental illness to violent crimes is only about 3%. When these crimes are examined in detail, an even smaller percentage of them are found to involve firearms.

☑ Laws intended to reduce gun violence that focus on a population representing less than 3% of all gun violence will be extremely low yield, ineffective, and wasteful of scarce resources. Perpetrators of mass shootings are unlikely to have a history of involuntary psychiatric hospitalization. Thus, databases intended to restrict access to guns and established by guns laws that broadly target people with mental illness will not capture this group of individuals.

☑ Gun restriction laws focusing on people with mental illness perpetuate the myth that mental illness leads to violence, as well as the misperception that gun violence and mental illness are strongly linked. Stigma represents a major barrier to access and treatment of mental illness, which in turn increases the public health burden.

Mass shootings understandably create outpourings of public horror and outrage. Nevertheless, and contrary to common media depictions and the general public's beliefs, mass shootings are extremely rare events. These tragedies are influenced by multiple complex factors, many of which are still poorly understood. However, the lay public and the media typically assume that the perpetrator has a mental illness and that the mental illness is the cause of these highly violent acts of horrific desperation. Although some mass shooters are found to have a history of psychiatric illness, no reliable research has suggested that a majority of perpetrators are primarily influenced by serious mental illness as opposed to, for example, psychological turmoil flowing from other sources. As a result, debate on how to prevent mass shootings has focused heavily on issues that are 1) highly politicized, 2) grossly oversimplified, and 3) unlikely to result in productive solutions.

In this chapter, we discuss the existing research, limited though it may be, on mass shootings and then examine the nature of the link between gun violence and mental illness. We consider the value of gun laws focusing on mental illness, with attention to their potential efficacy in preventing future mass shootings. We conclude by proposing that instead of the focus on mental illness, increased attention should be paid to sociocultural factors associated with mass shootings and exploring other interventions and areas for further research.

Mass Murder in the United States

Because of frequent and sensational media coverage, it may appear that the era of mass shootings began in 1966, atop the tower at the University of Texas in Austin, and became a part of American life in subsequent decades (Associated Press 2007). However, cases of mass murder, of which mass shootings are a subset, have been recorded over time long before mass shootings captured public attention. For example, in the Bath school disaster of 1927, to this day the deadliest mass murder in a school in United States history, one man killed 38 Michigan elementary school children and 6 adults and injured at least 58 other people.

The farmer who perpetrated these attacks had run into financial trouble. His wife was seriously ill with tuberculosis. He reportedly became angry after an increase in taxes and losing an election in which he had run for town clerk. He first killed his wife, then firebombed his farm, and then detonated explosives in the Bath Consolidated School, before committing suicide by detonating a final explosion in his truck. Like many modern-day mass murderers, he left a final communication. Stenciled and painted on a board outside his property, his message read, "Criminals are made, not born"—a statement suggestive of externalization of blame and long-held grievance. Many "premodern" cases of mass murder often involved a depressed and angry male who killed his family and then himself. Such cases did not capture much media attention because they were regarded primarily as "family business" and were "too close for comfort" (Dietz 1986, p. 481). In contrast, mass shootings beginning in the 1990s and covered intensely by the media appeared to be a different type of violence, at least in the eyes of the public. Heavily armed individuals who had meticulously planned a public massacre in which they intended to spread as much destruction as possible and then kill themselves seemed a new phenomenon. Compared with depressed and despairing familicide-suicides, these "modern" cases seemed distant enough from the average person's experience to capture the public's attention with morbid fascination over prolonged periods of time.

Mass shootings cause endless public speculation regarding causes and motives. However, high-profile cases of mass shootings, which typically receive the most intense media coverage, are in fact the least representative of mass killings. In reality, such rare cases are the result of many complex factors. Nevertheless, the news media have heavily influenced the public's perception of mass murders (Duwe 2005), offering simplified explanations that assume the perpetrator is either "mad or bad." After all, who but a madman would execute innocent people in broad daylight, while planning to commit suicide or be killed by police?

Such simplistic explanations are easier for the media to report, as well as easier for the public to accept. Nevertheless, these explanations are often inaccurate and based on little or no evidence. In addition, they stoke the political fires surrounding debates concerning regulation of firearms while providing no constructive suggestions to prevent future tragedies. Psychiatric illness, although present in some mass murderers and mass shooters, is far from the most significant or consistent finding from attempts to investigate the nature of these deeply troubling events.

Mass Shootings: What Is Known

A mass shooting is a specific type of mass murder. *Mass murder* is defined as the killing of three or more victims at one location within one event (Burgess 2006). The motives of mass murderers typically involve the desire to kill as many as possible; such a motive does not limit a perpetrator to a particular means (e.g., guns, bombs, arson). Those who commit mass murder may use more than one means to achieve this goal. For example, the mass shooting at an Aurora, Colorado, movie theater in 2012 involved a perpetrator who also booby-trapped his apartment with multiple bombs in an attempt to kill more people in addition to those killed in the shooting. The Norwegian man who committed a mass shooting on Utøya in 2011 set off a bomb in Oslo prior to the shooting. Nevertheless, guns are an efficient and often accessible means to carry out the goal of killing multiple victims. Because of this fact, and given the difficulty of neatly categorizing specific mass murder events as shootings versus murder by other means, the study of mass shootings benefits from an examination of mass murder.

As noted, mass shootings are a subset of mass murders; mass murder is also a catastrophic but rare phenomenon (Burgess 2006; Investigative Assistance for Violent Crimes Act of 2012, Pub. L. No. 112-265, 28 U.S.C. § 530C[b][1][M][i]). Given its extremely low base rate, mass murder (and thus mass shootings) cannot be predicted, especially by persons outside the perpetrator's social circle (Saleva et al. 2007). Little research exists that would serve to better inform mental health professionals or law enforcement regarding the problems that lead individuals to commit mass murder.

For example, in a clinical study of 144 individuals who had threatened some form of violence against others, 8 were found to have threatened mass homicide (Warren et al. 2011). All 8 subjects said they had intended to kill as many people as possible, and all cases involved targeting a specific group against whom the would-be perpetrator held a grievance. Over the 12-month study period, none of the 8 subjects carried out or attempted to carry out their plans. However, 2 of the 8 assaulted a person unrelated to the targeted group. Future research may enhance awareness of the presence of "identification warning behaviors" (Meloy et al. 2011).

Factors common among individuals who commit mass murder include extreme feelings of anger and revenge, the lack of an accomplice (when the perpetrator is an adult), feelings of social alienation, and planning well in advance of the offense. Many mass murderers do not plan to survive their own attacks and intend to commit suicide or to be killed by police after committing their assaults. However, in a detailed case study of five mass murderers who did survive, a number of common traits and historical factors were found. The subjects had all been bullied or isolated during childhood and subsequently became loners who felt despair over their social alienation. They demonstrated paranoid traits such as suspiciousness and grudge holding. Their worldview suggested a paranoid mind-set; they believed others to be generally rejecting and uncaring. As a result, they spent a great deal of time feeling resentful and ruminating on past humiliations. The ruminations subsequently evolved into fantasies of violent revenge (Mullen 2004).

The Federal Bureau of Investigation (FBI) studied 160 cases of active shooter incidents between 2000 and 2013 (Blair and Schweit 2014). An *active shooter* as defined by the FBI and other federal agencies is "an individual actively engaged in killing or attempting to kill people in a confined and populated area. Implicit in this definition is that the subject's criminal activities involve the use of firearms" (Blair and Schweit 2014, p. 5). An average of 11.4 incidents of mass shooting occurred annually, and the trend over the study period showed a steady rise in incidents. The main findings of the FBI study included the following:

- The vast majority of shootings (70%) occurred in either a place of business or an educational environment.
- All but two of the shootings were carried out by a single individual.
- The shooter committed suicide in 64 (40%) of the cases.
- Most incidents (67%) ended before police even arrived and could engage the perpetrator.
- Of the 160 incidents, 64 (40%) qualified as mass murder.
- Only 6 (3.8%) of the 160 cases involved a female perpetrator.

The U.S. Secret Service and the U.S. Department of Education conducted a study focused on targeted school violence in the United States from 1974 to 2000 (Vossekuil et al. 2002). Therefore, this study involved shootings that had occurred prior to the FBI study's findings suggesting a trend of increased mass shooting incidents from 2000 to 2013. Secret Service researchers analyzed 37 incidents of targeted school violence (most of them involving guns) perpetrated by 41 attackers during this time period. Key findings regarding school shooters included the following:

- A majority of perpetrators (68%, $n=28$) acquired guns used from their own or a relative's home.
- Perpetrators had easy access to family-owned firearms.
- Perpetrators often "leaked" their intent to peers.
- Perpetrators often engaged in behavior prior to the incident that caused others concern (e.g., weapon seeking, disturbing writings).
- Perpetrators had often considered or attempted suicide.

Chapter 5, "School Shootings and Mental Illness," provides a more detailed discussion of school shootings.

From an etiological standpoint, the factors contributing to mass murder are broad, and therefore analysis of any single incident should be approached using a model that addresses individual biological, social, and psychological factors (Aitken et al. 2008). Biological factors include possible brain pathology, as well as psychiatric illnesses such as depression and psychosis. Psychological factors include a negative or fragile self-image, paranoid dynamics, and retreat into violent and omnipotent revenge fantasies. Social factors include isolation, possible ostracism by peers, and an absence of prosocial supports. In sum, the extant research on mass murders suggests that these events are caused by a complex interaction of emotional turmoil, psychopathology, traumatic life events, and other precipitating factors unique to each case (Declercq and Audenaert 2011).

Careful study of individual cases of mass murder frequently reveals that the offender felt compelled to leave some type of final message (Hempel et al. 1999; Knoll 2010). These messages may be written, videotaped, or posted on the Internet or social media networks (Aitken et al. 2008). The communications often have great meaning to the perpetrators, who realize it will be the only "living" testament to their motivations and inner struggle (Knoll 2010). These messages are rich sources of data that provide a more complete understanding of the perpetrator's motive, mental state, and psychological disturbances (Smith and Shuy 2002).

Available research has not produced a widely accepted typology of mass murderers or mass shooters (Knoll 2012), and detailed examination of incidents indicates that not all perpetrators are alike in their motivations and psychology. Although no research has reliably established that most mass murderers and mass shooters are psychotic or even suffering from a serious mental illness, individual case studies often reveal paranoid themes in these persons' cognitions (Knoll and Meloy 2014). The paranoia may not rise to the level of psychosis; however, many are found to have been preoccupied with feelings of social persecution and fantasies of revenge against their perceived tormentors. Some appear to be driven by strong feelings of revenge born of social alienation or a perceived injustice. For example, one 15-year-old who shot and killed his two parents and two high school students and wounded another 25 students in 1998 in Springfield, Oregon (Frontline 2000) suffered intolerable anguish over feelings of social rejection. His peers described him as morbid and preoccupied with violence.

Others may in fact suffer from severe depression or, rarely, psychosis. For example, in 2009, a 41-year-old naturalized Vietnamese immigrant killed 14 people, wounded another 4, and then killed himself at the Binghamton, New York, American Civic Association. The man's father reported that in the 2 weeks leading up to the tragedy, his son had stopped eating dinner, stopped watching television, and become increasingly isolative (Chen 2009). A few days after the shooting, a local television news station received a letter composed by the shooter and postmarked the day of the shootings. Careful analysis of the letter revealed long-standing paranoid and persecutory delusions, as well as hallucinations (Knoll 2010). The shooter described his extreme resentment at being systematically persecuted in a bizarre manner by "undercover cops," whom he believed had destroyed his chances of assimilating and working successfully in the United States.

To date, the phenomenon of mass murder has also eluded classification in a broadly accepted system. One proposed system is based on the concept of homicide-suicide, derived from the work of Marzuk et al. (1992) and further adapted by Knoll (2012). *Homicide-suicide,* an event in which an individual commits a homicide and subsequently (usually within 24 hours) commits suicide (Bossarte et al. 2006; Felthous and Hempel 1995), is a distinct category of homicide with features that differ from other forms of killing. Homicide-suicide is also a rare event, estimated to occur at a rate of 0.20–0.38 per 100,000 persons annually (Bossarte et al. 2006; Coid 1983). The majority of homicide-suicides are carefully planned by the perpetrator as a two-stage sequential act. Marzuk et al. (1992) proposed classifying homicide-suicides by the *relationship* the perpetrator had to the victim (e.g., spousal, familial), along with the perpetrator's *motive* (e.g., jealousy, altruism, revenge) (Marzuk et al. 1992). Given that mass murder often ends in the suicide of the perpetrator and has been described as "suicide with hostile intent" (Preti 2008), a classification system similar to that used for homicide-suicide would seem to make sense. An accepted classification system for mass murder would be helpful in coordinating future research efforts. Table 4–1 gives a proposed classification system for mass murder based on the homicide-suicide classification system of Marzuk et al. (1992). In this proposed system, *relationship* is defined as "relationship *or link* between victims and perpetrator" to emphasize the fact that some perpetrators may have no meaningful interpersonal relationship with their victims but instead may have only a connection (link) via some mutually shared activity such as work or school.

This relationship link-motive classification scheme allows for multiple permutations that can be applied to best describe each individual case. Notably, mental illness does not appear consistently as a factor except in two of the six classification groups. For example, in this system, the *School-Resentful* type of mass murderer includes offenders who target schoolmates and have the motive of hostile revenge. Depression and/or suicidal threats are likely to be present prior to the offense, but not necessarily. These individuals are often described as bullied, disaffected, or socially alienated students who are motivated by feelings of rejection or humiliation by peers. The perpetrator often communicates intent to third-party peers (Knoll 2012; Vossekuil et al. 2002). Examples of murderers who fit this description include the shooters at Virginia Tech and Columbine, Colorado (Cullen 2010).

The *Workplace-Resentful* type describes the aggrieved or disgruntled employee or ex-employee who is upset with a supervisor, coworker(s), or some

TABLE 4–1. Proposed classification system for incidents of mass murder

Type	Victim	Relationship	Motive	Offense location	Paranoid cognitions	SMI
School-Resentful	Peers, teachers	Yes	Resentment/revenge	Educational environment	+	+/–
Workplace-Resentful	Coworkers, supervisors	Yes	Resentment/revenge	Place of business	+	+/–
Indiscriminate-Resentful	Arbitrary	No	Resentment/anger	Variable, place of easy access to many victims	+	+/–
Specific Community–Resentful	Identifiable group, culture, or political movement	Variable	Resentment/revenge	Variable according to location of targeted group	+	+/–
Pseudocommunity-Psychotic	Misperceived persecutors	Variable	Paranoid delusions	Variable according to persecutory delusion	+	+
Familial-Depressed	Family, spouse, or ex-spouse	Yes	Severe depression Possible psychosis Revenge	Family domicile	+	+

Note. Classification scheme: relationship (relationship or link between victims and perpetrator) + motive (primary rationale driving the perpetrator). SMI = serious mental illness, defined as psychosis or delusional disorder meeting DSM-5 diagnostic criteria (American Psychiatric Association 2013).
Source. Adapted from Knoll 2012 and Marzuk et al. 1992.

aspect of the work environment and who commits murder in the workplace. These individuals typically externalize blame for their problem onto others and feel they have been wronged. They are very likely to have depression, as well as paranoid and/or narcissistic traits. Persecutory delusions may sometimes be seen; however, mental illness is not necessarily present. An example of this category is the Atlanta day trader who shot and killed 9 people and injured 13 more in 1999. He entered two adjacent Atlanta day-trading firms, stating, "I hope this doesn't ruin your trading day" before carrying out the shootings. Shortly afterward, he shot himself. This individual was motivated by depression and anger, as well as serious financial and marital troubles. He had developed a highly resentful, hopeless attitude about his life and career. His suicide note stated, "I don't plan to live very much longer, just long enough to kill as many of the people that greedily sought my destruction" (Barton 1999; Cohen 1999).

The *Indiscriminate-Resentful* type describes the generally rageful, depressed, and often paranoid individual who vents anger arbitrarily in some public place. The victim group may be chosen randomly or on the basis of convenience or ease of access to large numbers of people. An example of this category is the man who shot and killed 22 and injured 19 others at a San Diego, California, McDonald's restaurant in 1984 (Mitchell 2002). This angry but nonpsychotic man told his wife immediately prior to the offense that "society had their chance" and that he was leaving to go "hunting humans." No evidence indicated that he felt particularly aggrieved by that specific McDonald's restaurant or its employees. Rather, the evidence indicated that he had chosen the location due to his familiarity with his target and his knowledge that large numbers of potential victims were likely to be present.

In a seminal paper on mass, serial, and sensational homicides, Park Dietz (1986) described a type of mass murderer he termed the "pseudocommando," who plans out the offense ritualistically and comes prepared with a powerful arsenal of weapons. The proposed classification system includes two types of pseudocommando-style mass murderers: the Specific Community–Resentful type and the Pseudocommunity-Psychotic type. Both categories include individuals who have paranoid character traits and are driven by strong feelings of anger and resentment.

The *Specific Community–Resentful* type may include disgruntled clients or others harboring deep resentment toward an identifiable group, culture, or political movement. In contrast, the *Pseudocommunity-Psychotic* type includes only those experiencing paranoid or persecutory delusions flowing from a psychotic disorder. In terms of the relationship to the victims, the pseudocommando-psychotic mass murderer focuses on a group that he delusionally believes is persecuting him. Dietz noted that the pseudocommando may focus his resentment on a specific community based in reality or on a "pseudocommunity" that he defines on the basis of psychosis or strong paranoid cognitions.

Finally, the *Familial-Depressed* type involves a member of a family unit who is suffering from severe depression with possible psychotic features. Motives may flow from cognitions distorted by depression and hopelessness, psychosis, and/or resentment toward an estranged spouse. A typical scenario involves a depressed father who kills his entire family, viewing the act as a delivery of his family from what he perceives to be continued hardship or stressors (Selkin 1976).

Mass Shootings and Mental Illness: Is There a Connection?

The publicity regarding mass shootings unfortunately overshadows another public health tragedy that affects exponentially more people: the daily toll of morbidity and mortality due to the more common types of gun violence, including suicide. Rarely, if ever, do these events receive the same media attention as mass shootings (Pinals et al. 2014). As discussed in Chapter 2, "Firearms and Suicide in the United States," evidence overwhelmingly demonstrates that suicide, not homicide, is the most significant public health concern in terms of guns and mental illness. Indeed, the small amount of research on firearm removal laws suggests that removal by police "was rarely a result of psychosis; instead, risk of suicide was the leading reason" (Parker 2010, p. 241).

Even if one assumes a direct association between violence against others and serious mental illness, the focus must be narrowed to the population of individuals with serious mental illness associated with less than 3% of all violence (Fazel and Grann 2006). Furthermore, current research suggests that in general there is a minimal relationship between psychiatric disorders and violence in the absence of substance abuse (Martone et al. 2013). Thus, the assumption that all persons with mental illness are a "high-risk" population relative to violence generally and gun violence in particular lacks supportive evidence. The likelihood of error and oversimplification is substantial when mental illness is considered on "the aggregate level" such that a "vast and diverse population of persons diagnosed with psychiatric conditions" is considered to uniformly represent people who are at risk of committing gun violence against others (Metzl and Macleish 2015, p. 241).

Some research has identified a small but higher fraction of homicides (not specific to those involving firearms) committed by individuals with schizophrenia than by those in the general population (Bennett et al. 2011; Schanda et al. 2004). Despite this small but elevated risk, the rate of stranger homicides committed by individuals with schizophrenia or chronic psychosis is extremely low. On the basis of a meta-analysis from 1999, one stranger homicide is perpetrated by someone with a psychotic illness per year in a population of 14.3 million (Nielssen et al. 2011). Assuming a U.S. population of 320 million, approximately 23 people a year on average are killed by an individual with a psychotic illness. In contrast, an average of about 330 people in the United States are struck by lightning per year (Jensenius 2014). A person is about 15 times more likely to be struck by lightning in a given year than to be killed by a stranger with a diagnosis of schizophrenia or chronic psychosis.

Few perpetrators of mass shootings have had verified histories of being in psychiatric treatment for serious mental illness. Rather, detailed case analyses reveal that individuals who commit mass shootings often feel aggrieved, are extremely angry, and have nurtured fantasies of violent revenge (Knoll 2010). Such individuals function (perhaps marginally) in society and do not typically seek out mental health treatment. Thus, in most cases, it cannot fairly be said that a perpetrator "fell through the cracks" of the mental health system. Rather, these individuals typically plan their actions well outside the awareness of mental health professionals.

Salient Yet Underexplored Sociocultural Factors in Mass Shootings

The majority of attention following mass shootings focuses on the role of mental illness, and sociocultural factors have received comparatively little examination. Gun violence "in all its forms has a social context," which is not meaningfully captured by psychiatric diagnoses in isolation (Metzl and Macleish 2015, p. 247). Mass shootings by disgruntled individuals have occurred in Western civilization since the invention of the gun. Alienation and social rejection are social phenomena that undoubtedly existed even before recorded history. Nevertheless, mass shootings over the past two to three decades have led to speculation about whether these differ from mass shootings of the past or whether they represent the same phenomenon in a more modern age. Another salient concern is whether the powerful social influence of today's media and Internet technology plays a significant role.

As noted above (see "Mass Shootings: What Is Known"), the FBI study finding that the incidence of mass shootings has increased over the past decade hints at other, possibly more relevant factors associated with these events relative to mental illness or psychiatric diagnosis. Since the 1990s, mass murders, and especially mass shootings, have arguably taken on a different quality, influenced by a cultural shift, social media, and expansive news coverage of the tragedies. Mullen (2004) described the results of his detailed forensic evaluations of five pseudocommando mass shooters who were captured before they were killed or could commit suicide. Most perpetrators acknowledged being influenced by previous mass killers who received significant media exposure. This led Mullen to propose the concept of a Western cultural "script" as one of several factors that contribute to the propagation of these tragic events.

Certain psychosocial characteristics are common among perpetrators of mass shootings. These include problems with self-esteem, a persecutory/paranoid outlook, narcissism, depression, suicidality, and a perception of being socially rejected (Knoll 2012; Modzeleski et al. 2008; Mullen 2004; O'Toole 2000). In a review of school-associated homicides in K–12 settings, Flannery et al. (2013) noted that "[a] need remains for researchers and commentators to examine other factors beyond the individual that may explain school shootings, including culture, the social ecology of the school or other community factors" (Flannery et al. 2013, p. 6). They cited studies (Brown et al. 2009; Flannery et al. 2001) suggesting differences between urban and suburban school shootings, and proposed that some acts are related to the perpetrator's perception of threats to his social identity. Suburban and rural shootings may be characterized by social alienation, whereas urban incidents are typically associated with interpersonal violence, often in the context of different kinds of relationships (see Chapter 3, "Gun Violence, Urban Youth, and Mental Illness"). Social marginalization and familial dysfunction are other common findings among mass shooters (Newman et al. 2005).

The call to investigate cultural and community factors seems particularly meaningful when attention is paid to the messages perpetrators leave behind. For example, one mass shooter from Montreal, Quebec, in 2006 wrote, "It's society's fault.... Society disgusts me" (Langan 2006). The Sandy Hook Elementary School (Newtown, Connecticut) shooter posted online in late 2011, "[You know what I hate]... Culture. I've been pissed out of my mind all night thinking about it" (Sandy Hook Lighthouse 2014). The Isla Vista, California, shooter posted a manuscript online in 2014 stating, "Humanity is a cruel and brutal species" (Rodger 2014). Further investigation of sociocultural factors of mass shootings, particularly in Western society, necessitates a consideration of the issues of narcissism and media responsibility.

Narcissism and Mass Shootings

Narcissism may be considered the classic American pathology (Twenge et al. 2008), but concern is growing that it may be proliferating "virally" and gaining momentum (Twenge and Campbell 2009). Is the changing character of mass shootings over the past few decades due, in part, to our society's increasingly narcissistic values (Twenge et al. 2012)? Narcissism has been demonstrated in the motivations and statements made by certain mass shooters since the 1990s. In 2007, a man who shot nine people in an Omaha, Nebraska, mall before killing himself left a suicide note that stated, "Just think tho [*sic*] I'm gonna be famous" (Kluger 2007; Nichols 2007). A similar message was communicated by the Columbine offenders, who stated on a preshooting video, "Isn't it fun to get the respect we're going to deserve?" (Twenge and Campbell 2003, p. 261).

Twenge and Campbell (2009) noted that crime has dropped overall since the 1990s due to a variety of factors, but crimes related to narcissism (or a wounded ego) have not had a corresponding drop and are directly relevant to mass shootings. These authors further noted that "narcissism and social rejection were two risk factors that worked together to cause aggressive behavior" (p. 199), and these factors have certainly been apparent in the histories of mass shooters. They concluded, "Given the upswing in the narcissistic values of American culture since the '90s, it may be no coincidence that mass shootings became a national plague around the same time" (p. 200).

Similarly, Pinker (2011) has laid out a comprehensive overview of how violence among *Homo sapiens* has greatly declined over the centuries due to a "civilizing process," but speculates that humans might have reached a point of limited returns. He indicates that further gains, which may be harder to attain, arguably also lie in the realm of attenuating the problem of narcissism.

Extensive media attention in the 1990s may have propagated the Western "script" described by Mullen (2004), resulting in a perverse glamorization of the act of mass killing, particularly in the eyes of subsequent perpetrators. The study of individual cases of mass shootings that have occurred since the 1990s suggests that perpetrators often felt socially rejected and perceived society as continually denouncing them as unnecessary, ineffectual, and pathetic. Instead of bearing the burden of the humiliation, they plan a surprise attack to prove their hidden "value."

Narcissism is strengthened and rigidified by obsessive ruminations along the lines of "I am right and I've been treated badly or wronged (by other people or by life)." It could be said that the mass shooter's persecutory and narcissistic mindset seeks a form of reverse specialness. By becoming a lone protestor against an "unjust" reality, the mass shooter creates and assumes a powerful victim role in which he can "win"—even by losing. This interest in the narcissistic antihero has conspicuously permeated Western fiction and popular culture, in which followers thrill to the exploits of characters who possess the "dark triad" of personality: narcissism, psychopathy, and Machiavellianism (Jonason et al. 2012). Western society in particular has had a long-standing fascination with the antihero, the outlaw, the Bonnies and Clydes and John Dillingers of American history (Kunhardt and Kunhardt 1995; Spillane 1999). Their short, violent lives became the stuff of romanticized, tragic legend.

Western culture has also come to include a vast and powerfully influential value system devoted to celebrity and fame. In place of what should be profound shame, an aura of undeserved notoriety and infamy is often accorded to certain individuals who commit horrible crimes (Brin 2012). The very public, dramatic, and at times theatrical nature of mass murder seems to speak to a "need for recognition from an audience" (Neuman 2012, p. 2). The staged and exposed act of revenge has the function of establishing a connection with spectators who will not soon forget what they have seen.

It might be theorized that the Internet and social media have amplified the high value placed on celebrity and the Western cultural script of the tragic antihero. The use of video-sharing Web sites and other Internet platforms perpetuates the alienated loner's conflict: his wish for social connection versus his deep-seated mistrust of others. This can create an isolating virtual socialization that is sustained well into young adulthood, leaving the individual without real experience in developing healthy social attachments, and resulting ultimately in feelings of being unwanted. The final written communication of the Isla Vista shooter reflects precisely such a pattern of alienation and malignant envy, culminating in a violent bid for fame and validation: "Humanity has rejected me.... Exacting my Retribution is my way of proving my true worth to the world" (Rodger 2014).

Media Coverage: Responsible Reporting and Stigma

After the Sandy Hook tragedy in 2012, a senator announced that he supported measures to keep guns "out of the hands of criminals and the mentally ill" (Strauss 2012). Shortly thereafter, a National Rifle Association official stated in a press conference that "our society is populated by an unknown number of genuine monsters. People that are so deranged, so evil, so possessed by voices and driven by demons, that no sane person can even possibly comprehend them.... How can we possibly even guess how many, given our nation's refusal to create an active national database of the mentally ill?" (The Washington Post 2012). Such statements, widely disseminated by the media, reinforce the existing societal presumptive association between "criminals," "evil," and "the mentally ill." In fact, such misguided associations need no further reinforcement. The lay public requires little persuasion to associate mental illness with criminality and evil (Coulter 2013).

Significant research data indicate that erroneous and negative attitudes toward persons with mental illness are widespread in society (Bizer et al. 2012). The term *stigma* is synonymous with *shame, disgrace,* and *humiliation.* To *stigmatize* means to brand, slur, or defame. Fear, anxiety, and the need to find quick and clear-cut solutions lead to common but mistaken beliefs that reinforce the stigmatization of individuals with mental illness. These myths include beliefs that people with mental illness (Link et al. 1999) are more dangerous than people without mental illness, are personally to blame for their illness, and have no "self-control."

Approximately 50 years after deinstitutionalization of individuals with mental illness, the misconception that these persons are "ticking time bombs, ready to explode into violence" remains a deeply ingrained societal belief (Appelbaum 2004). Research by Link et al. (1999) demonstrated strong stereotypes of these individuals' dangerousness and the desire for social distance from those with mental illness. Comparing the research from 1950 with that of 1996 further indicates that perceptions of persons with mental illness as violent or frightening have *substantially increased* rather than decreased. In short, persons with serious mental illness are more feared today than they were half a century ago (Phelan et al. 2000). One of the most problematic results of laws that perpetuate the myth that mental illness is linked to gun violence is the reinforcement of such negative stereotypes. Such reinforcement adds to the considerable stigma associated with mental illness, while having no appreciable effects on the incidence of mass killings that often drive the policy interventions.

Early news media coverage after a mass shooting may refer to the shooter as "mentally unstable" or "mentally ill," often prior to gathering any definitive information. News debate shows often feature speakers who call for measures such as creating a database of individuals with mental illness in an effort to prevent further tragedies. Such dialogue is unhelpful and further strengthens erroneous public views about mental illness and gun violence. Media coverage following collective traumas has been observed to have public health effects, particularly in terms of stress-related symptoms (Holman et al. 2014). With increasing reliance on social media as a source of news, media errors may easily exacerbate public stress, as well as exacerbate the problem of sensationalizing tragedies (Berkowitz and Liu 2014).

Thus, interventions designed to improve media responsibility should dissuade this and similar dialogue in the aftermath of a mass shooting. Efforts to develop a universal reporting code that would appropriately cover the tragedy and reduce the impact of the "copycat" effect have been recommended; these generally include avoiding emphasis on perpetrators and neither glorifying nor demonizing them (Etzersdorfer and Sonneck 1998). Media should consider avoiding much emphasis on the perpetrator while emphasizing victim and community recovery efforts. Future research should focus more distinctly on which elements of media coverage are problematic and which are more effective in promoting public health goals (Schildkraut and Muschert 2013).

Interventions to Prevent Mass Shootings

Gun Laws Focusing on Mental Illness

Equating mental illness and gun violence toward others in an effort to solve the overall problem of gun violence in the United States is an example of what the Greek philosopher Epictetus described as grasping a problem "by the wrong handle" (Gutheil et al. 2005; Pies 2008). In the wake of a frightening tragedy, reactive attempts to reduce gun violence by focusing on people with mental illness represent an intervention with no supportive evidence of practical efficacy.

From 2007 to 2013, as a result of the National Instant Criminal Background Check System (NICS) Improvement Act of 2008, mental health record submissions to NICS increased tenfold (Federal Bureau of Investigation 2013, 2014). Less than 1% of all firearm purchase denials were based on these records (Swanson et al. 2015). However, during this same period, the FBI's study of active shooters reflected an *increasing* trend of mass shooting incidents (Blair and Schweit 2014). The NICS background check system requires, for reporting regarding mental health, that the individual have a history of prior civil commitment, a legal adjudication of not guilty by reason of insanity, or an adjudication of not competent to stand trial. Thus, for a background check to deny firearm purchase to a potential mass shooter, that individual would have to 1) have a history of prior civil commitment (and that history would have had to have been reported to NICS) and 2) attempt to purchase a gun legally. The existing body of research on mass shooters suggests that a history of civil commitment or legal adjudication of criminal insanity or incompetence to stand trial is practically unheard of among perpetrators of mass homicide and mass homicide-suicide.

Recalling the very low percentage of violent acts that are attributable to serious mental illness, and considering that most of these acts do not involve guns, it becomes difficult to avoid the conclusion that the contribution to public safety of laws directed toward individuals with mental illness in preventing gun violence is likely to be small (Appelbaum and Swanson 2010). In addition, these special laws require resources and funding when cost-effective use of resources is a pressing matter. It would seem imperative to "question whether a comprehensive registry [of individuals with mental illness] would have prevented *any* of the mass killings in recent years, and whether the expenditures of the more than one hundred million dollars needed to create and maintain the registries for persons with mental health histories could be better spent on broader public-safety targeted interventions that might yield greater overall benefits to society" (Pinals et al. 2014, p. 2).

Efforts to Identify Effective Interventions

Mass shootings are multidetermined, extremely rare events with no simple preventive solution. The fact that they occur "too infrequently to allow for statistical modeling" suggests that a focus on mass shootings will serve as a questionable "jumping-off" point for "effective public health interventions" (Metzl and Macleish 2015, p. 426). Although research suggests that in recent years the incidence of these events may be increasing (see earlier section "Mass Shootings: What Is Known"), mass shootings are still relatively infrequent, making these tragedies exceptionally hard to anticipate and avert (Blair and Schweit 2014; Saleva et al. 2007). Given the extremely low base rate of mass murder in general and of mass shootings in particular, psychiatric efforts will be best spent in directions other than prediction (Dressing and Meyer-Lindenberg 2010).

Prevention efforts must rely on multiple approaches used in conjunction to provide the widest possible safety net. For example, third parties, particularly family members, have important roles because they are the most likely to have preoffense knowledge or significant concerns (Associated Press 2007). In addition, potential mass murderers often leak their intent to third parties who may not report violent threats or plans to authorities for various reasons (Katsavdakis et al. 2011; Kluger 2007), including not recognizing the seriousness of the potential threat.

Nevertheless, as Aitken et al. (2008) note, "prevention may only be possible when somebody warns that such behavior may occur.... Acquaintances often acknowledge concerns prior to the incident" (p. 265). Messages or leaked intent may be communicated verbally, or in writing via Internet pages, or through social media outlets such as YouTube. Family members or social contacts may be the only people in a position to take steps to have the potential offender evaluated and treated (Orange 2011). Therefore, family members of individuals who may present with increased risk of gun violence, with or without mental illness, should be provided with information about existing help and resources. They should be provided with support for notifying authorities and understand that doing so is a potentially heroic and compassionate act that may save the lives of others as well as their loved one's.

The FBI study of active shooters concluded that training and exercises for both police and citizens were indicated, especially given the brief period over which the shootings unfold (Blair and Schweit 2014). However, the FBI study placed primary emphasis on prevention efforts from a community standpoint. Future research should consider mass shootings that were prevented and/or aborted, with an eye toward identifying crucial preventive factors. Specialized threat assessment teams in Australia and the United Kingdom have been helpful in terms of enhancing prevention of low-frequency, high-intensity events (Meloy and Hoffmann 2014). Similar multidisciplinary teams in the United States should be explored, with a focus on the two areas of greatest concern noted in the FBI study: places of education and workplace violence.

For general mental health professionals, careful clinical risk assessment and management may be stressed as a part of overall competent psychiatric patient care (Mills et al. 2011; Swanson 2008). Future research will undoubtedly enhance awareness of "warning behaviors" for targeted violence, and mental health clinicians will best serve patients at risk by crafting a risk management plan at clinically relevant or critical times (Meloy et al. 2011). Special attention should be given to "availability of means, planning, preparation, and the acknowledged commitment to put the words into action irrespective of consequences" (Warren et al. 2011, p. 151). Risk assessments of individuals with strong revenge fantasies will need to consider the intensity and quality of these fantasies, vulnerability to ego threats, and relevant biopsychosocial variables (Baumeister et al. 1996).

Public education regarding mental illness and effective interventions can serve to lessen fears of those with serious mental illness and decrease the stigma attached to serious mental illness. For many decades, sexual health education has been taught to teens and adolescents. However, a similar focus on mental health education is rare in children's early education. Well-informed and compassionate education on mental health and mental wellness may not only reduce future stigma but also serve as a beneficial public health intervention. Such education could become increasingly sophisticated as children progress through school. In particular, this education may serve as an early preventive effort, while encouraging more open discussion in schools about important mental health issues.

Conclusion

Mass shootings by people with serious mental illness remain exceedingly rare events and represent a fraction of a percent of all yearly gun-related homicides. In contrast, firearm deaths by suicide account for the majority of yearly gun-related deaths. Although gun restriction laws that focus broadly on mental illness are an understandable initial reaction, they will be extremely low yield and wasteful of scant resources. Furthermore, such laws perpetuate the myth that mental illness leads to violence and gives the public the incorrect message that mental illness is significantly associated with gun violence directed toward others.

The problem of mass shootings and the motives of the shooters in present-day society stand apart from mental illness generally. The recent phenomenon of mass shootings in the United States is likely a result of a combination of factors, including sociocultural ones that must be better understood if these tragedies are to be prevented. Mental health clinicians will best serve patients at risk of harm to themselves and/or others by crafting a risk management plan at clinically relevant or critical times. As opposed to prediction, structured clinical risk assessment and management may be stressed as part of an overall competent psychiatric patient care effort (Knoll 2009; Swanson 2008; Webster et al. 2013).

Whether or not individuals who perpetrate mass shootings suffer from a diagnosable serious mental illness, they do have an ill-defined trouble of the mind for which the mental health field has no immediate, quick-acting "treatment." That said, if such individuals were motivated to overcome long-standing, pervasive feelings of anger, persecution, revenge, and egotism rather than act on them, they would presumably be more likely to improve their circumstances in nonviolent ways. Psychiatry may be able to assist individuals who are determined and willing to engage in treatment, form healthy social connections, and pursue other prosocial interventions. For these individuals, more resources need to be made available, as discussed elsewhere in this volume.

Unfortunately, some disturbed individuals are likely to remain inaccessible to whatever interventions mental health professionals have to offer. This situation accounts, at least in part, for the fact that measures such as screening for prior psychiatric treatment (often in the distant past) among individuals who want to *legally* purchase firearms do not represent meaningful interventions (Brady Handgun Violence Prevention Act of 1993, Pub. L. No. 103-159, 18 U.S.C. § 922 [s1–s6]; Norris et al. 2006; Simpson 2007). Experience and research have demonstrated that more promising, higher-yield interventions include both 1) third-party reporting of warning behaviors or leaked intent and 2) social and media responsibility (Meloy and O'Toole 2011; Meloy et al. 2011; O'Toole 2014).

On a fundamental level, the behavior and motives of mass shooters must be distinguished from psychiatric diagnoses. The belief that these categories overlap or have a direct causal association is not supported by available evidence. More importantly, interventions to decrease the morbidity and mortality of gun violence based on such overgeneralized views are not likely to be successful and may cause more harm than good.

Suggested Interventions

- Policies and laws should focus on those individuals whose behaviors identify them as having increased risk for committing gun violence, rather than on broad categories such as mental illness or psychiatric diagnoses.
- Public health educational campaigns should emphasize the need for third-party reporting of intent or concerning warning behaviors to law enforcement.
- Institutions and communities should develop specialized forensic threat assessment teams to evaluate third-party reports of potential dangerousness.
- Resources should be increased to provide enhanced education, beginning in elementary school, with a focus on constructive coping skills for anger and conflict resolution, mental health, and mental wellness education.

References

Aitken L, Oosthuizen P, Emsley R, et al: Mass murders: implications for mental health professionals. Int J Psychiatry Med 38(3):261–269, 2008 19069571

American Psychiatric Association: Diagnostic and Statistical Manual of Mental Disorders, 5th Edition. Arlington, VA, American Psychiatric Association, 2013

Appelbaum PS: Law and psychiatry: "One madman keeping loaded guns": misconceptions of mental illness and their legal consequences. Psychiatr Serv 55(10):1105–1106, 2004 15494320

Appelbaum PS, Swanson JW: Law and psychiatry: gun laws and mental illness: how sensible are the current restrictions? Psychiatr Serv 61(7):652–654, 2010 20591996

Associated Press: Mass public shootings on the rise, but why? Massacre at Virginia Tech on NBC News, April 21, 2007. Available at: http://www.msnbc.msn.com/id/18249724/. Accessed January 8, 2015.

Barton MO: Shootings in Atlanta: The Notes. New York Times, July 31, 1999. Available at: http://www.nytimes.com/1999/07/31/us/shootings-in-atlanta-the-notes-there-is-no-reason-for-me-to-lie-now.html. Accessed January 8, 2015.

Baumeister RF, Smart L, Boden JM: Relation of threatened egotism to violence and aggression: the dark side of high self-esteem. Psychol Rev 103(1):5–33, 1996 8650299

Bennett DJ, Ogloff JR, Mullen PE, et al: Schizophrenia disorders, substance abuse and prior offending in a sequential series of 435 homicides. Acta Psychiatr Scand 124(3):226–233, 2011 21644942

Berkowitz D, Liu ZM: Media errors and the "nutty professor": riding the journalistic boundaries of the Sandy Hook shootings. Journalism, October 9, 2014 doi:10.1177/1464884914552266

Bizer G, Hart J, Jekogian A: Belief in a just world and social dominance orientation: evidence for a mediational pathway predicting negative attitudes and discrimination against individuals with mental illness. Pers Individ Dif 52(3):428–432, 2012

Blair J, Schweit K: A Study of Active Shooter Incidents in the United States Between 2000 and 2013. Washington, DC, Federal Bureau of Investigation, 2014

Bossarte RM, Simon TR, Barker L: Characteristics of homicide followed by suicide incidents in multiple states, 2003–04. Inj Prev 12 (suppl 2):ii33–ii38, 2006 17170169

Brin D: Names of infamy: deny killers the notoriety they seek. Contrary Brin, July 21, 2012. Available at: http://davidbrin.blogspot.com/2012/07/names-of-infamy-deny-killers-notoreity.html. Accessed January 8, 2015.

Brown RP, Osterman LL, Barnes CD: School violence and the culture of honor. Psychol Sci 20(11):1400–1405, 2009 19843260

Burgess AW: Mass, spree and serial homicide, in Crime Classification Manual, 2nd Edition. Edited by Douglas J, Burgess AW, Burgess AG, et al. San Francisco, CA, Jossey-Bass, 2006

Chen P: Jiverly Wong's father: what prompted mass killing in Binghamton remains a mystery. The Post Standard, April 13, 2009. Available at: http://www.syracuse.com/news/index.ssf/2009/04/jiverly_wongs_father_our_son_w.html. Accessed August 4, 2015.

Cohen A: A portrait of the killer. Time, August 9, 1999. Available at: http://www.time.com/time/magazine/article/0,9171,991676,00.html?promoid=googlep. Accessed January 8, 2015.

Coid J: The epidemiology of abnormal homicide and murder followed by suicide. Psychol Med 13(4):855–860, 1983 6607479

Coulter A: Guns don't kill people, the mentally ill do. MRC NewsBusters, January 16, 2013. Available at: http://www.anncoulter.com/columns/2013-01-16.html. Accessed August 4, 2015.

Cullen D: Columbine. Lebanon, IN, Twelve, 2010

Declercq F, Audenaert K: Predatory violence aiming at relief in a case of mass murder: Meloy's criteria for applied forensic practice. Behav Sci Law 29(4):578–591, 2011 21748789

Dietz PE: Mass, serial and sensational homicides. Bull NY Acad Med 62(5):477–491, 1986 3461857

Dressing H, Meyer-Lindenberg A: Risk assessment of threatened amok: new responsibilities for psychiatry? [in German] Nervenarzt 81(5):594–601, 2010 20221743

Duwe G: A circle of distortion: the social construction of mass murder in the United States. West Crim Rev 6(1):59–78, 2005

Etzersdorfer E, Sonneck G: Preventing suicide by influencing the mass media reporting: the Viennese experience, 1980–1996. Arch Suicide Res 4(1):67–74, 1998

Fazel S, Grann M: The population impact of severe mental illness on violent crime. Am J Psychiatry 163(8):1397–1403, 2006 16877653

Federal Bureau of Investigation: National Instant Criminal Background Check System, Operations Report: 2012. Washington, DC, Federal Bureau of Investigation, 2013. Available at: www.fbi.gov/about-us/cjis/nics/reports/2012-operations-report. Accessed January 8, 2015.

Federal Bureau of Investigation: National Instant Criminal Background Check System, Operations Report: 2013. Washington, DC, Federal Bureau of Investigation, 2014. Available at: www.fbi.gov/about-us/cjis/nics/reports/2013-operations-report. Accessed January 8, 2015.

Felthous AR, Hempel A: Combined homicide-suicides: a review. J Forensic Sci 40(5):846–857, 1995 7595329

Flannery DJ, Singer MI, Wester K: Violence exposure, psychological trauma, and suicide risk in a community sample of dangerously violent adolescents. J Am Acad Child Adolesc Psychiatry 40(4):435–442, 2001 11314569

Flannery DJ, Modzeleski W, Kretschmar JM: Violence and school shootings. Curr Psychiatry Rep 15(1):331–337, 2013 23254623

Frontline: The killer at Thurston High. January 18, 2000. Available at: http://www.pbs.org/wgbh/pages/frontline/shows/kinkel/kip/cron.html. Accessed January 27, 2015.

Gutheil TG, Simon RI, Hilliard JT: "The wrong handle": flawed fixes of medicolegal problems in psychiatry and the law. J Am Acad Psychiatry Law 33(4):432–436, 2005 16394218

Hempel AG, Meloy JR, Richards TC: Offender and offense characteristics of a nonrandom sample of mass murderers. J Am Acad Psychiatry Law 27(2):213–225, 1999 10400430

Holman EA, Garfin DR, Silver RC: Media's role in broadcasting acute stress following the Boston Marathon bombings. Proc Natl Acad Sci USA 111(1):93–98, 2014 24324161

Jensenius JS Jr: National Weather Service Lightning Safety: Understanding Lightning. Silver Spring, MD, National Oceanic and Atmospheric Administration, 2014. Available at: http://www.lightningsafety.noaa.gov/science/scienceintro.htm. Accessed January 8, 2015.

Jonason P, Webster G, Schmitt D, et al: The antihero in popular culture: life history theory and the dark triad personality traits. Rev Gen Psychol 16(2):192–199, 2012

Katsavdakis KA, Meloy JR, White SG: A female mass murder. J Forensic Sci 56(3):813–818, 2011 21291471

Kluger J: Inside a mass murderer's mind. Time, April 19, 2007. Available at: http://www.time.com/time/magazine/article/0,9171,1612694,00.html. Accessed January 8, 2015.

Knoll JL IV: Violence risk assessment for mental health professionals, in Wiley Encyclopedia of Forensic Science. Edited by Jamieson A, Moenssens A. Chichester, UK, Wiley, 2009, pp 2597–2602

Knoll JL IV: The "pseudocommando" mass murderer, part II: the language of revenge. J Am Acad Psychiatry Law 38(2):263–272, 2010 20542949

Knoll JL IV: Mass murder: causes, classification, and prevention. Psychiatr Clin North Am 35(4):757–780, 2012 23107562

Knoll J IV, Meloy JR: Mass murder and the violent paranoid spectrum. Psychiatr Ann 44(5):236–243, 2014

Kunhardt P, Kunhardt P III: Violence: An American Tradition (video). Rockville, MD, National Criminal Justice Reference Service, 1995. Available at: http://www.ncjrs.gov/App/publications/abstract.aspx?ID=164419. Accessed August 4, 2015.

Langan A: I am Angel of Death, warned college killer. Daily Telegraph, September 15, 2006. Available at: http://www.telegraph.co.uk/news/worldnews/1528946/I-am-Angel-of-Death-warned-college-killer.html. Accessed January 8, 2015.

Link BG, Phelan JC, Bresnahan M, et al: Public conceptions of mental illness: labels, causes, dangerousness, and social distance. Am J Public Health 89(9):1328–1333, 1999 10474548

Martone CA, Mulvey EP, Yang S, et al: Psychiatric characteristics of homicide defendants. Am J Psychiatry 170(9):994–1002, 2013 23896859

Marzuk PM, Tardiff K, Hirsch CS: The epidemiology of murder-suicide. JAMA 267(23): 3179–3183, 1992 1593740

Meloy JR, Hoffmann J (eds): International Handbook of Threat Assessment. New York, Oxford University Press, 2014

Meloy JR, O'Toole ME: The concept of leakage in threat assessment. Behav Sci Law 29(4):513–527, 2011 21710573

Meloy JR, Hoffman J, Guldimann A, et al: The role of warning behaviors in threat assessment: an exploration and suggested typology. Behav Sci Law 30(3):256–279, 2011

Metzl J, Macleish K: Mental illness, mass shootings, and the policies of American firearms. Am J Public Health 105(2):240–249, 2015

Mills J, Kroner D, Morgan R: Clinician's Guide to Violence Risk Assessment. New York, Guilford, 2011

Mitchell R: Dancing at Armageddon: Survivalism and Chaos in Modern Times. Chicago, IL, University of Chicago Press, 2002

Modzeleski W, Feucht T, Rand M, et al: School-associated student homicides—United States, 1992–2006. MMWR Morb Mortal Wkly Rep 57(2):33–36, 2008 18199965

Mullen PE: The autogenic (self-generated) massacre. Behav Sci Law 22(3):311–323, 2004 15211554

Neuman Y: On revenge. Psychoanalysis, Culture & Society 17:1–15, 2012

Newman KS, Fox C, Roth J, et al: Rampage: The Social Roots of School Shootings. New York, Basic Books, 2005

Nichols A: Camera catches Omaha mall shooter. Daily News, December 8, 2007. Available at: http://www.nydailynews.com/news/world/camera-catches-omaha-mall-shooter-article-1.273367. Accessed January 8, 2015.

Nielssen O, Bourget D, Laajasalo T, et al: Homicide of strangers by people with a psychotic illness. Schizophr Bull 37(3):572–579, 2011 19822580

Norris D, Price M, Gutheil T, et al: Firearm laws, patients, and the roles of psychiatrists. Am J Psychiatry 163(8):1392–1396, 2006 16877652

Orange R: Anders Behring Breivik's sister warned mother about his behaviour two years ago. Daily Telegraph, December 4, 2011. Available at: http://www.telegraph.co.uk/news/worldnews/europe/norway/8934136/Anders-Behring-Breiviks-sister-warned-mother-about-his-behaviour-two-years-ago.html. Accessed January 8, 2015.

O'Toole ME: The School Shooter: A Threat Assessment Perspective. Quantico, VA, National Center for the Analysis of Violent Crime, Federal Bureau of Investigation, 2000

O'Toole ME: A different perspective on the UCSB mass murder. Violence and Gender 1(2):49–50, 2014

Parker GF: Application of a firearm seizure law aimed at dangerous persons: outcomes from the first two years. Psychiatr Serv 61(5):478–482, 2010 20439368

Phelan J, Link B, Stueve A, et al: Public conceptions of mental illness in 1950 and 1996: what is mental illness and is it to be feared? J Health Soc Behav 41(2):188–207, 2000

Pies R: Everything Has Two Handles: The Stoic's Guide to the Art of Living. Lanham, MD, Hamilton Books, 2008

Pinals D, Appelbaum P, Bonnie R, et al: Resource Document on Access to Firearms by People With Mental Illness. Arlington, VA, American Psychiatric Association, 2014

Pinker S: The Better Angels of Our Nature: Why Violence Has Declined. New York, Viking Press, 2011

Preti A: School shooting as a culturally enforced way of expressing suicidal hostile intentions. J Am Acad Psychiatry Law 36(4):544–550, 2008 19092074

Rodger E: My Twisted World (online), 2014. Available at: http://www.documentcloud.org/documents/1173808-elliot-rodger-manifesto.html. Accessed January 8, 2015.

Saleva O, Putkonen H, Kiviruusu O, et al: Homicide-suicide—an event hard to prevent and separate from homicide or suicide. Forensic Sci Int 166(2–3):204–208, 2007 16806773

Sandy Hook Lighthouse: Adam Lanza posted about "depression" on the day his mother bought him a gun. Sandy Hook Lighthouse, January 18, 2014. Available at: http://sandyhooklighthouse.wordpress.com/2014/01/18/adam-lanza-posted-about-depression-on-the-day-his-mother-bought-him-a-gun/. Accessed January 8, 2015.

Schanda H, Knecht G, Schreinzer D, et al: Homicide and major mental disorders: a 25-year study. Acta Psychiatr Scand 110(2):98–107, 2004 15233710

Schildkraut J, Muschert G: Media salience and the framing of mass murder in schools: a comparison of the Columbine and Sandy Hook massacres. Homicide Stud 18(1):23–43, 2013

Selkin J: Rescue fantasies in homicide-suicide. Suicide Life Threat Behav 6(2):79–85, 1976 941206

Simpson JR: Bad risk? An overview of laws prohibiting possession of firearms by individuals with a history of treatment for mental illness. J Am Acad Psychiatry Law 35(3):330–338, 2007 17872555

Smith S, Shuy R: Forensic psycholinguistics: using language analysis for identifying and assessing offenders. FBI Law Enforcement Bulletin 71(4):16–21, 2002

Spillane J: Myth, memory, and the American outlaw. Oral Hist Rev 26(1):113–117, 1999

Strauss D: Rubio supports "comprehensive study" of gun laws. The Hill, December 17, 2012. Available at: http://thehill.com/blogs/blog-briefing-room/news/273273-rubio-supports-comprehensive-study-of-gun-laws. Accessed January 8, 2015.

Swanson JW: Preventing the unpredicted: managing violence risk in mental health care. Psychiatr Serv 59(2):191–193, 2008 18245162

Swanson JW, McGinty EE, Fazel S, et al: Mental illness and reduction of gun violence and suicide: bringing epidemiologic research to policy. Ann Epidemiol 25(5):366–376, 2015 24861430

Twenge JM, Campbell WK: "Isn't it fun to get the respect that we're going to deserve?" Narcissism, social rejection, and aggression. Pers Soc Psychol Bull 29(2):261–272, 2003 15272953

Twenge J, Campbell WK: The Narcissism Epidemic: Living in the Age of Entitlement. New York, Atria Books, 2009

Twenge JM, Konrath S, Foster JD, et al: Egos inflating over time: a cross-temporal meta-analysis of the Narcissistic Personality Inventory. J Pers 76(4):875–902, discussion 903–928, 2008 18507710

Twenge JM, Campbell WK, Freeman EC: Generational differences in young adults' life goals, concern for others, and civic orientation, 1966–2009. J Pers Soc Psychol 102(5):1045–1062, 2012 22390226

Vossekuil B, Fein R, Reddy M, et al: The Final Report and Findings of the Safe School Initiative: Implications for the Prevention of School Attacks in the United States. Washington, DC, U.S. Department of Education, Office of Elementary and Secondary Education, Safe and Drug-Free Schools Program, and U.S. Secret Service, National Threat Assessment Center, 2002

Warren LJ, Mullen PE, Ogloff JR: A clinical study of those who utter threats to kill. Behav Sci Law 29(2):141–154, 2011 21374705

The Washington Post: Remarks from the NRA press conference on Sandy Hook school shooting, delivered on Dec. 21, 2012 (transcript). WashingtonPost.com, December 21, 2012. Available at: http://www.washingtonpost.com/politics/remarks-from-the-nra-press-conference-on-sandy-hook-school-shooting-delivered-on-dec-21-2012-transcript/2012/12/21/bd1841fe-4b88-11e2-a6a6-aabac85e8036_story.html. Accessed January 8, 2015.

Webster C, Haque Q, Hucker S: Violence Risk—Assessment and Management: Advances Through Structured Professional Judgment and Sequential Redirections, 2nd Edition. London, Wiley-Blackwell, 2013

5

School Shootings and Mental Illness

Peter Ash, M.D.

Common Misperceptions

☒ Shootings in K–12 schools and in institutions of higher education are a major source of gun violence morbidity and mortality.

☒ There is a profile of a "lone commando" gunman who is responsible for mass shootings at schools and institutions of higher education.

☒ School gun violence is caused by people with severe mental illness "snapping."

Evidence-Based Facts

☑ Only a very small percentage of gun-related homicides and injuries to young people take place in schools or at colleges or universities.

☑ There is no known profile that allows the early identification of a mass killer.

☑ Only a small proportion of school shooters have a psychotic mental illness. Mass shootings at schools are not impulsive acts, but rather the product of careful planning.

Columbine, Virginia Tech, and Sandy Hook are schools whose names have been burned into the public consciousness because they were sites of massacre and tragedy. Schools are supposed to be safe places, full of innocent children and young people studying in a peaceful haven away from the hurly-burly of adult life. The murder of students while engaged in peaceful learning is horrifying, and mass shootings of students unsurprisingly receive enormous publicity and prompt calls for interventions that will prevent such horrors in the future. People are too used to hearing about street violence, gang-related homicides, and even accidental firearm injuries to children, but the mass shootings of students who are not personally known to the shooter stand out from other types of firearm violence as especially sad and senseless. The search for understanding is all too often elusive. Many mass shooters commit suicide after killing others, preventing authorities from being able to reconstruct their thinking and motives before or during the killing spree.

Mass Shootings and Gun Violence: The Statistics

Mass shootings at schools are defined for purposes of this chapter as shootings at a school or institution of higher education (IHE) that fit the Federal Bureau of Investigation (FBI) definition of *mass murder:* four or more murders occurring during a particular event with no cooling-off period between the murders (Morton and Hilts 2005). Typically, the majority of the victims were not specifically targeted by the shooter prior to the rampage, and in most of these events, the shooter also died, usually by suicide.

Although mass shootings are clearly not the only instances of gun violence at schools, they are the events that have provoked the most discussion and calls for intervention. Mass shootings of youths at schools and campuses are statistically an exceedingly small, though highly visible, component of the problems associated with youth morbidity and mortality due to firearms. Unfortunately, the rates of death and injury of youth due to firearms, even without mass shootings, are demonstrative of an enormous public health problem. In the period 1999–2010, homicide typically involving firearms was the second leading cause of death, after accidents, among youth ages 14–18 years (roughly the high school age group), although beginning in 2011, falling homicide rates and increasing suicide rates resulted in suicide rising to the second leading cause (Centers for Disease Control and Prevention 2015).

Only about 1.3% of all youth homicides occur at school, a rate that has remained fairly stable over the past 20 years (Planty and Truman 2013). The majority of these homicides arise out of disputes that cause the shooter to specifically target an individual student or teacher. The good news is that firearm violent deaths among youth ages 12–17 years have dropped by almost two-thirds, from a high of 8 per 100,000 in 1993 to 2.8 per 100,000 in 2010. For nonfatal firearm violence, the improvement has been even greater, from a rate of 1,100 per 100,000 in 1993 to 60 per 100,000 in 2010, a drop of over 90% (Planty and Truman 2013). In the 2010–2011 school year, only 11 of the 1,336 homicides (0.8%) of school-age children ages 5–18 occurred at school (Robers et al. 2014).

The federal Jeanne Clery Disclosure of Campus Security Policy and Campus Crime Statistics Act of 1990 (Pub. L. No. 101-542, 20 U.S.C. § 1092[f]) requires colleges and universities to maintain and report crime statistics, and the data on college crime are quite good. Overall crime on college campuses decreased by almost half from 2001 to 2011, dropping from a rate of 35.6 crimes per 10,000 students in 2001 to 19.7 per 10,000 students in 2011 (Robers et al. 2014). In the same period, arrests for possession of illegal weapons dropped about 4%. Homicides on college campuses were quite rare, typically between 10 and 20 per year in the period 2001–2012, except in 2007, the year of the shootings at Virginia Polytechnic Institute and State University, better known as Virginia Tech (Office of Postsecondary Education 2014). This low number of homicides represents a rate of less than 1 per million of enrolled students, far less than the homicide rate of more than 200 per million in the general population ages 20–24 (Centers for Disease Control and Prevention 2015).

Suicides at school can also involve firearms. Although suicides are relatively rare, about 1–10 students in grades K–12 commit suicide each year at school, representing less than 1% of all youth suicides (Robers et al. 2014). However, suicide is the third leading cause of death among individuals ages 18–22 (Centers for Disease Control and Prevention 2015). Most college students live at college, where the rate of suicides is between 6.5 and 7.5 per 100,000—a rate higher than the rate in lower-level schools but about half the rate for nonstudent college-age adults (Schwartz 2006, 2011). College students who commit suicide use firearms as their lethal method about half as often as do same-age noncollege individuals (Schwartz 2011).

Violence directed at specifically identified individuals and suicides raise a host of issues related to street violence and suicide generally that are not specific to schools. These issues are beyond the scope of this chapter and are covered elsewhere in this volume (see Chapter 2, "Firearms and Suicide in the United States," and Chapter 3, "Gun Violence, Urban Youth, and Mental Illness"). Although mass shootings have garnered a great deal of media attention, it is important to maintain the perspective that such deaths represent only a very small percentage of youth deaths due to firearms.

School Shootings: Targets, Perpetrators, and Interventions

School shootings differ in significant ways. The following discussion is organized into three different categories that vary by target and perpetrators: middle school and high school shootings by students, college and university shootings by enrolled students, and school shootings perpetrated by nonstudents. This typology is used because for each of these groups, the school has a markedly different relationship with the perpetrator, and each relationship has important implications for the identification of and interventions with possible perpetrators. In addition, the developmental stage of each group of perpetrators is relatively distinct, which means that their motivations and their risks for particular types of mental illness are different.

K–12 School Shootings by Students

School shootings have been rare in the United States throughout history. The first mass killing by a student in a K–12 school appears to have occurred at the Frontier Middle School in Moses Lake, Washington, in February 1996. A 14-year-old boy shot and killed a teacher and two students and wounded another in his algebra class. In the next 4 years, six additional incidents of mass killings by students in K–12 schools took place. The most deadly of these was the mass shooting at Columbine High School in Littleton, Colorado, in which 12 students and 1 teacher were killed, 24 people were wounded, and the 2 student shooters committed suicide. These tragedies generated enormous publicity and concern. It was obvious that these killings did not fall into the usual pattern of youth violence (see Chapter 3, "Gun Violence, Urban Youth, and Mental Illness"): none took place in inner-city schools, none of the shooters were black, few of the shooters had a prior history of violence, and school shootings were increasing during the years when overall youth homicide rates were dropping significantly.

A number of studies of school shootings (Reddy et al. 2001; Verlinden et al. 2000), the influential FBI report in 1999 (O'Toole 1999), and the reports of the U.S. Secret Service and the Department of Education's Safe School Initiative in 2000 and 2002 (Fein et al. 2002; Vossekuil et al. 2000, 2002) were consistent in finding that there was *no* profile of a school shooter that was helpful in prospectively identifying the perpetrators. Except for the fact that all were male, the perpetrators were quite varied: few attackers had no close friends, only about one-third were characterized as loners, and the majority had never been in disciplinary trouble at school or had a history of violence. Many attackers had felt bullied or persecuted at school. Of the 37 school shootings investigated by the Safe School Initiative, only one-third of the attackers had ever received a mental health evaluation and only 7 (17%) had ever been diagnosed with a mental health or behavioral disorder (Vossekuil et al. 2002).

Of central importance, the studies found that in almost all cases, the shooters had made comments that communicated their plans to other students, but the other students had not taken the threats seriously and had not reported them. This finding led to an emphasis on threat surveillance and threat assessment:

students and staff were encouraged to report all threats, even joking ones, to school authorities, who would then institute a threat investigation.

Building on earlier work of the U.S. Secret Service in evaluating threats to the president (Fein and Vossekuil 1999), threat investigation of people with or without mental illness has moved away from profiling the subject to evaluating the pathways that lead to violent action (Borum et al. 1999). Put another way, threat assessment looks less at characteristics of the subject (stated intent, psychopathology, access to weapons) and more at recent behavior suggesting that the subject is moving on a path toward violence. This path typically begins with ideation, such as interest in mass killing or assassination; progresses through fantasies of killing; moves to a discreet planning stage (scouting out locations, selecting targets) and means acquisition (obtaining weapons); and culminates in offensive action. Because an individual in a psychiatric interview may deny recently engaging in such actions, a comprehensive evaluation involves obtaining collateral information (e.g., from peers and perhaps computer records, such as Internet browsing history).

The FBI report (O'Toole 1999) recommended assessment in four domains: personality characteristics, family dynamics, school dynamics, and social dynamics. A key concept is "leakage," referring to fantasy material of a violent nature that leaks out in behavior, such as reported fantasies to other students, written stories that involve mass homicide, or preoccupation with Internet sites regarding assassinations or mass murder.

A number of protocols have been developed to assist schools in implementing threat assessment protocols in the school environment (Cornell and Sheras 2006; Fein et al. 2002). These protocols emphasize developing multidisciplinary teams and detail the process of threat assessments. Teams typically consist of school administrators, law enforcement personnel, and mental health professionals.

An assessment typically begins with a triage process that considers the seriousness of the threat. Not all threats are serious. A study of the Virginia Student Threat Assessment program (Cornell et al. 2004) found that 70% of threats were transient and could be resolved quickly. The remaining substantive threats required more extensive evaluation and development of a safety plan to ensure the safety of the school and meet the educational needs of the threatening student. In one study, students who underwent assessment by threat assessment teams were more likely to receive supportive and mental health services and less likely to be suspended than students in schools that did not have such teams (Cornell et al. 2012).

The approach of encouraging students and staff to report threats, and then actively investigating such threats, appears to have been effective in significantly reducing mass shootings in K–12 schools. In the 15 years since the Columbine shootings, only two instances of mass shootings by students at K–12 schools have occurred that resulted in four or more deaths, not including the suicide of the shooter. Although national statistics regarding the number of attacks thwarted by threat investigations are not available, numerous anecdotal accounts and news reports indicate the success of these interventions (Associated Press 2014; Bowman 2012).

The assessment of planned predatory mass violence is quite a different process from the assessment of suicidality that mental health clinicians commonly make. In districts that have not instituted formal threat assessment teams, school administrators who have concern about a student's behavior based on one discrete piece of behavior, such as a reported joke about school shootings or a story with violent content, commonly suspend a student pending the completion of a clearance letter from a mental health professional.

The youth involved then often presents to an emergency department or to a mental health clinician asking for a clearance letter that documents that the student is not likely to commit an act of violence. Except in straightforward cases where a threat is clearly not serious, individual clinicians and those working in emergency departments are well advised to resist writing a clearance letter based solely on an individual or even family interview. Information from school personnel clarifying their concern as well as information from peers who may have heard expressed threats is almost always required. Unless a clinician is able to conduct this more extensive evaluation, emergency room clinicians and mental health clinicians asked to provide such documentation should generally refer the student and his or her family to a mental health professional with expertise in violence risk assessment.

The assessment of risk for predatory, planned violence requires specialized expertise. Many mental health clinicians have considerable training and experience in assessing suicide risk and may view assessing homicide risk as a parallel process. However, training and experience in suicide risk assessment does not translate into expertise in conducting violence risk assessments. Suicide assessment emphasizes the presence of suicidal ideation and a plan with identified means; individuals planning predatory violence more often deny their intent and hide their preparatory behaviors. Suicide assessment is conducted predominantly through clinical interview of the individual; threat assessment relies heavily on collateral information. Many clinicians know that prior violence, with or without mental illness, is the leading risk factor in predicting future violence; however, school mass shooters often have no prior history of violence (Vossekuil et al. 2002). Thus, a comprehensive violence risk assessment of someone referred for possibly planning to commit acts of violence relies heavily on collateral information obtained from peers, family, and even computer records, such as Internet browsing history.

Gun law reform is often discussed as a policy solution for firearm violence, but this approach is largely irrelevant in addressing the problem of K–12 shooters. Most K–12 mass shooters use handguns, and federal law already prohibits a youth under age 18 from owning a handgun. The Youth Handgun Safety Act of

1996 also prohibits anyone from selling a handgun to a minor, whether at a gun store, at a gun show, or in a private sale. The Gun-Free Schools Act of 1994 requires any school receiving federal funds to expel, for a period of at least 1 year, any student found to be in possession of a weapon or firearm at school. No major pro-gun organization is lobbying to change these statutes.

Despite these federal and similar state laws, youth appear to have little difficulty obtaining handguns. In one study of gun acquisition by juveniles, all the male subjects in a sample in juvenile detention were found to own a handgun (Ash et al. 1996). Although efforts have been made to educate parents who own firearms to secure them so that their children do not have access to them, the evidence demonstrates that parents frequently do not appreciate the risk that an adolescent might use a parent's gun. For example, in one study of suicidal adolescents, parents were given a strong recommendation to remove their guns from the home. Less than one-third of parents of suicidal adolescents were compliant with the recommendation, and about one-sixth of the parents who did not own a gun at the outset of the study purchased one in the following 2-year period (Brent et al. 2000).

The fact that many of the K–12 shootings by students occurred over a relatively brief span of years gave rise to theories about contagion and modeling effects. Cantor et al. (1999), in a study of mass shootings in Australia, New Zealand, and the United Kingdom, proposed that the widespread media coverage and attendant fame of the perpetrators exacerbated the problem, a pattern that appeared to resonate in the United States. For example, clear evidence indicates that the Columbine shooters wanted to do more damage than any previous school shooter. These concerns have led to an ongoing discussion about journalistic ethics in an attempt to balance the powerful appetite of the public for detailed information against the risk that such coverage might add to the risk of future attacks (Sullivan 2014).

The finding that many but by no means all student shooters had suffered from bullying has drawn added attention to bullying prevention programs. Bullying has been shown to be associated with later acts of violence against others (Nansel et al. 2003), and bullying prevention programs have been developed and studied (Twemlow and Sacco 2012; Vreeman and Carroll 2007). Various approaches have been demonstrated to be effective in reducing bullying in both general and specific populations of youth in schools (Khoury 2014; Kyriakides et al. 2014; Menard and Grotpeter 2014).

Driven in part by concerns about youth violence and youth suicide, a variety of programs have been developed to help schools identify mental illness in children (Hampton 2013). For example, the American Psychiatric Foundation has developed the *Typical or Troubled?* program, a curriculum for educating parents and teachers who interact with teens to recognize mental illness in teens and to help the adults intervene with troubled youth (American Psychiatric Foundation 2014). Although the program was evidence based in the development of its curriculum, its effect on rates of youth violence is unknown.

The Columbine shooting and the ensuing investigations also changed the nature of school and police responses to mass shootings, with an increased focus on decreasing the risk of injuries and fatalities when such incidents occur. Despite prompt law enforcement responses, most shooting incidents were stopped by means other than law enforcement intervention (Vossekuil et al. 2002). In the Columbine incident, police arrived promptly and, following the protocols then in place, spent time securing the perimeter prior to entering the school. Since Columbine, police departments have increasingly been provided with up-to-date school floor plans and alarm codes. Current standard "active shooter" protocols call for entering the scene of a mass shooting quickly, generally in four-person teams advancing in a diamond-shaped wedge toward the shooting and walking past wounded students so as to get to the shooter and end the carnage as quickly as possible (U.S. Department of Homeland Security 2008). This tactic has been credited with significantly shortening the rampage of the Virginia Tech shooter in 2007.

In the decade after 1999, many schools implemented additional security and safety measures. For example, children and teachers are drilled on lockdowns and evacuations. In addition, according to the federal report *Indicators of School Safety: 2011* (Robers et al. 2012), in the decade after 1999 there was an increase in the percentage of public schools reporting controlling access to the building during school hours (from 75% to 92%), controlling access to school grounds during school hours (from 34% to 46%), requiring faculty to wear badges or picture IDs (from 25% to 63%), and using security cameras to monitor the school (from 19% to 61%). In the 2009–2010 school year, 28% of schools reported that security personnel routinely carried firearms (Robers et al. 2014). The deterrent effect of these measures is unknown.

College and University Shootings by Students

On August 1, 1966, a 25-year-old engineering student at the University of Texas in Austin killed his mother and his wife, and then ascended to the twenty-eighth-floor observation deck of the Tower on the university campus heavily armed with rifles and other firearms. He killed 3 people inside the Tower, and proceeded sniper-style to randomly shoot people below, ultimately killing 16 and wounding another 32, before police were able to enter the observation deck 96 minutes later and stop the attack by killing him. The evening before, he composed a letter/suicide note that included the following:

> I do not really understand myself these days. I am supposed to be an average reasonable and intelligent young man. However, lately (I cannot recall when it started) I have been a victim of many unusual and irrational thoughts....I con-

> sulted a Dr. Cochrum at the University Health Center and asked him to recommend someone that I could consult with about some psychiatric disorders I felt I had. I talked with a Doctor once for about two hours and tried to convey to him my fears that I felt come [*sic*] overwhelming violent impulses. After one session I never saw the Doctor again, and since then I have been fighting my mental turmoil alone, and seemingly to no avail. After my death I wish that an autopsy would be performed on me to see if there is any visible physical disorder. (Whitman 1966)

His letter went on to discuss his intent to kill his wife and mother but did not include his plan to shoot people from the Tower. The autopsy he requested was performed and revealed a glioblastoma multiforme, the most common and most aggressive malignant primary brain tumor in humans, near the amygdala. This may have played a role in the shooter's mental functioning, but its significance in regard to his violent behavior is unclear (Governor's Committee 1966).

The Tower shooting, the first highly publicized mass shooting of its type in the United States, received a great deal of media attention and investigation. In part because the Tower mass shooting was the first of its kind, generalizing from this unique act of violence in order to develop intervention strategies to prevent future incidents is difficult. However, the planning and heavily armed commando aspects of the Tower shooting case were to be repeated in many later mass shootings. The tactical difficulties encountered by the Austin Police Department in reaching a concealed sniper who was more heavily armed than the police contributed significantly to the founding of the Los Angeles SWAT (special weapons and tactics) team the following year and the rapid spread of the SWAT team concept thereafter (Snow 1996).

The Tower shooting would remain the deadliest shooting on a U.S. college campus until the April 16, 2007, Virginia Tech massacre in Blacksburg, Virginia. The Virginia Tech shooter engaged in a murderous rampage that killed 32 people and wounded 17 before the shooter shot and killed himself. The publicity surrounding the University of Texas and the Virginia Tech shootings, as well as other mass shootings on or near college campuses, has given many the impression that college students perpetrating mass murder of other college students is a serious danger. In fact, however, the Texas Tower and Virginia Tech shootings are the only two incidents of mass murder committed by enrolled college or university students on other students through the time of this writing (for a comprehensive list of school shootings, see Blair and Schweit 2014; Wikipedia 2015). Mass murders of university students by nonstudents have occurred (see next section, "School Violence Perpetrated by Nonstudents"), as have incidents of disgruntled students killing several professors, but such incidents present very different problems with regard to surveillance, identification, and intervention. The fact that only two mass killing incidents on campuses by enrolled college or university students have taken place makes it difficult to generalize about them.

Unlike the K–12 mass killer students, neither the Texas Tower shooter nor the Virginia Tech shooter communicated his intentions to others. In large part, the threat assessment teams in K–12 schools have been effective because they have received notice of threats. With adult killers who do not communicate threats, the threat surveillance problem is far more complex. As is well known, the Virginia Tech shooter was thought to be dangerous by some staff, students, campus police, and mental health personnel more than a year before the killings. He was briefly held involuntarily in a psychiatric hospital for evaluation, but he was then released and committed to outpatient treatment. Although he never attended this court-ordered mental health treatment, in the 15 months prior to his murder spree, the Virginia Tech shooter managed to avoid coming to the attention of the authorities.

However, because the Virginia Tech shooter had come to the attention of the school administration in 2005, attention became focused on the issue of a college administration's response to a general notice of dangerousness. President George W. Bush convened a federal panel to address issues raised by the Virginia Tech shootings. This panel found that not only at Virginia Tech but across the nation, communication between college administrators, college mental health services, and law enforcement was impaired, which seriously interfered with coordinating a response to a problematic student (U.S. Department of Health and Human Services et al. 2007). Much of this impaired communication derived from misunderstandings of relevant federal and state privacy laws that created a common belief among college officials with relevant information that they could not divulge this information to others. College mental health services felt constrained by their understanding of confidentiality mandated by the Health Insurance Portability and Accountability Act of 1996 (HIPAA; Pub. L. No. 104-191, 110 Stat. 1936) and state confidentiality laws, and college administrators felt constrained by their understanding of the confidentiality requirements of the Family Educational Rights and Privacy Act of 1974 (Pub. L. No. 93-380, 20 U.S.C. § 1232[g]; 34 C.F.R. Part 99). The panel, which found that much of the concern of both mental health service providers and administrators stemmed from misunderstandings of the laws, recommended interventions at both the state and national levels to educate college administrators and improve communication about potentially threatening students. In K–12 schools, because parents can consent to release of information, administrators are far less constrained by concerns regarding privacy and confidentiality.

K–12 assessment teams often become involved when a student makes a threat. In contrast, neither the Texas Tower shooter nor the Virginia Tech shooter made direct threats, although both had been seen by mental health professionals prior to their attacks. The Virginia Tech shooter had also come to the attention of the campus police after stalking complaints were made against him. Had a threat assessment team been in place at Virginia Tech, the shooter's behavior, which had come to the notice of administrators and campus security, would likely have triggered a more complete investigation of his mental status and potential dangerousness, although whether such an investigation would have prevented the attacks is impossible to know.

After the Virginia Tech shootings, a multidisciplinary task force involving the FBI, Secret Service, and U.S. Department of Education, similar to the Safe School Initiative group formed following the Columbine shootings, was appointed and charged with researching the scope of the problem of targeted violence at IHEs. The task force report (Drysdale et al. 2010) identified and examined 272 incidents of targeted violence that occurred at IHEs between 1900 and 2008. The task force found that 27% of the perpetrators of these 272 incidents were active students at the time of their crimes, and another 33% were prior students. Firearms were used in 54% of the incidents. The most common motivation involved issues with an intimate relationship (33.9%). Notably, only 7.9% of the perpetrators were thought to be psychotic, and in only 13% of all cases were prior threats identified. Stalking or harassing behaviors were more common (19%) than serious mental illness or prior threats, and prior physically aggressive acts (10%) were less common than prior threats but more common than serious mental illness.

In addition, in the wake of the Virginia Tech shooting, many IHEs created threat assessment teams, although the low reporting of threats by college and university students complicates identifying prospective offenders. IHE threat assessment teams vary widely in their mission scope: some focus only on identifying actual threats, whereas others take on a more expansive role of fostering campus safety (Higher Education Mental Health Alliance 2013).

Prior to the Virginia Tech tragedy, considerable concern regarding problems with civil commitment procedures and follow-up care had been expressed in the Commonwealth of Virginia. This concern led the Virginia Supreme Court to establish a Commission on Mental Health Reform about 7 months prior to the Virginia Tech shootings. After the shootings occurred, the fact that the shooter had previously been involuntarily committed to outpatient care but had never engaged in mental health treatment despite the court order was widely publicized. The commission therefore conducted detailed examinations of the shooter's involvement with the mental health system, as well as of larger systems issues regarding access to mental health care and involuntary commitment procedures.

Public concern about the Virginia Tech shootings helped draw attention to the commission's recommendations, which focused on four main goals: improving access to voluntary mental health services, utilizing a recovery paradigm, reducing criminalization of mental illness, and redesigning the civil commitment process (Bonnie et al. 2009). In response to the commission's report, the Virginia legislature passed a number of civil commitment reforms in 2008, allocating money to help close gaps in services and to create an organizational structure to oversee the commitment process.

Unfortunately, the 2008 economic downturn slowed much of the funding for these reforms. Richard Bonnie, a law professor and mental health law expert, served on the commission. In 2013, at a hearing before a panel tasked with recommending policy reforms in the wake of the Sandy Hook Elementary School (Newtown, Connecticut) shootings, Bonnie testified that "the [Virginia] General Assembly made a 'down payment' on the necessary investment in fiscal year 2009, but then the recession began and we have just been holding on since then" (Bonnie 2013).

In the majority of cases of mass shootings, the police arrive after the perpetrator has committed suicide. As a result, pro-gun groups have called for allowing adult students to carry guns on campus so students can defend themselves with their own firearms from a rampaging shooter. No evidence exists to support this proposal. For example, a study published by *Mother Jones* surveying 62 incidents of mass murder found that in none of them was the shooter stopped by a civilian with a gun (Follman 2012). Colleges and universities generally have resisted such suggestions, arguing that the protective value of allowing students to carry firearms is low because mass shootings are so rare. In addition, IHE authorities have raised concerns that increasing student access to firearms would lower the threshold for students using guns in circumstances other than those of stopping a rampaging mass shooter. College students present a number of elevated risks for irresponsible gun use. By virtue of their young age, college students are developmentally more impulsive than older adults, increasing the risk that the students might use guns during common interpersonal conflicts or arguments. The high rates of alcohol use on campus and alcohol's effect of lowering inhibitions raise additional concerns about elevated risk of inappropriate and dangerous use of firearms. Student suicide is also a major concern on college campuses, and access to guns has been widely demonstrated to increase the risk of suicide (see Chapter 2, "Firearms and Suicide in the United States," and Chapter 10, "Decreasing Suicide Mortality").

The concept of students carrying firearms remains controversial, and state laws regarding firearms on campuses vary. At the time of this writing, seven states have provisions that allow students with a concealed carry permit to carry guns on college campuses (National Conference of State Legislatures 2014).

School Violence Perpetrated by Nonstudents

On December 14, 2012, a 20-year-old man dressed himself in commando-style clothes, shot and killed his mother, and then drove to Sandy Hook Elementary School, which he had attended briefly as a youngster. He entered the school with a semiautomatic rifle and two semiautomatic handguns, shot and killed 20 children and 6 adult staff, and then, as police arrived, committed suicide. The shooting was the second deadliest mass shooting by an individual in U.S. history. Because so many of the victims were young children, the killings seemed especially horrific and intensified the national debate over reform of firearm laws.

The official report of the Office of the State's Attorney, Judicial District of Danbury (2013), noted that the shooter had been obsessed with mass murders and had planned his actions, including his suicide. The report indicated that the shooter had "significant mental health issues that affected his ability to live a normal life and to interact with others" (p. 3) but also noted that the connection between his mental health problems and his actions was unclear. In an extensive report, the Connecticut Office of the Child Advocate, State of Connecticut (2014), reviewed the shooter's mental health history, noting that he had received extensive evaluation in his early life and had been diagnosed with an autism spectrum disorder, as well as anxiety and obsessive-compulsive disorder. Services had been recommended during his adolescence, but he was resistant to treatment, and his parents accommodated his wish to withdraw from school and not engage in treatment.

As discussed in the previous two subsections, school-based threat assessment teams, formed in response to mass shootings in schools and colleges by students, can often obtain information from other members of the school community. Such teams have minimal value, however, when it comes to preventing violence perpetrated by those who are not part of the school community. Not only do such teams lack access to information about possible perpetrators outside the school community, but they also lack any legal authority or jurisdiction over those who might be identified as threats even if teams received such information.

Therefore, prevention strategies for non-school-affiliated school shooters are limited to primary prevention strategies applicable to the public in general. These include various forms of firearm regulation and risk assessments of dangerous behavior in individuals, with or without mental illness, through the mental health, law enforcement, and judicial systems. Prevention may also include other strategies, such as target hardening or police active shooter protocols, which are intended to minimize damage when an attack is under way.

The adult mass murderer who attacks schools, whether a student or a member of the general public, bears considerable resemblance to mass killers who operate in other settings, such as in workplace and public settings (see Chapter 3, "Gun Violence, Urban Youth, and Mental Illness"). For example, a man who shot six people at his workplace and then shot himself was found to have previously considered and planned an attack on a school (Stevens 2014). In these cases, the risk that a school or IHE will be subjected to a mass shooting is similar to the risk at any other public site, such as a movie theater or shopping mall, where many people gather at the same time in the same place to engage in similar activities together.

Studies evaluating adult mass killers have identified a constellation of characteristics typical of many but by no means all such murderers (Dietz 1986; Knoll 2010; Meloy et al. 2004; Mullen 2004) (see also Chapter 4, "Mass Shootings and Mental Illness"). This constellation includes the behaviors of careful planning of the attack, dressing in paramilitary clothing, arriving armed with multiple weapons, killing as many people as possible, and expecting to die or commit suicide at the end of the attack. Most commando-style killers are not psychotic but instead feel wronged by a rejecting world and want revenge. This pattern fits the individuals in the specific examples discussed in this chapter.

The data about the internal life of the killers who fit this pattern are limited because most die at the end of the attack. Mullen (2004), who was able to interview five mass murderers who survived their attacks, found that they had personality disorders characterized by suspiciousness, obsessional traits, and grandiosity. Their personality disorders may bring them to the attention of mental health clinicians at some point in their lives, but at those times these individuals may not be planning attacks or, if they are, do not communicate their plans to clinicians. Therefore, identifying future mass shooters in the planning stage is extremely difficult.

In the wake of the Sandy Hook shootings, Governor Malloy of Connecticut convened a commission to make recommendations to prevent future school violence. The Sandy Hook Advisory Commission's (2015) final report includes recommendations in multiple areas, including firearm regulation, school target hardening, and improvement of the mental health system. The proposed firearm regulations focused on background checks for all sales and transfers of firearms, with tightening of the screening process and a ban on civilian use of weapons that could fire more than 10 shots without reloading. The commission called for hardening school targets by setting state standards on physical security through such means as installing lockable doors to all classrooms and providing schools with hardware that would allow a rapid lockdown of the perimeter.

The commission's recommendations on mental health problems were fairly general, focusing on such issues as the fragmentation of the mental health system, funding and payment issues, and the reduction of stigma. The commission did recommend some school-specific interventions, including implementing social-emotional curricula, antibullying strategies, and multidisciplinary threat assessment teams. As discussed in this chapter and throughout this volume, the public perceives a strong causal association between serious mental illness and violence, including gun violence. However, the data consistently indicate that serious mental illness is not of itself a major risk factor for violent behavior, including gun violence, unless the behavior under consideration is that of suicide alone.

Preventive Intervention Strategies: Challenges and Evidence Base

Mass shootings in schools and colleges are just the tip of the iceberg of school-related violence. The horrific nature of such incidents results in enormous publicity and leads to calls for interventions, such as limiting mentally ill people from owning a firearm, that have effects on many more people than the small number of prospective mass shooters. Preventive interventions for school shootings can be conceptualized as occurring at three different levels: primary prevention aims to reduce the risk of someone ever moving to the stage of planning an attack on a school, secondary prevention efforts focus on identifying and managing those persons planning an attack, and tertiary prevention interventions reduce the carnage once an attack is under way.

Primary Prevention Efforts

Primary prevention efforts center on understanding the course of the development of a problem. Although perpetrators of mass shootings, and indeed of most criminal acts, may have emotional problems, these shootings are seldom the result of serious mental illness. Actual psychosis with delusional motives is fairly rare in school violence. As noted, mass violence is not impulsive but rather is carefully planned. Careful planning requires the ability to sustain organized thinking, a capacity that most acutely psychotic individuals lack. Rather than acting on delusional motives, perpetrators more commonly feel rejected by the world and desire revenge, and are often prepared to commit suicide and thereby die in a blaze of infamy. Moreover, the base rate of mass shooting incidents is so low that assessing the efficacy of any type of intervention presents problems in designing studies and interpreting results.

Therefore, in assessing the evidence base for the effectiveness of preventive interventions for mass shootings, one needs to keep a number of general points in mind. First, because the frequency of mass shootings is extremely low, the methodology employed in studies of these events is typically that of a case study or a small case series, with the limitations inherent in those methodologies when compared to studies using control groups or large samples. Second, the time delay between a primary prevention effort and a rare outcome allows for so many intervening variables to occur that drawing strong causal conclusions is difficult. For example, some evidence indicates that many school shooters were bullied as youngsters (Vossekuil et al. 2002). However, if schools implemented programs that significantly reduced the frequency of bullying, and a decade later somewhat fewer mass shootings had taken place, it would be difficult to conclude that the intervention and the outcome were causally linked.

That said, a number of possible evidence-based preventive interventions with some demonstrated although varied degrees of efficacy have been discussed in this chapter and are organized by school and shooter categories in Table 5–1. Just as school shootings fall into different categories depending on the type of school or IHE and the affiliation of the perpetrator with the school or IHE, suggested interventions also have to take the specific circumstances associated with each category of school shooting into account.

Primary prevention efforts to reduce violence through improved mental health services, school-based antiviolence education, and the reduction of bullying, although likely to be helpful for the general population in multiple ways (Kyriakides et al. 2014), are likely to have low specificity for reducing mass murder in schools or on college campuses. Nevertheless, the extent to which such programs reduce violence generally and gun violence in particular is unknown.

Even with the availability of such resources, predicting who among the significant number of resentful, angry young men is likely to become a mass murderer remains a challenge. The rarity of mass shootings, combined with the difficulty of identifying those who might commit such crimes, renders attempts at primary prevention a significant challenge. The current knowledge base limits the ability to accurately assess the risk of future dangerousness of a troubled youth or young adult who has no prior history of violence, denies homicidal ideation, and demonstrates no extrinsic evidence of planning a homicide. Although most of the mass shooters discussed in this chapter had seen mental health professionals multiple times in their lives, they had not been identified as constituting a serious danger to others.

Moreover, because adults report their intentions to others with considerably less frequency than youth under age 18, adults planning violence or mass murder are much more difficult to identify. The fact that many school mass killers are not students at all, but instead are members of the general public who choose a school or college as the site for their rampage, adds to the difficulty of identification. Additionally, it must be acknowledged that mental health professionals have few evidence-based treatments for treating youth who feel wronged by the world and feel angry and vengeful toward it.

Secondary Prevention Efforts

Secondary prevention efforts rely on the identification of imminently dangerous persons. As discussed above in the subsection "K–12 School Shootings by Students," school surveillance through increased reporting of threats has been helpful in identifying students at risk for mass violence. The establishment of school-based threat assessment teams appears to have been effective in reducing mass shootings by K–12 students. Such multidisciplinary teams provide a coordinated response to threats of other types of violence as well, and anecdotal evidence

TABLE 5–1. Evidence-based intervention strategies

<table>
<tr><th rowspan="2">Intervention timing</th><th colspan="3">Site and perpetrator</th></tr>
<tr><th>K–12 shooting by student</th><th>College shooting by student</th><th>School shootings by nonstudent</th></tr>
<tr><td>Primary prevention:
Prior to considering mass murder</td><td>Reduce bullying in schools*</td><td>Improve integration of student mental health centers with college administration*</td><td></td></tr>
<tr><td></td><td>Teach antiviolence coping skills</td><td colspan="2">Do not allow those with mental illness to purchase guns*
Restrict access to firearms for those individuals, with or without mental illness, who have risk factors indicating increased potential for dangerous behavior**</td></tr>
<tr><td></td><td colspan="3">Provide better access to mental health treatment*</td></tr>
<tr><td>Secondary prevention:
During planning stage</td><td colspan="2">Increase surveillance by encouraging reporting of threats to education officials**</td><td></td></tr>
<tr><td></td><td colspan="2">Implement multidisciplinary threat assessment teams**</td><td></td></tr>
<tr><td>Tertiary prevention:
During attack</td><td>Increase school presence of and access to school resource officers*</td><td colspan="2">Increase security personnel training and availability at institutions of higher education*</td></tr>
<tr><td></td><td colspan="3">Improve building security measures (cameras, metal detectors, armed security)**</td></tr>
<tr><td></td><td colspan="3">Improve staff and student preparedness by increasing access to communication/lockdown procedures and drills**</td></tr>
<tr><td></td><td colspan="3">Implement SWAT teams and “active shooter” police policies**</td></tr>
</table>

Note. Strength of supporting evidence: *indirect: some evidence that intervention affects variables associated with violence; **direct evidence for reducing violence. SWAT=special weapons and tactics.

indicates that they have successfully managed risk across a wide domain of problematic behaviors. Limiting civilian availability of assault rifles and other high-capacity weapons, another type of secondary intervention, might reduce the number of deaths in an attack by slowing down the rate at which people are killed. However, both youth and adults have little difficulty in obtaining firearms, legally or otherwise, and this appears unlikely to change in the foreseeable future.

Tertiary Prevention Efforts

Tertiary prevention has evolved with experience of mass shootings. As noted in the section "School Shootings: Targets, Perpetrators, and Interventions" above, improvements in police response tactics have been shown to reduce the carnage in some cases, but most violent incidents have ended by the time the police arrive. Target hardening through such means as restricting access to K–12 schools and classrooms, practicing lockdown procedures, and arming staff make it more difficult for a shooter to kill large numbers, and might decrease the death toll, at some cost to the ambience of schools as calm, peaceful places for learning. At the college level, strategies to increase the number of armed students so they can act in their own defense run the unintended risk that the ready availability of guns would increase the lethality of impulsive violence, which is much more common than mass murder or predatory violence.

Conclusion

Schools have become safer places over the past two decades. Crime rates at schools and campuses have dropped significantly. In part, this decline likely reflects the decreasing homicide rates in the general population among both youth and adults over the last 20 years, a decrease about which many theories have been proposed but no generally accepted consensus of understanding exists. In the 4 years preceding the Columbine shootings, mass shootings by students at K–12 schools went from being practically unheard of to a frequency of more than one a year, and then such shootings dropped off markedly. In other settings—colleges, the workplace, and public spaces—a large number of mass shootings appear to follow the script of an angry and vengeful young man outfitting himself in paramilitary garb with multiple weapons and shooting as many strangers as possible before committing suicide, a script that was essentially unknown before the University of Texas Tower shooting.

These patterns do not reflect marked changes in rates of bullying, mental illness, gun availability, or other factors that are the targets of various interventions, but point instead to the importance of poorly understood social trends as underlying causes. The methodologies for studying such systemic factors may be quite different from the methodologies used thus far in the study of mass violence. Such research will likely need to be multidisciplinary, will need to take into account a wider array of social factors than have thus far been studied, and may require a structured institutional approach. For example, a standing structure similar to the National Transportation Safety Board, which investigates both airline crashes and near misses using a multidisciplinary team, has been proposed (Harris and Harris 2012) to organize future research. Much remains to be learned.

Suggested Interventions

- Screening and mental health resources for troubled youth in grades K–12 should be increased. Although this intervention is not likely to have a direct, measurable effect on school mass shootings, indirect evidence suggests that improving access to mental health resources will have a significant effect on other problematic public health mental disorder issues, such as use of drugs and alcohol by youth, learning disabilities, youth suicide, and school violence.
- Antibullying programs should be supported in grades K–12.
- More threat assessment teams, in both K–12 schools and institutions of higher education (IHEs), need to be funded and implemented. These will vary in structure, access to information, and authority to intervene, depending on various school factors (e.g., school size, student ages).
- Students at all levels, in grades K–12 and in IHEs, should be educated to take all threats or threatening behavior seriously and report it to appropriate personnel: "If you hear something, say something."
- Efforts should be made to improve communication between school administration and security, threat assessment teams, law enforcement, and mental health services.
- School and IHE campuses should improve target hardening to reduce damage during an attack.

References

American Psychiatric Foundation: Typical or Troubled? School Mental Health Education Program. Arlington, VA, American Psychiatric Association, 2014. Available at: http://www.americanpsychiatricfoundation.org/what-we-do/public-education/typical-or-troubled/typical-or-troubled. Accessed September 13, 2014.

Ash P, Kellermann AL, Fuqua-Whitley D, et al: Gun acquisition and use by juvenile offenders. JAMA 275(22):1754–1758, 1996 8637174

Associated Press: School shooting thwarted: teens arrested after making plans to kill as many students as possible, police say. Huffington Post, August 19, 2014. Available at: http://www.huffingtonpost.com/2014/08/19/school-shooting-thwarted-south-pasadena-high-school_n_5690163.html. Accessed November 23, 2014.

Blair J, Schweit K: A Study of Active Shooter Incidents in the United States Between 2000 and 2013. Washington, DC, U.S. Department of Justice, Federal Bureau of Investigation, 2014

Bonnie RJ: UVA law professor Richard Bonnie testifies before Sandy Hook Panel. University of Virginia School of Law News & Events, January 25, 2013. Available at: http://www.law.virginia.edu/html/news/2013_spr/bonnie_sandy_hook.htm. Accessed August 26, 2014.

Bonnie RJ, Reinhard JS, Hamilton P, et al: Mental health system transformation after the Virginia Tech tragedy. Health Aff (Millwood) 28(3):793–804, 2009 19414889

Borum R, Fein R, Vossekuil B, et al: Threat assessment: defining an approach for evaluating risk of targeted violence. Behav Sci Law 17(3):323–337, 1999 10481132

Bowman L: More than 120 school shooting plots thwarted in U.S. KHSB Kansas City Channel 41, December 18, 2012. Available at: http://www.kshb.com/news/national/more-than-120-school-shooting-plots-thwarted-in-us. Accessed November 23, 2014.

Brent DA, Baugher M, Birmaher B, et al: Compliance with recommendations to remove firearms in families participating in a clinical trial for adolescent depression. J Am Acad Child Adolesc Psychiatry 39(10):1220–1226, 2000 11026174

Cantor CH, Sheehan P, Alpers P, et al: Media and mass homicides. Arch Suicide Res 5:283–290, 1999

Centers for Disease Control and Prevention: WISQARS Fatal Injury Reports, National and Regional, 1999–2013. Atlanta, GA, Centers for Disease Control and Prevention, 2015. Available at: http://webappa.cdc.gov/sasweb/ncipc/mortrate10_us.html. Accessed August 11, 2015.

Cornell DG, Sheras P: Guidelines for Responding to Student Threats of Violence. Longmont, CO, Sopris West, 2006

Cornell DG, Sheras PL, Kaplan S, et al: Guidelines for student threat assessment: field-test findings. School Psych Rev 33(4):527–546, 2004

Cornell DG, Allen K, Fan X: A randomized controlled study of the Virginia Student Threat Assessment Guidelines in kindergarten through grade 12. School Psych Rev 41(1):100–115, 2012

Dietz PE: Mass, serial and sensational homicides. Bull NY Acad Med 62(5):477–491, 1986 3461857

Drysdale D, Modzeleski W, Simons A: Campus Attacks: Targeted Violence Affecting Institutions of Higher Education. Washington, DC, U.S. Secret Service, U.S. Department of Education, and Federal Bureau of Investigation, 2010

Fein RA, Vossekuil B: Assassination in the United States: an operational study of recent assassins, attackers, and near-lethal approachers. J Forensic Sci 44(2):321–333, 1999 10097356

Fein R, Vossekuil B, Pollack WS, et al: Threat Assessment in Schools: A Guide to Managing Threatening Situations and to Creating Safe School Climates. Washington, DC, U.S. Secret Service and U.S. Department of Education, 2002

Follman M: Do armed civilians stop mass shooters? Actually, no. Mother Jones, December 19, 2012. Available at: http://www.motherjones.com/politics/2012/12/armed-civilians-do-not-stop-mass-shootings. Accessed August 11, 2015.

Governor's Committee: Report to the Governor: Medical Aspects, Charles J. Whitman Catastrophe. Austin, TX, The Whitman Archives, September 8, 1966. Available at: http://alt.cimedia.com/statesman/specialreports/whitman/findings.pdf. Accessed November 13, 2014.

Hampton T: Programs aim to help schools identify and address mental illness in children. JAMA 309(17):1761–1762, 2013 23632696

Harris JM Jr, Harris RB: Rampage violence requires a new type of research. Am J Public Health 102(6):1054–1057, 2012 22515868

Higher Education Mental Health Alliance: Balancing safety and support on campus. 2013. Available at: http://www.jedfoundation.org/campus_teams_guide.pdf. Accessed December 4, 2014.

Khoury L: Bullying prevention and intervention: realistic strategies for schools. J LGBT Youth 11(2):176–181, 2014

Knoll JL IV: The "pseudocommando" mass murderer, Part I: the psychology of revenge and obliteration. J Am Acad Psychiatry Law 38(1):87–94, 2010 20305080

Kyriakides L, Creemers BPM, Muijs D, et al: Using the dynamic model of educational effectiveness to design strategies and actions to face bullying. School Effectiveness and School Improvement 25(1):83–104, 2014

Meloy JR, Hempel AG, Gray BT, et al: A comparative analysis of North American adolescent and adult mass murderers. Behav Sci Law 22(3):291–309, 2004 15211553

Menard S, Grotpeter JK: Evaluation of bully proofing your school as an elementary school antibullying intervention. J Sch Violence 13(2):188–209, 2014

Morton RJ, Hilts MA (eds): Serial Murder: Multi-Disciplinary Perspectives for Investigators. Washington, DC, Federal Bureau of Investigation, 2005

Mullen PE: The autogenic (self-generated) massacre. Behav Sci Law 22(3):311–323, 2004 15211554

Nansel TR, Overpeck MD, Haynie DL, et al: Relationships between bullying and violence among U.S. youth. Arch Pediatr Adolesc Med 157(4):348–353, 2003 12695230

National Conference of State Legislatures: Guns on Campus: Overview. Denver, CO, National Conference of State Legislatures, 2014. Available at: http://www.ncsl.org/research/education/guns-on-campus-overview.aspx. Accessed December 4, 2014.

Office of Postsecondary Education: The Campus Safety and Security Data Analysis Cutting Tool. Washington, DC, U.S. Department of Education, 2014. Available at: http://www.ope.ed.gov/security/. Accessed September 15, 2014.

Office of the Child Advocate, State of Connecticut: Shooting at Sandy Hook Elementary School: Report of the Office of the Child Advocate. Hartford, CT, Office of the Child Advocate, November 21, 2014. Available at: http://www.ct.gov/oca/lib/oca/sandyhook11212014.pdf. Accessed November 22, 2014.

Office of the State's Attorney, Judicial District of Danbury: Report of the State's Attorney for the Judicial District of Danbury on the Shootings at Sandy Hook Elementary School and 36 Yogananda Street, Newtown, Connecticut on December 14, 2012. Danbury, CT, Office of the State's Attorney, 2013

O'Toole ME: The School Shooter: A Threat Assessment Perspective. Washington, DC, Federal Bureau of Investigation, 1999

Planty M, Truman JL: Special Report: Firearm Violence, 1993–2011 (NCJ 241730). Washington, DC, Bureau of Justice Statistics, 2013

Reddy M, Borum R, Berglund J, et al: Evaluating risk for targeted violence in schools: comparing risk assessment, threat assessment, and other approaches. Psychol Sch 38(2):157–172, 2001

Robers S, Zhang J, Truman J, et al: Indicators of School Crime and Safety: 2011. NCES 2012-004/NCJ 236021. Washington, DC, National Center for Education Statistics, 2012

Robers S, Kemp J, Rathbun A, et al: Indicators of School Crime and Safety: 2013. NCES 2014-042/NCJ 243299. Washington, DC, National Center for Education Statistics, 2014

Sandy Hook Advisory Commission: Final Report of the Sandy Hook Advisory Commission. Hartford, CT, Office of the Governor, 2015. Available at: http://www.shac.ct.gov/SHAC_Final_Report_3-6-2015.pdf. Accessed August 11, 2015.

Schwartz AJ: College student suicide in the United States: 1990–1991 through 2003–2004. J Am Coll Health 54(6):341–352, 2006 16789650

Schwartz AJ: Rate, relative risk, and method of suicide by students at 4-year colleges and universities in the United States, 2004–2005 through 2008–2009. Suicide Life Threat Behav 41(4):353–371, 2011 21535095

Snow RL: SWAT Teams: Explosive Face-Offs With America's Deadliest Criminals. New York, Da Capo Press, 1996

Stevens A: Cops: FedEx shooter had deadly plans. Atlanta Journal-Constitution, September 12, 2014, B1

Sullivan M: Giving killers coverage, not platforms. New York Times, May 31, 2014. Available at: http://www.nytimes.com/2014/06/01/public-editor/giving-killers-coverage-not-platforms.html?_r=0. Accessed December 4, 2014.

Twemlow SW, Sacco FC: Preventing Bullying and School Violence. Washington, DC, American Psychiatric Publishing, 2012

U.S. Department of Health and Human Services, U.S. Department of Education, U.S. Department of Justice: Report to the President on Issues Raised by the Virginia Tech Tragedy. Washington, DC, U.S. Department of Justice, June 13, 2007. Available at: http://www.justice.gov/opa/pr/2007/June/vt_report_061307.pdf. Accessed August 31, 2014.

U.S. Department of Homeland Security: Active Shooter: How to Respond. Washington, DC, U.S. Department of Homeland Security, 2008

Verlinden S, Hersen M, Thomas J: Risk factors in school shootings. Clin Psychol Rev 20(1):3–56, 2000 10660827

Vossekuil B, Reddy M, Fein R, et al: Safe School Initiative: An Interim Report on the Prevention of Targeted Violence in Schools. Washington, DC, U.S. Secret Service National Threat Assessment Center and U.S. Department of Education, 2000

Vossekuil B, Fein R, Reddy M, et al: The Final Report and Findings of the Safe School Initiative: Implications for the Prevention of School Attacks in the United States. Washington, DC, U.S. Secret Service and U.S. Department of Education, 2002

Vreeman RC, Carroll AE: A systematic review of school-based interventions to prevent bullying. Arch Pediatr Adolesc Med 161(1):78–88, 2007 17199071

Whitman C: "Whitman Letter," July 31, 1966. Austin, TX, Austin American-Statesman: The Whitman Archives, 1966

Wikipedia: List of school shootings in the United States. Wikipedia.org, 2014. Available at: http://en.wikipedia.org/wiki/List_of_school_shootings_in_the_United_States. Accessed July 21, 2014.

6

Mental Illness and the National Instant Criminal Background Check System

Marilyn Price, M.D., C.M.
Patricia R. Recupero, J.D., M.D.
Donna M. Norris, M.D.

Common Misperceptions

- ☒ People with mental illness are automatically reported to the National Instant Criminal Background Check System (NICS).
- ☒ States are required to report prohibited individuals to the NICS and routinely comply with NICS reporting requirements.
- ☒ When people are reported to NICS, they lose their access to firearms and no longer pose a danger.
- ☒ States are not particularly interested in improving record reporting to NICS.
- ☒ Gun laws that restrict persons with mental illness from acquiring firearms will prevent future tragedies from mass shootings.

Evidence-Based Facts

- ☑ Having a history of a mental health diagnosis does not lead to automatic inclusion in the NICS databases.
- ☑ States cannot be required by law to participate in NICS. Many states do not comply with reporting all categories of prohibited people, including people who have met criteria for mental health prohibitions.
- ☑ When people are reported to NICS, they often are able to retain any firearms they already own, and they may still acquire new firearms through secondary channels.
- ☑ Since 2011, many states have passed new legislation to improve NICS reporting, although reporting remains incomplete.
- ☑ Laws that seek to restrict firearm acquisition through background checks and increased reporting of persons with mental illness may help to reduce rates of suicide by firearms but are unlikely to achieve the desired aim of preventing future acts of mass violence.

The intent of the National Instant Criminal Background Check System (NICS) is, in the interest of public safety, to prevent people considered dangerous from purchasing or possessing firearms. The strategy of existing federal laws has been to identify and focus on classes of persons who are considered at increased risk to themselves and others and then to prohibit those individuals from being able to possess, register, license, retain, or carry a firearm. The NICS database, maintained by the Federal Bureau of Investigation's (FBI's) NICS Section, was intended to serve as a central repository of the names of prohibited persons. Persons seeking to purchase a firearm from a federally licensed dealer would be required to undergo a check through NICS to verify eligibility.

Empirical evidence of increased risk of violence supports the inclusion of classes of persons such as those convicted of a felony or those who are subject to a restraining order for harassing, stalking, or threatening an intimate partner. Evidence also indicates that legislation restricting access to firearms may be effective in reducing rates of suicide for persons with mental illness. However, scant evidence supports the belief that such legislation would be effective in reducing the incidence of homicide by firearms, particularly the incidence of mass shootings, by persons with mental illness.

Public perception that persons with mental illness pose an increased risk of violence, including gun violence, toward others is widespread. The media coverage following high-profile shootings reinforces this misperception and has led to calls for passage of additional restrictions on persons with mental illness at both state and federal levels. In fact, persons "adjudicated as a mental defective" (as per 18 U.S.C. § 922[d][4]) already constitute a federally prohibited class. Many states have expanded the definition of persons with mental illness beyond that included in federal legislation, in an effort to reduce violence. In this chapter, we focus primarily on the federal background check system. States may have tighter restrictions and databases separate from NICS; however, when states do not have their own mental health firearm prohibitions, federal prohibitions apply.

Firearms and Firearm-Related Death in the United States

As of 2005, roughly 2.5 million new firearms were sold each year in the United States—a number that does not include thefts or sales of used weapons (Hahn et al. 2005). Much of the trade in firearms in the United States is through loosely regulated channels (Wintemute 2013). Firearms accounted for more than 31,000 fatalities in the United States each year between 2007 and 2010 (Fleegler et al. 2013). In recent years, the rate of firearm homicides has declined (Centers for Disease Control and Prevention 2013a), as did violent crime from the early 1990s to 2011 (Bjelopera et al. 2013), but firearm-related violent crime increased 26% between 2008 and 2011 (Wintemute 2013b).

Although firearm homicides have been decreasing in recent years, the firearm suicide rate has been increasing (Centers for Disease Control and Prevention 2013a). In 2010, suicide accounted for 61% of firearm deaths in the United States (Centers for Disease Control and Prevention 2013b), and firearms are used in over half of all suicides in the United States (Rodríguez Andrés and Hempstead 2011). Firearm ownership appears to function as an independent risk factor for suicide, regardless of suicidal behavior; Miller et al. (2013) found that across all 50 states, "higher rates of firearm ownership…were strongly associated with higher rates of overall [completed] suicide" (p. 948), after controlling for rates of suicidal attempts overall.

In a systematic review and meta-analysis of 16 studies evaluating the odds of death (including both homicide and suicide) associated with the presence of a firearm in the home, "[a]ll but 1 of the 16 studies…reported significantly increased odds of death associated with firearm access" (Anglemyer et al. 2014, p. 105), and the evidence was particularly strong for risk of death by suicide. Because of the high lethality of firearms as a suicide method, fatality rates in suicide attempts by firearm are estimated to be around 85% (Vyrostek et al. 2004).

Creation of NICS

NICS was introduced in the context of a series of federal legislative reforms intended to reduce gun violence. The first of these reforms that specifically mentioned individuals with mental impairment was the Omnibus Crime Control and Safe Streets Act of 1968 (Pub. L. No. 90-351, 82 Stat. 197; Simpson 2007a). This was followed shortly thereafter by the Gun Control Act of 1968 (Pub. L. No. 90-618, 82 Stat. 1213, codified at 18 U.S.C. §§ 922–931), enforced by the Bureau of Alcohol, Tobacco, Firearms and Explosives (ATF) and inspired in part by the assassinations of Martin Luther King Jr. and Robert F. Kennedy (Wiehl 2013). The Gun Control Act prohibits firearm purchases by classes of persons considered at increased risk for committing gun violence, including persons with certain criminal convictions; fugitives; illegal aliens; dishonorably discharged military; persons subject to court orders for harassment, stalking, or domestic violence; and persons using or addicted to controlled substances (Price and Norris 2008).

The Gun Control Act also prohibits the sale or transfer of firearms or ammunition to anyone previously "'tadjudicated as a mental defective' or 'committed to any mental institution.'" Under the Gun Control Act, "adjudicated as a mental defective" is defined as a determination by a court, board, commission, or other lawful authority that a person, as a result of marked subnormal intelligence, or mental illness, incompetency, condition, or disease, is a danger to himself or herself or others or lacks the mental capacity to contract or manage his or her own affairs (Meaning of Terms, 27 C.F.R. § 478.11, 2014). Affected persons include those found insane by a court in a criminal case and those found either incompetent to stand trial or not guilty by reason of lack of mental responsibility. "Committed to any mental institution" refers to a formal commitment to a mental institution by a court, board, commission, or other lawful authority and includes involuntary commitment to a mental institution for mental "defectiveness" or mental illness as well as for other reasons (e.g., drug use). The term specifically does not include a person in a mental institution for observation, such as an individual involuntarily held on a temporary detention order, or a person voluntarily admitted to a mental institution.

However, despite defining classes of persons who were prohibited from purchasing or owning firearms, the Gun Control Act did not provide a process for ensuring or enforcing these prohibited classes of individuals from purchasing firearms. In 1993, Congress passed the Brady Handgun Violence Prevention Act (Pub. L. No. 103-159, 107 Stat. 1536) following the attempted assassination of President Reagan and the wounding of several of his staff members, including press secretary James Brady. The Brady Act required the U.S. Attorney General to establish the NICS, the permanent provisions of which went into effect in 1998 (Hahn et al. 2005; Price and Norris 2008, 2010; Wiehl 2013). Under this system, a person seeking to purchase firearms, including long guns, from a federally licensed firearm dealer is subject to an instant background check using the NICS databases (American Psychiatric Association 2014). If the NICS check is positive, the dealer is informed that the request is denied but is not informed why (Lewis 2011; Price and Norris 2010).

NICS comprises three databases administered by the FBI (Price and Norris 2010): 1) the Interstate Identification Index, which contains state and federal criminal history record information, including felony convictions and individuals who have been adjudicated as not guilty by reason of insanity or incompetent to stand trial; 2) the National Crime Information Center, which includes persons subject to civil protection orders and arrest warrants; and 3) the NICS Index, which contains information from federal and state agencies about prohibited purchasers not identified in the other databases (Price and Norris 2010). The Interstate Identification Index and the NICS Index thus contain the names of individuals who are prohibited by law from purchasing or owning a firearm because of a judicial finding of mental impairment (Legal Community Against Violence 2008).

The purpose of the NICS background check is to ensure that prospective gun buyers are not prohibited by federal and/or state law from purchasing or owning a firearm. On April 16, 2012, the NICS Index was expanded to include state-prohibiting records. This expansion provides the NICS Section and state users with the ability to effectively and efficiently identify people prohibited from possessing guns by state as well as federal law through NICS, provided states have reported those records to the NICS Index (Federal Bureau of Investigation 2015a). Over the 1990s, additional legislation created new categories of federally prohibited gun purchasers. The federal Violent Crime Control and Law Enforcement Act of 1994 prohibits a person from possessing or receiving a firearm while subject to a permanent restraining order in the context of intimate partner violence or child protection (Price and Norris 2010). In 1996, the Lautenberg Amendment added those convicted of misdemeanor domestic violence offenses to the prohibited purchaser category (Gun Ban for Individuals Convicted of a Misdemeanor Crime of Domestic Violence, Pub. L. No. 104-208, 18 U.S.C. § 922[g][9], 1996).

NICS and Mental Health Prohibitors

In the years following passage of the Brady Act, several highly publicized multiple shootings raised public concern about the effectiveness of the NICS background check system and firearm restrictions in the United States. Many of these incidents involved individuals with mental illness, such as the 1993 Long Island RailRoad shooting, in which 6 people were killed and 19 were wounded (Dowd 1993); the 1998 U.S. Capitol shooting, in which 2 officers were killed (Lewis 2011; Price and Norris 2008); the 2007 Virginia Tech shooting, in which 32 people were killed and 17 wounded before the shooter killed himself; and the worst mass shooting in U.S. history, at Sandy Hook Elementary School in Newtown, Connecticut, in 2012, in which 20 children and 6 adults were killed, in addition to the shooter and his mother (Mayors Against Illegal Guns 2011; Wiehl 2013).

These and other high-profile incidents are often invoked to bolster support for further gun legislation reform. A review of three of these incidents highlights the problems inherent in relying on NICS to prevent mass shootings. The person who killed two officers at the U.S. Capitol in 1998 did have a history of involuntary commitment, but the state failed to report his disqualification for firearm purchase to NICS. The Long Island RailRoad shooter had not been involuntarily committed for a mental illness and therefore would not have met the federal criteria for inclusion in NICS. Finally, the person responsible for the deaths in Newtown, Connecticut, would not have met federal mental health prohibitors, because he had never been involuntarily committed or adjudicated with mental illness. Moreover, he was able to access his mother's legally acquired firearms, an indication that persons with mental illness can obtain firearms through family and friends or the secondary market.

The NICS Improvement Amendments Act of 2007 (Pub. L. No. 110-180, 121 Stat. 2559, codified at 18 U.S.C. § 922, 2008) was at least in part a reaction to the revelation that the perpetrator of the Virginia Tech shootings had purchased guns through licensed dealers after passing background checks, despite having been subject to a court order for involuntary outpatient mental health treatment (Price and Norris 2010). In *Printz v. United States* (521 U.S. 898, 1997), a case challenging the constitutionality of some of the provisions of the 1993 Brady Act, the Supreme Court ruled that the federal government may not mandate that state officials administer or enforce a federal regulatory program. States therefore could not be required to participate in the federal NICS system.

The NICS Improvement Amendments Act of 2007 was intended to increase reporting to the NICS by offering financial incentives to states for providing NICS with information on persons in prohibited categories, including mental health–related prohibited purchasers, and financial disincentives for not participating (Parker 2010). This legislation also instituted requirements for the restoration of firearm ownership rights specifically for those barred from purchasing or owning firearms due to the mental health disqualifications through a federal "relief from disabilities" program, although the requirements of a restoration process were not specified (Price and Norris 2010; also see Chapter 13, "Relief From Disabilities: Firearm Rights Restoration for Persons Under Mental Health Prohibitions").

The process by which someone who is a prohibited purchaser for mental health reasons is reported to the NICS databases varies from state to state. In many states, court orders, such as involuntary commitments, are automatically reported to NICS. However, other aspects of the reporting requirements vary widely across states. In addition, as per the Supreme Court's decision in *Printz,* state participation in the NICS database remains voluntary, and not all states participate to the same degree. State laws vary regarding the exact definition of which people must be reported, the person who is responsible for making the report, the length of time a prohibition is active, the firearms that are included in the prohibition, confidentiality protections for records that are reported, the existence or maintenance of a state-based mental health database, and the process for appealing a prohibition (Price and Norris 2010).

Do Firearm Legislation, NICS, and Background Checks Reduce Morbidity and Mortality From Gun Violence?

Few published research studies investigating whether firearm laws result in decreases in firearm morbidity and mortality are available. More and better data are clearly needed. Nevertheless, a review of some of the available empirical data can help to inform the debate over the efficacy of an approach to firearm prohibition based on classes of persons considered dangerous. Researchers for the Centers for Disease Control and Prevention–supported Task Force on Community Preventive Services reviewed a variety of different types of firearm laws, including those banning specific weapons or ammunition, prohibiting certain purchasers, mandating waiting periods, and specifying registration and licensing requirements; concealed carry laws; laws relating to child protection and schools; and laws that combined different types of provisions (Hahn et al. 2005). The task force's ultimate finding was inconclusive. More recently, Webster and Wintemute (2015) summarized studies published between 1999 and August 2014 on effects of policies designed to keep firearms from high-risk persons.

Fleegler et al.'s (2013) compared rates of reported firearm-related deaths to the number and strength of firearm laws in states throughout the United States. They found a correlation between higher numbers of firearm laws in a state and lower rates of overall firearm fatalities in that state; the relationship also held true when testing for homicides and suicides individually. However, the authors noted the necessity for further research to determine the reason for this association, because they were unable to determine causation. Wintemute (2013b) suggests that the lower rates of firearm fatalities in the Fleegler et al.'s (2013) study could have been due to confounding variables.

Another recent study found that firearm injury rates among children were lower in states characterized as having strict firearm laws (Safavi et al. 2014). Some literature suggests that more restrictive firearm laws have reduced rates of firearm injuries and deaths in Australia and the United Kingdom (Chapman et al. 2006; Record and Gostin 2013), which lends some support to Fleegler et al.'s (2013) findings. In Australia, a 1996 law that drastically reduced access to firearms resulted in a dramatic decrease in the incidence of public mass shootings and gun suicides (Chapman et al. 2006).

A study from Norway found a correlation between a decreased risk of firearm-related mortality among men and the passage of several firearm laws, but the data were inconclusive; the authors indicated that the firearm laws in question may have had no effect (Gjertsen et al. 2014). Reisch et al. (2013) compared suicide rates before (1995–2003) and after (2004–2008) a reform that halved the number of army soldiers in Switzerland, thereby decreasing the availability of firearms in the homes of men ages 18–43 years. The overall suicide rate as well as the firearm suicide rate decreased. This group estimated that 22% of the reduction in firearm suicides was substituted by other suicide methods. Nevertheless, the overall suicide rate remained lower than rates of suicide prior to the decrease in firearm availability.

Using data from the National Center for Health Statistics for a period overlapping the implementation of the Brady Act, Ludwig and Cook (2000) investigated whether the Brady Act was associated with any changes in the rates of homicide and suicide. They found an apparent reduction in firearm suicides among persons age 55 years and older but no reduction in homicide or suicide rates overall (Ludwig and Cook 2000). Some empirical data suggest that denial of an application to purchase a handgun may be associated with a reduced risk of subsequent violent crime (Wintemute 2014), but much of these data were collected in the years prior to developments such as the increasing availability of and trade in individual firearm components.

Parker (2010) evaluated outcomes following Indiana's implementation of a law authorizing the removal of firearms by police officers without a warrant from individuals reasonably believed to be mentally ill and dangerous. He found that removals were most commonly due to the firearm owner's risk for suicide or substance abuse; over time, court hearings increasingly led to weapons being returned to their original owners. Parker concluded that the overall effect of the law was "minimal," because of the large percentage of the population owning firearms and the comparatively small number of firearms that were removed.

Rodríguez Andrés and Hempstead (2011) investigated the effect of state-level firearm permit and licensing restrictions and found that broad restrictions of public access resulted in a significantly lower rate of firearm suicide among men. They also found that regulations restricting firearm ownership specifically among high-risk persons have less effect (Rodríguez Andrés and Hempstead 2011). The most effective measures included requirements for permits and regulations that ban the sale of firearms to minors. They noted the extreme heterogeneity of gun laws across states in the United States and the fact that a number of states continue to allow the purchase of long guns (as opposed to handguns) by minors. An earlier study by Loftin et al. (1991) lends support to these findings; these authors found that the passage of a law in the mid-1970s highly restricting handgun licensing in the District of Columbia preceded a 25% reduction in firearm homicides and a 23% reduction in firearm suicides in that area.

Finally, Swanson et al. (2013) examined the effectiveness of NICS background checks and mental health disqualifiers in the state of Connecticut. They found that expanded NICS reporting after 2007 legislation was associated with a slight decrease in the risk of violent crime among persons who had been disqualified from purchasing a gun, but a minimal effect (<0.5%) on violent crime overall (Swanson et al. 2015). Furthermore, persons with a gun-disqualifying criminal history were found to have an *increased* risk for future perpetration of violent crime (Swanson et al. 2013).

The NICS System and the Mental Health Prohibition: Does It Work as Intended?

NICS has had some success in denying the purchase of firearms to certain prohibited categories of individuals associated with increased risk of firearm violence. As of July 31, 2015, the NICS Index had more than 13 million active records (Federal Bureau of Investigation 2015a). Between 1998 and July 31, 2015, the ATF denied more than 1.2 million firearm purchases based on these records (Federal Bureau of Investigation 2015b).

Of these denials, the largest number, 677,016, were based on a history of criminal convictions (Federal Bureau of Investigation 2015b). A significant body of evidence of the increased risk for potential firearm violence exists for this group of prohibited purchasers (American Psychological Association 2013; Swanson et al. 2013). The third and sixth largest numbers of denials, 116,874 and 49,461, were based on history of domestic violence, another category for which research has demonstrated an increased risk of firearm violence (Campbell et al. 2007; Vigdor and Mercy 2006). Research has also demonstrated that restricting access to firearms for this group decreases homicides due to intimate partner violence (Frattaroli and Vernick 2006; Zeoli and Frattaroli 2013).

In contrast, these statistics also indicate that the NICS is not denying firearm access to significant numbers of individuals with mental health prohibitors, regardless of whether these individuals are at increased risk for committing firearm violence. As of July 31, 2015, "adjudicated mental health" was the second largest category of active records in the NICS Index, with 4,087,528 (30%) of the total active records and almost twice as many records as those for a disqualifying criminal history (Federal Bureau of Investigation 2015a). However, only 19,010 firearm purchases were denied between 1998 and mid-2015 on the basis of the adjudicated mental health category, representing only 1.56% of total denials (Federal Bureau of Investigation 2015b). Overall, the adjudicated mental health category ranks eighth of the 12 categories listed, far behind denials based on criminal history or histories of domestic violence. These statistics indicate that 1) the NICS mental health prohibitors are overinclusive and 2) they are ineffective in decreasing firearm violence in regard to persons with mental illness.

As discussed in Chapter 1, "Gun Violence and Serious Mental Illness," the relationship between violence and mental illness is complex (Elbogen and Johnson 2009; Price and Norris 2010). However, most violence, including gun violence, is committed by persons who are *not* mentally ill (Appelbaum 2006), and most persons with mental illness are not violent (McGinty et al. 2014). Studies from the United States and other countries have estimated that no more than 5% of all violent crimes are committed by persons with severe mental illness (American Psychiatric Association 2014; Fazel and Grann 2006).

The fact that the number of denials based on mental health prohibitors makes up so small a percentage of the total number of active records is not surprising and is in fact predictable on the basis of the available research evidence. The few violent crimes committed by persons with mental illness alone, uncomplicated by comorbid substance abuse, typically do not involve guns (American Psychiatric Association 2014), and persons with mental illness are not statistically more likely to own firearms (Ilgen et al. 2008). In contrast, a strong relationship has been demonstrated between substance abuse and violence. Researchers suggest that this relationship is responsible for the increased risk of violent behavior often attributed to people with mental illness, who statistically have higher rates of substance abuse (Van Dorn et al. 2012).

Moreover, the FBI's statistics clearly indicate that the overall effectiveness of the NICS federal background check system has fallen far short of what was originally hoped for and intended in 1998. Of the nearly 214,603,597 firearm background checks conducted between 1998 and mid-2015 (Federal Bureau of Investigation 2015c), a total of 1,222,213 purchases were denied (Federal Bureau of Investigation 2015b), representing only 0.57% of all background checks run. The continuing morbidity and mortality due to firearm violence in the United States—far higher than those of any other comparable country (Masters and Council on Foreign Relations 2012)—demonstrate that NICS alone cannot be relied on to achieve the goal of effectively protecting the American public as a whole from injury or death due to firearms (Price and Norris 2010).

A background check system can only be effective if prohibited persons are unable to access firearms. Multiple and complicated reasons lie behind the failure of the NICS system to live up to expectations, including variable state participation, illegal firearm sales, the gun-show loophole, and so-called straw purchases (whereby someone purchases a firearm and transfers it to someone else to avoid NICS). In addition, NICS is designed to thwart gun acquisition among persons who pose a chronic risk. It is not equipped to address acute, high-risk scenarios, or to remove previously acquired firearms from persons who have recently been deemed dangerous. For example, evidence indicates that acts of firearm suicide are often impulsive (see Chapter 2, "Firearms and Suicide in the United States"). Most states lack a process for the swift, temporary removal of firearms from persons who pose an acute risk for violence or suicide, a fact of significant concern because over one-third of households in the United States contain firearms (Norris et al. 2006; Price and Norris 2008).

Negative press about the NICS system continued after the NICS Improvement Amendments Act of 2007. Many commentators focused on the apparently low rates of mental health reporting to NICS as cause for concern. For example, a widely cited report by the advocacy group Mayors Against Illegal Guns noted that as of October 2011, twenty-four states had each submitted fewer than 100 mental health records to NICS, 17 had submitted fewer than 10 each, and 4 had submitted no records at all (Mayors Against Illegal Guns 2011). As Swanson et al. (2015) noted, "[t]he not-so-implicit message was that states' spotty reporting of mental health records to the background check database is partly to blame for the senseless deaths in mass shootings" (p. 7).

However, the number of persons with mental illness who have been reported to the NICS databases has increased dramatically since 2007, and many states have expanded the scope and definition of persons prohibited by mental illness (Record and Gostin 2012). Researchers report a 700% increase in the number of mental health records in the NICS system between the Virginia Tech shooting in April 2007 and January 31, 2014 (Law Center to Prevent Gun Violence 2013). As noted earlier in this section, at the time of this writing, almost 4.1 million persons have been included in the NICS Index in the adjudicated mental health category (Federal Bureau of Investigation 2015a).

Despite these changes, overall rates of firearm-linked homicide and suicide have not decreased correspondingly (Record and Gostin 2012). "The very small proportion of people with mental illnesses who are inclined to be dangerous often do not seek treatment before they do something harmful" (Swanson et al. 2013, p. 36). Several researchers have noted that the mass shootings that many of the newer laws aim to prevent are statistically rare events and nearly impossible to predict (Swanson et al. 2013, 2015). An analysis of 43 such incidents in the United States between January 2009 and January 2013 suggests that most of the perpetrators would not have been barred through a NICS background check (Mayors Against Illegal Guns 2013).

Finally, the NICS background check system of course cannot work if it is not used. In states with less restrictive firearm laws overall and more permissive attitudes toward gun ownership, background checks are often conducted grudgingly, if at all. As of 2013, nineteen states issued "Brady permits," which allow licensed firearm sellers to waive background checks, and seven of these states do not exclude individuals with mental illness from purchasing firearms (Record and Gostin 2013). Moreover, scholars have characterized background check enforcement as "nearly nonexistent," noting that of 80,000 people caught falsifying applications, authorities prosecuted only 44 (Record and Gostin 2013, p. 1231).

Additional significant loopholes in firearm regulation laws have not been closed, and newer laws discussed in the remainder of this chapter have not addressed other problems in mental health reporting laws.

Efforts to Improve the Background Check System

Federal Initiatives

In January 2013, the White House announced more than 20 executive actions intended to reduce gun violence (U.S. Department of Health and Human Services 2013; The White House 2013), some of which directly addressed the issue of mental health reporting and the NICS database. Spurred in part by a July 2012 U.S. Government Accountability Office report noting that the Health Insurance Portability and Accountability Act (HIPAA) Privacy Rule could pose a barrier to NICS reporting in states that had not enacted laws to facilitate increased mental health reporting for firearm background checks (U.S. Government Accountability Office 2012), two notices of proposed rulemaking were published in the Federal Register on January 7, 2014. The first, issued by the Department of Health and Human Services (Office of Civil Rights), would "modify the [HIPAA] Privacy Rule to expressly permit certain HIPAA covered entities to disclose to [NICS] the identities of individuals who are subject to a Federal 'mental health prohibitor' that disqualifies them from shipping, transporting, possessing, or receiving a firearm" (U.S. Department of Health and Human Services 2014, p. 784).

The second notice, issued by the U.S. Department of Justice, Bureau of Alcohol, Tobacco, Firearms and Explosives (2014), proposed changes that would clarify the definition of who meets criteria under the 1968 Gun Control Act for NICS reporting purposes. One proposed change would expressly indicate that individuals court-ordered to outpatient treatment (such as the perpetrator of the Virginia Tech shootings) do fall under the "committed to a mental institution" definition in federal law. The proposed rule would also introduce several additional changes to the law's implementation by "clarifying" the definition of "mental defective." The notice acknowledged that although the term *mental defective* was outdated, the term had been included in the original statute and thus could not be amended by regulation (Levin 2014). The new regulation defining "mental defective" would include persons found incompetent to stand trial or not guilty by reason of mental disease or defect, lack of mental responsibility, or insanity, as well as persons found guilty but mentally ill. The amendment would also "clarify" that federal, state, local, and military courts are all authorized to declare persons incompetent to stand trial or not guilty by reason of insanity.

Public comment, to be submitted by April 2014, was sought regarding whether the term *committed to a mental institution* should include an involuntary commitment that occurred when the person was under age 18 years. It was proposed that ATF regulations be amended to clarify that the term does indeed include involuntary commitments of persons under age 18 (U.S. Department of Justice, Bureau of Alcohol, Tobacco, Firearms and Explosives 2014). The American

Psychiatric Association submitted a comment opposing any "clarification" that would result in reporting commitments or adjudications of juveniles to the NICS system (American Psychiatric Association 2014).

A number of other bills have been drafted or proposed at the federal level relating to NICS and mental health reporting (see McGinty et al. 2014), including proposals to cut federal funding to states with poor NICS reporting rates (Strengthening Background Checks Act of 2013, H.R. 329 113th Congress, 1st Session), to increase funding to support the removal of firearms from mentally ill prohibited purchasers (Armed Prohibited Persons Act of 2013, H.R. 848 113th Congress, 1st Session), and to implement other interventions to restrict firearm access among those who have sought or received mental health treatment.

State Initiatives

Increased Reporting to NICS

In recent years, many states have passed legislation or introduced bills intended to improve NICS reporting and the background check system. Following the Virginia Tech shooting in 2007 and subsequent mass shootings (e.g., Tucson, Arizona, in 2011; Aurora, Colorado, and Newtown, Connecticut, in 2012), roughly half of all states passed laws to improve NICS reporting (Law Center to Prevent Gun Violence 2013), spurred in part by the NICS Improvement Amendments Act of 2007 (Price and Norris 2010). According to Everytown for Gun Safety (2014), the following were reported to have occurred between 2011 and mid-2014:

- Eighteen states passed new legislation or amended their existing laws regarding reporting (at the time of this writing, 11 states are without reporting laws).
- Mental health records reported to NICS tripled.
- Only 12 states contributed fewer than 100 records to NICS.
- The number of persons with mental illness who are prohibited from purchasing firearms through dealers that use the background check system increased by 65%.

This report described the background check system as "markedly improved" (Everytown for Gun Safety 2014, p. 3).

In Illinois and Connecticut, state law requires specified state agencies to enter into a Memorandum of Understanding (MOU) with the FBI for the purpose of submitting records to the NICS system (Law Center to Prevent Gun Violence 2013). In Illinois, for example, the state police and the state Department of Human Services have MOUs with the FBI, which are essentially written agreements to provide information for the purpose of firearm background checks (Firearm

Owners Identification Card Act of 2014, 430 Ill. Comp. Stat. Ann. 65/3.1[e][2]). Any individual prohibited from purchasing or holding a firearm under federal or Illinois state law is reportable under the MOU. The law also has provisions for protecting the confidentiality and privacy of clinical information about the prohibited purchaser.

As of 2013, over 75% of the states had laws in place mandating the reporting of at least some limited mental health data to NICS or to a state database for background checks in gun purchasing (Law Center to Prevent Gun Violence 2013), and nearly all states had some firearm restrictions laws pertaining to mental illness (Wiehl 2013). An additional handful of states had laws that permit but do not mandate mental health reporting to NICS (Law Center to Prevent Gun Violence 2013). Some states also maintained state-based registries or databases analogous to NICS for the purpose of firearm purchase background checks (Law Center to Prevent Gun Violence 2013).

The scope of the mental health information that must be reported, either to NICS or to a state-run database, varies by state. This area of state law is dynamic: more than 400 *new* firearm regulation bills (proposing either tightening or loosening of restrictions) were introduced during the 2014 legislative session alone (Law Center to Prevent Gun Violence 2014).

Expansion by States of Prohibited Classes

Some states that previously had fairly restricted definitions of persons who must be reported amended their laws or regulations in response to the NICS Improvement Amendments Act of 2007. Prior to 2007, for example, Illinois only required reporting in the case of mental retardation, hospitalization at a mental institution within the past 5 years, or a finding of clear and present danger, and public hospitals were not required to file reports. In 2008, the state passed a law requiring public hospitals and mental health facilities to file reports on any person "who is an outpatient or provided services by a public or private hospital or mental health facility whose mental condition is of such a nature that it is manifested by violent, suicidal, threatening or assaultive behavior or reported behavior, for which there is a reasonable belief by a physician, clinical psychologist, or qualified examiner that the condition poses a clear and present or imminent danger to the patient, any other person or the community" (Illinois Publ. Act No. 095-0564, codified at 740 Ill. Comp. Stat. 110, § 12 [Ch. 91], 2008).

Similarly, Washington State revised its laws to clarify that a 14-day involuntary commitment is sufficient to trigger the obligation to report, whereas previously a patient had to have been involuntarily committed for at least a 90-day period (Petition for Involuntary Treatment or Alternative Treatment: Probable Cause Hearing, Rev. Code Wa. § 71.05.240, 2009).

States have enacted other laws specifying who must be reported, by whom, and how. For example, persons found not guilty by reason of insanity (or some similar language) and persons who have been found to lack competency to stand trial must be reported in approximately half of all states (Law Center to Prevent Gun Violence 2013). These laws echo the original provisions of the Gun Control Act of 1968. Other states, such as Washington (Petition for Involuntary Treatment or Alternative Treatment: Probable Cause Hearing, Rev. Code Wa. § 71.05.240, 2009), have shortened the minimum duration of involuntary hospitalization required before a psychiatric patient falls within the prohibited purchaser class (Price and Norris 2010).

Outpatient Commitment

Several states already authorize or require the reporting (to NICS or to state databases) of persons who have been mandated to receive outpatient mental health treatment. For example, following the Virginia Tech shootings, the governor of Virginia issued an executive order stating that involuntary outpatient treatment should be reported to the state database and to federal law enforcement (Price and Norris 2008). Consequently, in Virginia, persons ordered by a court to outpatient treatment are reported to a state criminal records database, and the names of prohibited purchasers from this database are in turn forwarded to the NICS system (Order of Involuntary Admission or Involuntary Outpatient Treatment Forwarded to CCRE [Virginia], Va. Code Ann. § 37.2–819, 2011).

Voluntary Admission to Psychiatric Hospital

In April 2013, Connecticut passed a law (Publ. Act No. 13-3 [SB 1160], 2013) amending portions of its mental health law to authorize and require the reporting of persons who have been voluntarily admitted to psychiatric hospitals to the state's commissioner of emergency services and public protection, in connection with applications for new or renewed firearm permits or certificates. Formerly, only persons who had been involuntarily committed, pursuant to an order of the probate court, would have been reported to the commissioner. As of July 1, 2013, Connecticut's Department of Mental Health and Addiction Services must now disclose the commitment status, *including* voluntary admissions "to a hospital for persons with psychiatric disabilities" within the past 6 months, of any person seeking renewal or new permits or certificates to carry firearms. The law does not appear to specify whether admission to a partial hospital or day program (as opposed to overnight/inpatient stays) would fall within the definition of a voluntary admission.

Other states have enacted laws with similar provisions. For example, Florida revised its definition of "committed to a mental institution" for purposes of firearm restrictions such that the term now includes the following voluntary patients (Sale and Delivery of Firearms, Fla. Stat. § 790.065 [2][a] 4.b, 2013):

- Those whom a physician found to constitute a danger to self or others
- Those for whom a petition for involuntary commitment would have been filed had the admission not been voluntary
- Those who acknowledged in writing (within a specified format) receipt of a certified finding that he or she might be prohibited from purchasing a firearm
- Those for whom a judge has reviewed the above elements and agreed, ordering the record to be submitted

New York's Secure Ammunition and Firearms Enforcement Act of 2013

One of the most controversial packages of firearm legislation enacted in recent years is New York's Secure Ammunition and Firearms Enforcement (SAFE) Act of 2013 (NY Penal Law §§ 265.00[22]–[23]; 265.45; 400.08[5]–[6]). The SAFE Act was passed rapidly in January 2013, largely in response to the December 2012 mass shooting at Sandy Hook Elementary School in Newtown, Connecticut (Appelbaum 2013; Swanson 2013). As amended in 2013, The Mental Hygiene Laws for New York (Section 9.46) now require mental health professionals to file reports on patients deemed to be "likely to engage in conduct that would result in serious harm." The determination that a patient falls into this "likely" category is made on the basis of "reasonable professional judgment." In addition, the SAFE Act requires reporting of persons who have been found "not guilty by reason of mental disease or defect" or incompetent to stand trial, as well as those who have been subject to involuntary commitment orders.

When a report is made to the Division of Criminal Justice Services (DCJS), the division determines whether the person possesses a firearm license; if so, the DCJS notifies a local licensing official, who is required to suspend or revoke the license "as soon as practicable." The individual who is the subject of the report is then required to surrender the license and all firearms to the licensing officer; if the person fails to comply, law enforcement officers are authorized (but presumably not required) to remove the weapons.

A recent report indicated that between March 16, 2013, when the law went into effect, and October 18, 2014, mental health professionals made almost 43,000 reports of potentially dangerous patients. Of these, the names of approximately 34,500 New York residents categorized as dangerous were entered into the state's database (Hartocollis 2014). However, of the people named in the newly created New York database, fewer than 300 were found to have a gun permit.

The effects of the SAFE Act have not yet been studied to determine its impact, if any, on rates of firearm morbidity and mortality. Nevertheless, from these numbers alone, the database is likely to be significantly overinclusive. The consequences of being officially categorized as potentially dangerous for those already in mental health treatment and for those who might need treatment but are not yet receiving it are also unknown. Nevertheless, consequences, if any, are unlikely to encourage those in need of treatment to seek mental health care. For those already in treatment, the consequences of the breach of confidentiality and of being reported as potentially dangerous are likely to have treatment repercussions.

Temporary Removal of Firearms

Some states, such as California, Indiana, and Connecticut, have enacted laws that allow the temporary removal of firearms from persons deemed to be dangerous (American Psychiatric Association 2014). Connecticut's law (Seizure of Firearms of Persons Posing Risk of Imminent Personal Injury to Self or Others of 2009, 529 Conn. Gen. Stat. § 29-38c) was among the first of its kind, authorizing removal of firearms in a crisis or emergency. It includes provisions for the issuance of a warrant, requirements to establish probable cause and evidence for the judge to consider, a requirement for an affidavit, documentation requirements (including a written inventory of any firearms removed), and provisions for a hearing within 14 days to determine whether the firearms should be returned or held by the state. The American Psychiatric Association (2014) praised the Connecticut law for addressing *dangerousness* rather than mental illness and for providing law enforcement authorities with the necessary authority to implement the law effectively.

In Indiana, a warrant is not required for police to confiscate firearms from an individual if that person is believed to be dangerous ("Dangerous" [Indiana], Ind. Code § 35-47-14, 2013; Parker 2010). Although this law might appear to infringe on persons' rights, Indiana, like Connecticut, requires a hearing to be held within 14 days to determine whether the evidence supports the gun removal or whether the firearms should be returned to the person. Because Indiana's law has been in place since 2005, some data investigating its use are available. Parker (2010) found that the most common reasons for firearm removal were (in order from most to least common) risk of suicide, substance abuse, violence risk, and "domestic disturbance." However, as noted by an investigative report in the *New York Times,* in many cases nothing in Indiana law prevents an individual whose guns were removed from purchasing new firearms (Luo and McIntire 2013).

In Connecticut, in contrast, the law requires gun removal records to be forwarded to the NICS system (Luo and McIntire 2013). Similar to the pattern in Indiana, the most common reasons for gun removal in Connecticut in 2013 were threats of suicide (over 50% of all removals) and substance abuse (34%); mental illness of some kind was noted in 42% of all cases (Luo and McIntire 2013). The latter number may reflect public fears of mental illness rather than objective evidence that an individual is dangerous and likely to be violent (McGinty et al. 2013).

Despite the existence of state laws allowing temporary gun removal, the legislation must be adequately funded to be effective. Removing firearms from persons added to the NICS system or to a similar state database is a costly and resource-intensive endeavor. In California, to address a backlog of cases, a law was passed in late April 2013 granting $24 million to the state's Department of Justice to supply the necessary funds and resources to law enforcement to remove guns from persons listed in the state's Armed Prohibited Persons system (Pinion-Whitt 2013).

Consequences of Legislative Reform Focusing on Persons With Mental Illness

Legislative efforts to reform firearm laws have often faced an uphill struggle because of the political influence of advocacy groups who oppose firearm reform (Goss 2008; Rodríguez Andrés and Hempstead 2011; Swanson et al. 2015). In contrast, bills that specifically focus on individuals with mental illness have received more public support (Barry et al. 2013; McGinty et al. 2014) and government support (U.S. Government Accountability Office 2012), including bipartisan political support (Talev 2014). Nevertheless, the belief that reporting large numbers of persons with mental illness to a massive federal database will result in lower rates of gun-related homicide and suicide has not been supported by empirical studies (Price and Norris 2008; Simpson 2007a).

Negative media representations of isolated incidents of violence committed by persons with mental illness can increase public perceptions of the dangerousness of persons with mental illness in general (McGinty et al. 2013). In a recent survey, 46% of Americans agreed with the statement that people with mental illness, in general, are "far more dangerous than the general population" (Barry et al. 2013). However, the public's fear of persons with mental illness is "generally disproportionate to the actual risk of harm" (Lewis 2011, p. 153). A number of commentators have argued that the broad public support for legislation specifically focusing on individuals with mental illness derives from the media's focus on the mental health of perpetrators of mass shootings, often without evidence to support speculations of mental illness (Appelbaum 2013; Swanson et al. 2015; Wiehl 2013).

Firearm policy focusing on mental illness represents a form of regulation based on public perceptions and beliefs, not facts and data (Gold 2013; Price and Norris 2008; Simpson 2007a). This approach reflects "a deeply irrational public policy" (Appelbaum 2006, p. 1320), especially given the evidence suggesting that current policy is unlikely to succeed in reducing the incidence of firearm violence, including the incidence of mass shootings. One of the most significant consequences of pursuing such policies is that they divert attention from and support for more evidence-based legislative interventions, while creating the mistaken perception that "something is being done" to decrease the morbidity and mortality of firearm violence.

This approach to public firearm policy may have additional unintended but serious consequences. First and foremost, the use of mental health registries as part of efforts to reduce gun violence is discriminatory because such registries utilize categorical exclusions as opposed to individual risk assessments (American Psychiatric Association 2014). The language employed in the statutes often further stigmatizes persons with psychiatric disorders (Swanson et al. 2013). For example, the outdated term *mental defective,* still in use in federal and many state laws, perpetuates a harmful stereotype and has been criticized as "plainly demeaning and offensive" (Norko and Dreisbach 2008, p. 269). Moreover, although access to NICS data is restricted, merely being listed in the database carries stigma. Corrigan et al. (2005) discuss the legal and ethical implications of structural stigma—that is, legislation that further stigmatizes persons with mental illness and restricts their civil liberties.

Some of the other salient problems with many of the recent legislative efforts to reduce gun violence by specifically focusing on persons with mental illness are discussed in the following subsections.

Intrusion Into the Therapist-Patient Relationship and Confidentiality Issues

A reporting mandate like that embodied in New York's SAFE Act requires mental health professionals to act as agents of the state. Commentators have expressed concern that laws such as the SAFE Act will have a chilling effect on treatment seeking and an adverse impact on the therapist-patient relationship (American Psychiatric Association 2009; Appelbaum 2013; Price and Norris 2008; Swanson 2013). Mandatory reporting laws may also make patients reluctant to be forthcoming about their access to guns, making it more difficult for clinicians to identify patients at higher risk of gun violence, especially firearm suicide. In addition, as discussed earlier in this chapter (see "Efforts to Improve the Background Check System"), conflicts with HIPAA have also been identified as significant problems for some of the newer state laws, such as the SAFE Act in New York.

Most states already have laws explicitly granting an exception to therapist-patient confidentiality when a patient is dangerous (Wiehl 2013). As even the U.S. Supreme Court has acknowledged, however, "[e]ffective psychotherapy . . . depends upon an atmosphere of confidence and trust" (*Jaffee v. Redmond*, 518 U.S. 1, 1996). State intrusions into therapist-patient confidentiality can threaten the efficacy of psychotherapy, thereby limiting clinicians' ability to help their patients. Similarly, mental health professionals already have an ethical duty and legal responsibility to take some protective action if they believe a patient is dangerous to self or others, and it is not always necessary for them to breach confidentiality to do so (Swanson 2013).

Additional concerns exist in regard to the privacy of individuals whose names and other identifying information are entered into the NICS as well as state databases. State-based systems may pose even higher risks to psychiatric patients' privacy if the state database contains more detailed information. Data breaches have become a frequent occurrence in recent years, and patients may justifiably worry about who might access their personal information.

Conflicts With Federal Law and Other Due Process Concerns

Prior to the SAFE Act, the removal of the right to possess firearms from those deemed mentally ill typically involved a formal process, such as commitment hearings or a criminal trial. Several legal scholars believe that legislation like the SAFE Act would not survive a challenge on substantive due process grounds (Wiehl 2013).

Tarasoff laws (*Tarasoff v. Regents of the University of California* 1976), which involve granting an exception to therapist-patient confidentiality when a therapist believes that a patient is dangerous to others, typically contain standards limiting disclosures to cases in which the threat or dangerousness is based on evidence, such as a specific threat, imminent danger, or an identifiable victim (Wiehl 2013). The SAFE Act, by contrast, removes these protective standards and even exempts mental health professionals from liability for making reports "in good faith." Thus, individuals who are reported by their therapists lose their gun permits immediately, without any hearing or opportunity to challenge the therapist's judgment before the permit loss becomes effective. If these individuals wish to regain their gun permits, they must then go through a lengthy and tedious process for the restoration of their rights.

No Process or Resources to Address Real Threats

Most of the recent bills and laws are intended to prevent future tragedies like those of the 2012 Sandy Hook shootings. However, many of them do not require or provide for immediate removal of firearms and other weapons from those who pose the greatest danger to others. Few states have an efficient process for the removal of weapons from persons who pose a high acute risk. The gun violence restraining order legislation (Consortium for Risk-Based Firearm Policy 2013b; also see Chapter 12, "Preventing Gun Violence") passed in California in 2014 (Calif. A.B. 1014) is, to date, an exception to this policy trend. At the time of this writing, California's gun violence restraining order legislation has not been put into practice but has the potential for addressing this problem common to most state firearm legislative initiatives.

In addition, in states that do have an immediate removal process, the guns often are returned to the owner with little to no monitoring or assessment to ensure that the individual does not become dangerous again. Even in cases where the weapons are not readily returned, often, as noted above (see "Efforts to Improve the Background Check System"), there is little to prevent the person from purchasing new firearms (Luo and McIntire 2013). More commonly, while the law may prevent certain people from legally purchasing a handgun in the future, it does not ensure that those individuals will not be able to use the guns acquired prior to the individuals' being added to the NICS databases.

A Focus on Persons for Whom No Evidence of Increased Risk of Firearm Violence Exists

When the reporting mandates do narrow the group to be reported, some specify that patients discharged from involuntary hospitalization be reported to NICS. For example, Delaware requires the reporting, upon their release, of persons who have been involuntarily committed (Information to be Supplied by Heads of Institutions, Del. Code Ann., Tit. 11, § 8509, 2014). Discharge from a psychiatric hospital arguably represents a consensus opinion held among the treating medical and other mental health clinicians that the person no longer poses an immediate danger to self or others.

As the American Psychiatric Association has stated, mandated reporting of all involuntary civil commitments is excessively broad and not justified by actuarial risk predictions (American Psychiatric Association 2009). Scant evidence exists to support the assumption that persons with a history of involuntary hospitalization are at a greater risk of perpetrating gun violence (Simpson 2007a). Some patients are hospitalized involuntarily for illnesses that have no demonstrable relationship to gun violence. Many of these patients pose little to no risk to society. "To date, 99% of mental health records in NICS have not resulted in a federal gun denial" (Swanson et al. 2015, p. 7), despite the fact that these constituted 30% of the active records in NICS as of July 31, 2015 (Federal Bureau of Investigation 2015a).

Firearm legislation that emphasizes dangerousness based on identified risk factors for firearm violence rather than placing an emphasis on mental illness is more likely to yield results in terms of decreasing morbidity and mortality. Wright and Wintemute (2014) note that persons convicted of violent misdemeanors are 9–15 times more likely to be arrested for future violent offenses, yet are not restricted from purchasing handguns under federal law. Research has identified a number of such risk factors, including alcohol abuse, drug abuse, conviction for prior violent offenses, and a history of domestic violence (Consortium for Risk-Based Firearm Policy 2013a, 2013b).

Overly Broad and Ineffective Administration

The trend of "crisis-driven" firearm reform legislation (Swanson 2013) in recent years has been toward expanding the class of prohibited purchasers (Norris et al. 2006; Price and Norris 2010). The net cast by some of these laws is so wide that the sheer numbers of persons who will be reported to the NICS or state databases are staggering. For example, as of 2013, the NICS system had mental health records for nearly 14,000 individuals from Connecticut alone (Swanson et al. 2013). Within a system such as that of the SAFE Act, few disincentives to excessive reporting exist, and the New York law as written will encourage overreporting of persons who do not pose a real threat (Hartocollis 2014). This may be especially problematic for persons such as law enforcement and military personnel, whose careers require that they be allowed to carry a firearm (Price and Norris 2010; Simpson 2007b).

Police departments often lack the resources or funding to properly investigate and address numbers of this magnitude (Hall and Friedman 2013). Instead of removing firearms from individuals who actually present a legitimate threat, the net cast by the SAFE Act covers many individuals who pose no actual threat. Many of the proposals fail to consider the lack of funding and resources that police departments and mental health departments charged with compliance with such overbroad mandates will encounter.

Problems NICS Cannot Address

The federal background check system is only required to be used when a purchaser seeks to buy a gun from a licensed gun retailer. Newer laws and proposed legislation fail to address other significant sources of legal and illegal access to guns, such as private sellers, theft, and illegal purchases. The secondary market for firearm sales—that is, transfers by unlicensed private parties, such as people who attend gun shows—accounts for approximately 40% of all firearm sales (Wintemute 2013). Prohibited purchasers and those with criminal intent have ready access to firearms through such sales. Selling a firearm to a prohibited person is illegal only if sellers know or have "reasonable cause to believe" that they are doing so (18 U.S.C. § 922[d]). If sellers do not ask, they do not know. Private party sales account for at least 80% of firearms used in the commission of crimes and are also an important component of firearm trafficking operations (Wintemute 2013a).

The availability of individual firearm components, such as unfinished receivers, is another significant and growing concern. Such components are currently unregulated and can be purchased through gun shops or online (Horwitz 2014). For example, the AR-15, a semiautomatic assault rifle that has been used in several mass shootings, can be assembled from parts purchased on the Internet (Baum 2013). Commentators predict that 3D printing will further increase the public's access to firearms outside federally licensed dealers (Greenberg 2014; Jensen-Haxel 2012). The June 2013 shootings in Santa Monica, California, underscore this growing problem (Horwitz 2014). The 23-year-old shooter had originally tried to purchase a firearm in 2011 but failed the background check (Allen 2013). The gun he used was assembled from individual components that he had purchased from several different sources throughout the country (Evans 2013).

Conclusion

Unfortunately, existing firearm laws will not prevent all prohibited persons from gaining access to firearms. Prohibited persons can still gain access to firearms owned by others and purchase firearms from the secondary market. Although state participation in the federal system has increased over past years, resulting in improved reporting of prohibited persons to NICS, participation remains incomplete. These factors limit the efficacy of using federal firearm laws as the primary tool for decreasing morbidity and mortality of gun violence. They also suggest that using background checks to restrict categories of people assumed, with or without evidence, to be dangerous may not be the best way to improve public safety and decrease the morbidity and mortality associated with firearms.

Multiple factors associated with increased risk of committing firearm violence have been identified through research studies. Although NICS includes some categories of persons with increased risk of dangerousness, individuals with mental illness are not one of those categories. Effective legislation that improves background checks based on evidence of dangerousness, with or without mental illness, and that does not stigmatize individuals with mental illness, as well as legislation that makes background checks comprehensive across all legal firearm sales, is needed to improve the federal background check system. Ultimately, decreasing the personal, family, community, and social tolls of gun violence will require broad-scale changes in public attitudes, social norms (Hemenway 2013), and policy approaches (Swanson et al. 2015), and not only additional legislation.

Suggested Interventions

- Future legislative efforts to improve the NICS system should focus on empirically proven actuarial risk factors rather than unsupported and stigmatizing public fears about mental illness. Recent efforts broadly focusing on persons with mental illness for inclusion in databases for background checks on gun purchases are not likely to have a significant impact on future rates of violent crime. Broadening the definition of *prohibited person* to include outpatients who suffer from mental illness may have the effect of discouraging patients from reporting and receiving treatment for suicidal or violent ideation, thereby undermining the purpose of mental health reporting laws. Instead, Swanson et al. (2015) recommend using epidemiological risk data to inform policy-making regarding guns and mental illness.

- To improve the NICS system and related background check processes in the states, lawmakers would do well to heed the advice of the American Psychiatric Association in their resource documents (American Psychiatric Association 2009, 2013, 2014). For states with mental health registries, the American Psychiatric Association stresses the critical importance of fairness; the focus should not be limited to people with a history of mental illness, but rather broadened to "actuarial risk factors proven to be significant predictors of violence, such as prior episodes of violence, documented incidents of loss of control while intoxicated, and so on" (American Psychiatric Association 2009, p. 2). For example, studies suggest that firearm prohibitions for violent misdemeanants, who are at markedly higher risk for committing future firearm violence, would likely receive broad support from the public, including firearm owners and the National Rifle Association (Barry et al. 2013; Wintemute 2014; Wright and Wintemute 2014). Further evidence-based factors to consider for future legislation (such as reporting substance use disorder records) are discussed in a recent policy paper from the American College of Physicians (Butkus et al. 2014).

- State and federal governments should follow the example of those states that have been recognized by experts for having well-thought-out legislation in the area of NICS and mental health reporting. These government entities should avoid reliance on "crisis-driven" legislation fueled by highly publicized tragedies. Swanson et al. (2013) held Indiana's and California's models as examples for other states to follow. Indiana's law is based on determinations that a person is dangerous, rather than a categorical inclusion of all persons with mental illness, and it contains provisions for immediate removal of firearms to which a person already has access (Parker 2010). Similarly, in California, temporary restraining orders can help to restrict firearm access in acute situations among persons believed to be at increased risk for violent behavior (Gun Violence Restraining Orders, A.B. 1014 [California], Ch. 872 [2013–2014], codified in Title 2 Part 6 of the CA Penal Code and § 8105 of the CA Welfare and Institutions Code, 2014; Mason 2014). The Consortium for

Risk-Based Firearm Policy (2013a, 2013b) also recommended policies that authorize law enforcement professionals to remove firearms from individuals who pose a credible and acute risk for harm. Laws such as those passed in California, Indiana, and Connecticut can provide models for other states to follow. Media-driven legislation proposed or passed in response to a highly publicized event often overlooks potential conflicts with other laws, including citizens' fundamental rights.

- The language of any new legislation pertaining to mental health reporting (to NICS or to other systems) should be very clear regarding conditions under which a person must be reported, can be reported, and should not be reported. Also, in all new legislation, a bill's interaction with (and potential conflicts with) existing state and federal laws should be considered before it is sent to the floor. Mental health clinicians' reluctance to report potentially dangerous patients due to concerns about potential HIPAA violations and the effects of reporting on treatment and the therapeutic alliance underscores the importance of carefully thought-out bills that anticipate potential conflicts with existing laws and clinicians' ethical responsibilities. Similarly, the failure to report patients under outpatient commitment orders demonstrates that the existing law was not clear enough regarding who should and should not be reported to the NICS system. The NICS definition does include a requirement for an *adjudication* of dangerousness, which is an objective measure. This is analogous to specific recommendations for driving restrictions by ophthalmologists, who can base recommendations for driving on a minimum visual acuity and visual field requirement, and by neurologists, who can base recommendations for driving following a neurological seizure on a specific requirement for seizure-free interval. These determinations for ophthalmologists and neurologists are simplified by the existence of objective criteria to guide determinations of which patients must be reported. The laws should provide mental health clinicians with similarly objective guidelines to help them determine whether or not a patient should be reported to NICS. *Tarasoff* statutes, for example, often have very specific definitions, whereas recently proposed or enacted state laws regarding firearms often allow a much broader interpretation.
- Physicians need education and guidance about the requirements of reporting under NICS and the expanded state laws and regulations. Clarity in the wording of the laws is insufficient if physicians and other mental health professionals are not provided with adequate education about how to comply with the laws in their daily

practice. As the scope of mandated reporting shifts to psychiatrists and therapists in outpatient settings, some guidance on who should or should not be reported must be provided. Training on how the clinical assessment of dangerousness should be made consistent with state reporting requirements is needed (Pierson et al. 2014). The American College of Physicians, for example, has noted that "[c]lear guidance should be issued on what mental and substance use records should be submitted to the [NICS]. This should include guidance on parameters for inclusion, exclusion, removal, and appeal" (Butkus et al. 2014, p. 859).

- Firearm legislation is needed that reduces access to certain types of firearms, closes loopholes, and requires safe storage of firearms and ammunition. The strategy of firearm legislation has been to focus on restricting access to firearms for classes of persons considered to be at higher risk of violence to self and others, such as persons with mental illness. Strategies that would decrease accessibility in general have had far less support (McGinty et al. 2013; Price and Norris 2010). Legislation to ban large-capacity magazines in the aftermath of recent high-profile shootings has failed (Barry et al. 2013), as has legislation that would close the gun-show loopholes. The availability of guns from secondary sources reduces the effectiveness of a category-focused approach such as NICS, even if such categories are expanded (Swanson et al. 2015). Similarly, reluctance has been shown to further tightening of safe gun-storage laws. One study, however, suggests that attitudes about gun legislation may be changing (Barry et al. 2013). Public support was high for measures prohibiting certain persons from having guns, enhancing background checks, and instituting greater oversight of gun dealers. Even banning the sale of military-style semiautomatic weapons and large-capacity ammunition magazines was supported by 65% of those surveyed, although gun owners were less supportive of these measures. Overall, 67.2% of survey respondents supported a law requiring firearm owners to lock up guns in the home when not in use and to prevent handling by children and teenagers without adult supervision.

References

Allen J: California shooting rampage death toll rises to five. Reuters, U.S. Edition, June 9, 2013. Available at: http://www.reuters.com/article/2013/06/09/us-usa-shooting-california-idUSBRE95615W20130609. Accessed March 26, 2014.

American Psychiatric Association: Resource Document on Access to Firearms by People With Mental Illness. Arlington, VA, American Psychiatric Association, June 2009

American Psychiatric Association: Resource Document on Firearm Access, Acts of Violence and the Relationship to Mental Illness and Mental Health Services. Arlington, VA, American Psychiatric Association, July 2013. Available at: http://www.psych.org/File%20Library/Learn/Archives/rd2013_Firearms.pdf. Accessed October 8, 2013.

American Psychiatric Association: Resource Document on Access to Firearms by People With Mental Illness. Arlington, VA, American Psychiatric Association, May 2014

American Psychological Association: Gun Violence: Prediction, Prevention, and Policy, 2013. Available at: http://www.apa.org/pubs/info/reports/gun-violence-prevention.aspx. Accessed January 7, 2015.

Anglemyer A, Horvath T, Rutherford G: The accessibility of firearms and risk for suicide and homicide victimization among household members: a systematic review and meta-analysis. Ann Intern Med 160(2):101–110, 2014 24592495

Appelbaum PS: Violence and mental disorders: data and public policy. Am J Psychiatry 163(8):1319–1321, 2006 16877640

Appelbaum PS: Public safety, mental disorders, and guns. JAMA Psychiatry 70(6):565–566, 2013 23553282

Barry CL, McGinty EE, Vernick JS, et al: After Newtown—public opinion on gun policy and mental illness. N Engl J Med 368(12):1077–1081, 2013 23356490

Baum D: How to make your own AR-15: the gun Congress can't ban. Harper's Magazine, June 2013, pp 32–38

Bjelopera JP, Bagalman E, Caldwell SW, et al: Public Mass Shootings in the United States: Selected Implications for Federal Public Health and Safety Policy. Washington, DC, Congressional Research Service, March 18, 2013

Butkus R, Doherty R, Daniel H, et al: Reducing firearm-related injuries and deaths in the United States: executive summary of a policy position paper from the American College of Physicians. Ann Intern Med 160(12):858–860, 2014 24722815

Campbell JC, Glass N, Sharps PW, et al: Intimate partner homicide: review and implications of research and policy. Trauma Violence Abuse 8(3):246–269, 2007 17596343

Centers for Disease Control and Prevention: Firearm homicides and suicides in major metropolitan areas—United States, 2006–2007 and 2009–2010. MMWR Morb Mortal Wkly Rep 62(30):597–602, 2013a 23903593

Centers for Disease Control and Prevention: Injury Prevention and Control: Data and Statistics (WISQARS): Fatal Injury Data. Atlanta, GA, Centers for Disease Control and Prevention, 2013b. Available at: http://www.cdc.gov/injury/wisqars/fatal.html. Accessed February 2, 2013.

Chapman S, Alpers P, Agho K, et al: Australia's 1996 gun law reforms: faster falls in firearm deaths, firearm suicides, and a decade without mass shootings. Inj Prev 12(6):365–372, 2006 17170183

Consortium for Risk-Based Firearm Policy: Guns, Public Health and Mental Illness: An Evidence-Based Approach for Federal Policy. Washington, DC, Consortium for Risk-Based Firearm Policy, December 11, 2013a. Available at: http://www.efsgv.org/wp-content/uploads/2014/10/Final-Federal-Report.pdf. Accessed March 6, 2014.

Consortium for Risk-Based Firearm Policy: Guns, Public Health and Mental Illness: An Evidence-Based Approach for State Policy. Washington, DC, Consortium for Risk-Based Firearm Policy, December 2, 2013b. Available at: http://www.efsgv.org/wp-content/uploads/2014/10/Final-State-Report.pdf. Accessed March 6, 2014.

Corrigan PW, Watson AC, Heyrman ML, et al: Structural stigma in state legislation. Psychiatr Serv 56(5):557–563, 2005 15872164

Dowd M: Death on the L.I.R.R.: The White House; Moved by killings, Clinton urges action on gun legislation. New York Times, New York Region, December 9, 1993. Available at: http://www.nytimes.com/1993/12/09/nyregion/death-lirr-white-house-moved-killings-clinton-urges-action-gun-legislation.html. Accessed May 19, 2014.

Elbogen EB, Johnson SC: The intricate link between violence and mental disorder: results from the National Epidemiologic Survey on Alcohol and Related Conditions. Arch Gen Psychiatry 66(2):152–161, 2009 19188537

Evans C: Santa Monica shooter built his own weapon. CBS News, June 14, 2013. Available at: http://www.cbsnews.com/news/santa-monica-shooter-built-his-own-weapon/. Accessed May 19, 2014.

Everytown for Gun Safety: Closing the Gaps: Strengthening the Background Check System to Keep Guns Away From the Dangerously Mentally Ill. New York, Everytown for Gun Safety, May 22, 2014. Available at: http://everytown.org/article/closing-the-gaps/. Accessed May 28, 2014.

Fazel S, Grann M: The population impact of severe mental illness on violent crime. Am J Psychiatry 163(8):1397–1403, 2006 16877653

Federal Bureau of Investigation: Active records in the NICS Index, July 31, 2015a. Available at: https://www.fbi.gov/about-us/cjis/nics/reports/active_records_in_the_nics-index.pdf. Accessed August 10, 2015.

Federal Bureau of Investigation: Federal denials: reasons why the NICS Section denies, November 30, 1998–July 31, 2015b. Available at: http://www.fbi.gov/about-us/cjis/nics/reports/federal_denials.pdf. Accessed January 7, 2015.

Federal Bureau of Investigation: NICS Firearm background checks: month/year, November 30–July 31, 2015c. Available at: https://www.fbi.gov/about-us/cjis/nics/reports/nics_firearm_checks_-_month_year.pdf. Accessed August 10, 2015.

Fleegler EW, Lee LK, Monuteaux MC, et al: Firearm legislation and firearm-related fatalities in the United States. JAMA Intern Med 173(9):732–740, 2013 23467753

Frattaroli S, Vernick JS: Separating batterers and guns: a review and analysis of gun removal laws in 50 states. Eval Rev 30(3):296–312, 2006 16679498

Gjertsen F, Leenaars A, Vollrath ME: Mixed impact of firearms restrictions on fatal firearm injuries in males: a national observational study. Int J Environ Res Public Health 11(1):487–506, 2014 24380979

Gold LH: Gun violence: psychiatry, risk assessment, and social policy. J Am Acad Psychiatry Law 41(3):337–343, 2013 24051585

Goss K: The Missing Movement for Gun Control in America. Princeton, NJ, Princeton University Press, 2008

Greenberg A: How 3-D printed guns evolved into serious weapons in just one year. Wired, May 15, 2014. Available at: http://www.wired.com/2014/05/3d-printed-guns/. Accessed May 15, 2014.

Hahn RA, Bilukha O, Crosby A, et al: Firearms laws and the reduction of violence: a systematic review. Am J Prev Med 28(2 suppl 1):40–71, 2005 15698747

Hall RCW, Friedman SH: Guns, schools, and mental illness: potential concerns for physicians and mental health professionals. Mayo Clin Proc 88(11):1272–1283, 2013 24138962

Hartocollis A: Mental health issues put 34,500 on New York's no-guns list. New York Times, NY Region, October 19, 2014. Available at: http://www.nytimes.com/2014/10/19/nyregion/mental-reports-put-34500-on-new-yorks-no-guns-list.html. Accessed October 20, 2014.

Hemenway D: Preventing gun violence by changing social norms. JAMA Intern Med 173(13):1167–1168, 2013 23609319

Horwitz S: "Unfinished receivers," a gun part that is sold separately, lets some people get around laws. The Washington Post, National Security, May 13, 2014. Available at: http://www.washingtonpost.com/world/national-security/unfinished-receivers-that-can-be-used-to-build-guns-pose-problems-for-law-enforcement/2014/05/13/8ec39e9e-da51-11e3-bda1-9b46b2066796_story.html. Accessed May 14, 2014.

Ilgen MA, Zivin K, McCammon RJ, et al: Mental illness, previous suicidality, and access to guns in the United States. Psychiatr Serv 59(2):198–200, 2008 18245165

Jensen-Haxel P: 3D printers, obsolete firearm supply controls, and the right to build self-defense weapons under Heller. Gold Gate Univ Law Rev 42(3):447–496, 2012

Law Center to Prevent Gun Violence: Mental Health Reporting Policy Summary. San Francisco, CA, Law Center to Prevent Gun Violence, updated September 16, 2013. Available at: http://smartgunlaws.org/mental-health-reporting-policy-summary/. Accessed February 5, 2014.

Law Center to Prevent Gun Violence: Tracking State Gun Laws: 2014 Developments. San Francisco, CA, Law Center to Prevent Gun Violence, February 3, 2014. Available at: http://smartgunlaws.org/tracking-state-gun-laws-2014-developments/. Accessed February 6, 2014.

Legal Community Against Violence: Regulating Guns in America: An Evaluation and Comparative Analysis of Federal, State and Selected Local Gun Laws. San Francisco, CA, Legal Community Against Violence, February 2008

Levin S: Letter to U.S. Attorney General Eric Holder, Re: Amended Definition of "Adjudicated as a Mental Defective" and "Committed to a Mental Institution." Arlington, VA, American Psychiatric Association, April 7, 2014. Available at: http://www.psychiatry.org/File Library/Advocacy and Newsroom/04-07-2014-APA-Comment_DOJ-HIPAA-NICS--3-.pdf. Accessed May 16, 2014.

Lewis L: Mental illness, propensity for violence, and the Gun Control Act. Houst J Health Law Policy 11:149–174, 2011

Loftin C, McDowall D, Wiersema B, et al: Effects of restrictive licensing of handguns on homicide and suicide in the District of Columbia. N Engl J Med 325(23):1615–1620, 1991 1669841

Ludwig J, Cook PJ: Homicide and suicide rates associated with implementation of the Brady Handgun Violence Prevention Act. JAMA 284(5):585–591, 2000 10918704

Luo M, McIntire M: When the right to bear arms includes the mentally ill (U.S. section). New York Times, December 21, 2013. Available at: http://www.nytimes.com/2013/12/22/us/when-the-right-to-bear-arms-includes-the-mentally-ill.html. Accessed December 24, 2013.

Mason M: Lawmakers seek "gun violence restraining order" after UCSB slayings (Local/Political section). Los Angeles Times, May 27, 2014. Available at: http://www.latimes.com/local/political/la-me-pc-gun-violence-restraining-order-20140527-story.html. Accessed May 28, 2014.

Masters J, Council on Foreign Relations: U.S. gun policy: global comparisons. The Rundown: PBS Newshour, December 21, 2012. Available at: http://www.pbs.org/newshour/rundown/2012/12/gun-policy.html. Accessed January 7, 2015.

Mayors Against Illegal Guns: Fatal Gaps: How Missing Records in the Federal Background Check System Put Guns in the Hands of Killers. New York, Mayors Against Illegal Guns, November 2011

Mayors Against Illegal Guns: Mass Shootings Since January 20, 2009. Survey Report. New York, Mayors Against Illegal Guns, January 2013. Available at: http://www.washingtonpost.com/blogs/wonkblog/files/2013/02/mass_shootings_2009-13_-_jan_29_12pm1.pdf. Accessed August 14, 2015.

McGinty EE, Webster DW, Barry CL: Effects of news media messages about mass shootings on attitudes toward persons with serious mental illness and public support for gun control policies. Am J Psychiatry 170(5):494–501, 2013 23511486

McGinty EE, Webster DW, Barry CL: Gun policy and serious mental illness: priorities for future research and policy. Psychiatr Serv 65(1):50–58, 2014 23852317

Miller M, Barber C, White RA, et al: Firearms and suicide in the United States: is risk independent of underlying suicidal behavior? Am J Epidemiol 178(6):946–955, 2013 23975641

Norko MA, Dreisbach VM: Concerns related to federal gun control legislation. J Am Acad Psychiatry Law 36(2):269–270, 2008 18583705

Norris DM, Price M, Gutheil T, et al: Firearm laws, patients, and the roles of psychiatrists. Am J Psychiatry 163(8):1392–1396, 2006 16877652

Parker GF: Application of a firearm seizure law aimed at dangerous persons: outcomes from the first two years. Psychiatr Serv 61(5):478–482, 2010 20439368

Pierson J, Viera AJ, Barnhouse KK, et al: Physician attitudes and experience with permit applications for concealed weapons. N Engl J Med 370(25):2453–2454, 2014 24941197

Pinion-Whitt M: Governor Brown signs firearms database bill. San Bernardino Sun, April 30, 2013. Available at: http://www.sbsun.com/general-news/20130501/governor-brown-signs-firearms-database-bill. Accessed May 28, 2014.

Price M, Norris DM: National Instant Criminal Background Check Improvement Act: implications for persons with mental illness. J Am Acad Psychiatry Law 36(1):123–130, 2008 18354133

Price M, Norris DM: Firearm laws: a primer for psychiatrists. Harv Rev Psychiatry 18(6):326–335, 2010 21080771

Record KL, Gostin LO: A robust individual right to bear arms versus the public's health: the court's reliance on firearm restrictions on the mentally ill. Charleston Law Review 6(2):371–384, 2012

Record KL, Gostin LO: A systematic plan for firearms law reform. JAMA 309(12):1231–1232, 2013 23392297

Reisch T, Steffen T, Habenstein A, et al: Change in suicide rates in Switzerland before and after firearm restriction resulting from the 2003 "Army XXI" reform. Am J Psychiatry 170(9):977–984, 2013 23897090

Rodríguez Andrés A, Hempstead K: Gun control and suicide: the impact of state firearm regulations in the United States, 1995–2004. Health Policy 101(1):95–103, 2011 21044804

Safavi A, Rhee P, Pandit V, et al: Children are safer in states with strict firearm laws: a National Inpatient Sample study. J Trauma Acute Care Surg 76(1):146–150, discussion 150–151, 2014 24368370

Simpson JR: Bad risk? An overview of laws prohibiting possession of firearms by individuals with a history of treatment for mental illness. J Am Acad Psychiatry Law 35(3):330–338, 2007a 17872555

Simpson JR: Issues related to possession of firearms by individuals with mental illness: an overview using California as an example. J Psychiatr Pract 13(2):109–114, 2007b 17414687

Swanson J: Mental illness and new gun law reforms: the promise and peril of crisis-driven policy. JAMA 309(12):1233–1234, 2013 23392291

Swanson JW, Robertson AG, Frisman LK, et al: Preventing gun violence involving people with serious mental illness, in Reducing Gun Violence in America: Informing Policy With Evidence and Analysis. Edited by Webster DW, Vernick JS. Baltimore, MD, Johns Hopkins University Press, 2013, pp 33–51

Swanson JW, McGinty EE, Fazel S, et al: Mental illness and reduction of gun violence and suicide: bringing epidemiologic research to policy. Ann Epidemiol 25(5):366–376, 2015 24861430

Talev M: Obama seeks tighter mental health restrictions on guns. Bloomberg, January 4, 2014. Available at: http://www.bloomberg.com/news/articles/2014-01-03/obama-seeks-tighter-mental-health-restrictions-on-guns. Accessed January 8, 2014.

Tarasoff v Regents of the University of California, 17 Cal3d 425, 131 CalRptr 14, 551 P2d 334 (1976)

U.S. Department of Health and Human Services: HIPAA Privacy Rule and the National Instant Criminal Background Check System (NICS): advance notice of proposed rulemaking. Fed Regist 78(78):23872–23876, 2013

U.S. Department of Health and Human Services: Health Insurance Portability and Accountability Act (HIPAA) Privacy Rule and the National Instant Criminal Background Check System (NICS): notice of proposed rulemaking. 45 CFR Part 164. Fed Regist 79(4):784–796, 2014

U.S. Department of Justice, Bureau of Alcohol, Tobacco, Firearms and Explosives: Amended definition of "adjudicated as a mental defective" and "committed to a mental institution" (2010R-21P): notice of proposed rulemaking. 27 CFR Part 478. Fed Regist 79(4):774–777, 2014

U.S. Government Accountability Office: Gun Control: Sharing Promising Practices and Assessing Incentives Could Better Position Justice to Assist States in Providing Records for Background Checks. Report to Congressional Requesters, GAO-12-684. Washington, DC, U.S. Government Accountability Office, July 2012

Van Dorn R, Volavka J, Johnson N: Mental disorder and violence: is there a relationship beyond substance use? Soc Psychiatry Psychiatr Epidemiol 47(3):487–503, 2012 21359532

Vigdor ER, Mercy JA: Do laws restricting access to firearms by domestic violence offenders prevent intimate partner homicide? Eval Rev 30(3):313–346, 2006 16679499

Vyrostek SB, Annest JL, Ryan GW: Surveillance for fatal and nonfatal injuries—United States, 2001. MMWR Surveill Summ 53(7):1–57, 2004 15343143

Webster DW, Wintemute GJ: Effects of policies designed to keep firearms from high risk individuals. Annu Rev Public Health 36:21–37, 2015

The White House: Now Is the Time: The President's Plan to Protect Our Children and Our Communities by Reducing Gun Violence. Washington, DC, The White House, January 16, 2013. Available at: http://www.whitehouse.gov/sites/default/files/docs/wh_now_is_the_time_full.pdf. Accessed May 19, 2014.

Wiehl T: The presumption of dangerousness: how New York's SAFE Act reflects our irrational fear of mental illness. Seton Hall Legis J 38(1):35–69, 2013

Wintemute GJ: Comprehensive background checks for firearm sales, in Reducing Gun Violence in America: Informing Policy With Evidence and Analysis. Edited by Webster DW, Vernick JS. Baltimore, MD, Johns Hopkins University Press, 2013a, pp 95–107

Wintemute GJ: Responding to the crisis of firearm violence in the United States: comment on "Firearm legislation and firearm-related fatalities in the United States." JAMA Intern Med 173(9):740–742, 2013b 23467768

Wintemute GJ: Support for a comprehensive background check requirement and expanded denial criteria for firearm transfers: findings from the Firearms Licensee Survey. J Urban Health 91(2):303–319, 2014 24203524

Wright MA, Wintemute GJ: Firearm prohibition for persons convicted of violent crimes: a potential non-legislative approach. Am J Prev Med 47(2):e3–e5, 2014 24923863

Zeoli AM, Frattaroli S: Evidence for optimism: policies to limit batterers' access to guns, in Reducing Gun Violence in America: Informing Policy With Evidence and Analysis. Edited by Webster DW, Vernick JS. Baltimore, MD, Johns Hopkins University Press, 2013, pp 53–63

7

Mental Illness, Dangerousness, and Involuntary Commitment

Eric Y. Drogin, J.D., Ph.D., ABPP (Forensic)
Carol Spaderna, L.L.B. (Hons.)

Common Misperceptions

☒ Most people with serious mental illness can be committed involuntarily without difficulty.

☒ The federal government and the states provide adequate acute inpatient hospital beds and other treatment resources for involuntarily committed individuals.

☒ After discharge, people who have been involuntarily committed are easily able to continue accessing mental health services.

Evidence-Based Facts

☑ Commitment criteria are in fact very narrowly defined, and many people with serious mental illness do not meet these criteria even when in obvious need of treatment.

☑ The federal government and the states do not provide adequate numbers of acute inpatient hospital beds and other treatment resources for involuntarily committed individuals.

☑ People who have been involuntarily committed often find it very difficult to continue accessing mental health services after discharge.

When we as a society periodically revisit the topic of gun violence, the ensuing discussion "is often precipitated by horrific but sensational mass shootings and focused on preventing individuals with severe mental illness from committing such crimes" (Gold 2013, p. 337). Once we reach the conclusion that gun violence and mental illness are prominently and inextricably intertwined—although, as discussed in preceding chapters of this volume, the most up-to-date social scientific evidence characterizes this notion as misinformed at best—we then attempt to determine who should be tasked with "solving" the problem.

Perhaps, we reason, prevention of such crimes should be the responsibility of the lawmakers. Can our elected representatives reform the gun laws, with reference to recently enhanced risk assessment strategies and techniques? Is the answer, for example, a statutory process enabling temporary gun removal at times of high risk (Frattaroli and Vernick 2006), such as the law recently passed in California (Gun Violence Restraining Orders, A.B. 1014, 2014; also see Chapter 12, "Preventing Gun Violence"), followed by the implementation of a carefully considered, clinically informed, and stepwise scheme for the restoration of gun rights (Nichols 2006; see also Chapter 13, "'Relief From Disabilities': Firearm Rights Restoration for Persons Under Mental Health Prohibitions")?

Legal interventions to decrease morbidity and mortality from gun violence by persons with or without mental illness have been difficult to enact, because of in large part what social scientists have termed an entrenched "gun culture" in the United States (Brown et al. 2014; Cooke and Puddifoot 2000). Our gun culture is legally protected by the Second Amendment of the Bill of Rights and is promoted socially and politically by powerful advocacy groups. These forces have often proved so resistant to reform of firearm laws (see, e.g., Draper 2014) that a decrease in the number of firearm deaths and injuries cannot be expected from a purely "legal" solution to the problem of gun violence.

One common response to the political, social, and legal forces arrayed against firearm reform focused on the guns themselves is to shift focus to the laws regarding persons with mental illness and the mental health professionals who treat them. Mental health professionals can be exhorted to function as effectively as possible within the existing framework, employing the best evidence-based techniques for risk assessment and clinical management, as discussed in Chapter 9, "Structured Violence Risk Assessment," and Chapter 10, "Decreasing Suicide

Mortality." If mental health professionals determine that someone with serious mental illness may become dangerous but is unwilling to seek treatment, then perhaps the process of involuntary psychiatric commitment could be invoked, confining the individual against his or her wishes to a psychiatric hospital in order to provide treatment and to keep the public safe. Perhaps, as discussed in Chapter 11, "Treatment Engagement, Access to Services, and Civil Commitment Reform," it might be possible to reform criteria for involuntary civil commitment to include a "need-for-treatment criterion" to prevent an individual with serious mental illness from decompensating and perhaps becoming dangerous to self or others.

In matters of potential gun violence, is it worth considering whether "prediction" is a realizable or even appropriate goal (American Psychological Association 2013)? As discussed throughout this volume, the relationship between serious mental illness, violence in general, and gun violence in particular is complex. Although many people believe that individuals with mental illness are dangerous to others, those with serious mental illness are responsible for only about 5% of all reported violent behavior—and a significantly smaller percentage of gun violence toward others (see Chapter 1, "Gun Violence and Serious Mental Illness"). In contrast, approximately 90%–95% of all individuals who commit suicide have a diagnosable mental illness, and more than half of all suicides in the United States are committed using firearms (see Chapter 2, "Firearms and Suicide in the United States").

Nevertheless, let us assume for the sake of this discussion that certain widely held misperceptions, such as those listed at the beginning of this and other chapters, are true: that individuals with serious mental illness are inherently more dangerous to others and more likely to commit gun violence than people without mental illness. Against this backdrop, the present chapter addresses the current status and implications of the core legal concepts of mental illness, dangerousness, and involuntary commitment in the context of gun violence, both separate from and in conjunction with lack of access to mental health treatment (which is discussed more fully in Chapter 8, "Accessing Mental Health Care").

Why does the law not allow our society to treat persons who refuse treatment until they have met commitment criteria? Why is it so legally difficult to commit individuals at high risk of violent behavior before they become actually, demonstrably, "imminently" dangerous to themselves or others? To what extent is the evolving legal concept of outpatient commitment (also known as assisted outpatient treatment) a viable option in these cases? Laypersons and professionals alike are often hampered in their understanding of these issues by the common misperceptions listed at the beginning of this chapter. The following discussion addresses these misperceptions and the data supporting the corresponding facts.

Involuntary Civil Commitment for Purposes of Mental Health Treatment

Legal Issues

The factors that inform and drive regulation of involuntary civil commitment differ significantly from those typically understood by the general public and the media, as the facts corresponding to the commonly held misperceptions listed above indicate. Each state has its own statutory regulations governing involuntary civil commitment (a review of the commitment statutes of all 50 states and the District of Columbia is available at the Web site of the Mental Illness Policy Organization [2011]).

Regardless of jurisdiction, involuntary psychiatric commitment criteria are in fact extremely narrow. For these criteria to be met, individuals must be found to be both mentally ill and dangerous to themselves or others. The mere need for treatment is not a sufficient criterion, in and of itself, for the deprivation of an individual's liberty that results from compelled hospitalization. The great majority of persons with serious mental illness fail to meet the dangerousness criteria even when in obvious need of clinical treatment. Moreover, both inpatient and outpatient mental health treatment resources are scarce, even when individuals with serious mental illness do meet commitment criteria (as discussed in Chapter 8), often resulting in inadequate treatment or denial of care even for those under a court order.

Civil Versus Criminal Psychiatric Commitment

The *civil* manifestation of involuntary commitment must be understood to differ legally from forms of confinement or other restrictions of liberty that are associated with criminal offenses or are styled as a punishment for criminal offenses. This distinction is emphasized in *Black's Law Dictionary* (Garner 2014), which specifies that such civil proceedings involve "a court-ordered commitment of a person who is ill, incompetent, drug-addicted, or the like, as contrasted with a criminal sentence" (p. 299), with the further observation that unlike a criminal confinement (also referred to at times as "commitment") to a correctional institution, the length of a civil commitment is indefinite because it depends on the person's recovery (p. 299).

However, indefinite commitment to a psychiatric hospital does occasionally occur as a *by-product* of criminal proceedings in three distinct contexts. First, defendants may be committed for mental health treatment during the pendency of a criminal case, so that they might attain competency to stand trial (Samuel and Michals 2011). Second, the postconviction disposition of persons found not guilty by reason of insanity or the posthearing disposition of those found irretrievably incompetent to stand trial may result, in some jurisdictions, in an automatic commitment to a mental hospital or in proceedings for such commitment (Mrad and Nabors 2007). The third, and often most controversial, circumstance that may give rise to civil commitment is occasioned by the perceived mental condition and potential continued dangerousness of individuals who have served their criminal sentences and are therefore deemed to be in need of inpatient psychiatric services (Metzner and Dvoskin 2010). These types of involuntary commitment may also be indefinite, because such individuals typically cannot be held unless they are both mentally ill and dangerous (*Foucha v. Louisiana,* 504 U.S. 71, 1992), and this finding is not based on the amount of time confined.

Involuntary Civil Commitment Criteria: The Legal Background

The focus in this section is on purely civil psychiatric commitments—that is, those that occur in the absence of a serious criminal offense. Each state has its own regulations governing these procedures, but all civil commitment processes share common elements. Civil commitment issues typically arise when an individual has demonstrated behavior that has raised the concern of family members, the community, or often the police. For example, an acutely psychotic individual swearing and shouting at passersby in a public place might be detained by the police, brought to a local hospital emergency room, and deemed to be potentially violent. Similarly, a severely depressed woman who expresses suicidal thoughts to her husband might be brought to a mental health treatment provider, who may become concerned that the risk of suicide is high enough to warrant immediate treatment.

Competence to Consent to Voluntary Treatment

Acutely ill individuals, such as those just described, are first offered the option of voluntary treatment, and this option is offered repeatedly throughout any involuntary detention and commitment process. However, a person who agrees to a voluntary admission must be competent to provide valid consent. If not, as the Supreme Court ruled in *Zinermon v. Burch* (494 U.S. 113, 1990), the person is entitled to the due process and protection of liberty interests provided by an involuntary commitment hearing.

Darrell Burch, appearing hurt and disoriented, was found wandering along a Florida highway. He was taken to a private mental health care facility, where he was described on arrival as "hallucinating, confused, and psychotic" (p. 118). Burch was diagnosed with paranoid schizophrenia. He signed forms consenting to admission and treatment and was given psychotropic medication. Three days later, when transferred to a state psychiatric hospital, Burch again signed forms consenting to admission and treatment. Doctors there described Burch on admission as "disoriented, semi-mute, confused and bizarre in appearance and thought," "not cooperative to the initial interview," and "extremely psychotic," and they observed that he "appeared to be paranoid and hallucinating" (pp. 119–120).

Burch later alleged that he was deprived of his liberty without due process of law when he was admitted as a "voluntary" mental patient because he was in fact incompetent to give informed consent to his admission. After a series of appeals, the Supreme Court held that in providing by law that a mental patient must give informed consent to hospitalization but then failing to make provision for the patient's competence to be examined at admission, Florida predictably violated the patient's rights. Justice Blackmun, writing for the five-to-four majority opinion, stated that Burch was "deprived of a substantial liberty interest without either valid consent or an involuntary placement hearing, by the very state officials charged with the power to deprive mental patients of their liberty and the duty to implement procedural safeguards" (p. 1380). Justice Blackmun further noted that "such a deprivation is foreseeable, due to the nature of mental illness, and will occur, if at all, at a predictable point in the admission process" (p. 139). The Court ruled that Florida's established procedure for involuntary placement needed to be applied "both to those patients who are unwilling and to those who are unable to give consent" (p. 114).

Therefore, individuals with acute mental illness who are offered and agree voluntarily to inpatient admission and treatment must be competent to do so. Under circumstances in which individuals either are not competent to consent to admission and treatment or refuse treatment despite indications that they might require treatment due to family, community, or police concerns that they might be dangerous, medical or mental health professionals contact authorities to begin the process of detaining acutely ill individuals. This process is undertaken in order to provide treatment and to keep both the persons and the community safe.

Involuntary Civil Commitment: The Legal Background

Some clinicians still practicing today can recall when the process for admitting persons to a psychiatric hospital against their will was a more medically based and legally straightforward undertaking. Until the mid-1960s, most states required only the presence of mental illness and a need for treatment to involuntarily commit a patient to a state mental hospital. In the wake of the civil rights movement of the 1960s and 1970s, activists and legal scholars began to look at the constitutional issues of due process and equal protection for groups that lacked the political strength to protect their own interests, including individuals with mental illness (Appelbaum 1994).

Legal trends began to favor a more libertarian approach to government intervention. A series of judicial decisions and legislative changes, combined with arguments regarding the benefits of community mental health treatment and the poor conditions in many state institutions, supported restricting the scope of commitment laws (Appelbaum 1994; Dain 1980; Lamb 2000; Schwartz et al. 2003). These legal changes also provided a framework that supported and further incentivized the already accelerating process of deinstitutionalization of patients with mental illness, as discussed in Chapter 8.

Four decades of progressive judicial and legislative innovation have resulted in case law and statutes that have vastly changed the process of compelling mental health treatment from a process based on mental health needs to one based on protection of legal rights. By the end of the 1970s, individuals with mental illness could not be involuntarily committed to a psychiatric hospital in any state absent a judicial or semi-judicial hearing in which they were found to be both mentally ill and dangerous to themselves or others (Appelbaum 1994). The need for treatment as a rationale for involuntary commitment did not entirely disappear but became more narrowly and strictly applied (Appelbaum and Gutheil 2007).

Many mental health professionals and patient advocates welcomed the increased autonomy and dignity these changes brought to individuals with mental illness. The strengthening of individuals' rights to autonomy decreased many abuses that had been associated with involuntary hospitalization. Nevertheless, the strict legal limitations on the involuntary commitment of individuals with severe mental illness have been a mixed blessing for those with such disorders. On the one hand, their civil liberties are unquestionably better protected. On the other hand, these limits have increased the difficulty of accessing mental health treatment for individuals who may desperately need it. Many clinicians have subscribed to the class notion that their patients are "dying with their rights on," a phrase coined in 1974 (see Appelbaum 1994, p. 30).

Involuntary Civil Commitment Procedures

Although involuntary civil commitment statutes and requirements vary from state to state, most share common legal and procedural elements. Civil commitment procedures typically begin with a temporary and statutorily time-limited detention in a mental health facility, followed by a hearing to determine whether the individual meets criteria for longer-term civil commitment in a psychiatric hospital, with subsequent periodic inpatient assessment for continuing need for involuntary detention. As discussed in several previous chapters, under federal law, individuals who have been involuntarily committed to a psychiatric institution are prohibited from purchasing or possessing firearms.

Commitment hearings are conducted by a judge or other court official, such as a magistrate, and require testimony and/or other evidence that a detained individual meets the state's criteria for involuntary commitment. The detained person has certain rights throughout this process, such as the right to be present at the hearing and the right to representation. Following is a brief review of some of the case law in this area, by which we can track the courts' evolving reasoning that has narrowed the circumstances and procedures required to involuntarily treat even those with acute psychiatric symptoms.

Due Process

Lessard v. Schmidt (349 F. Supp. 1078 [E.D. Wis.], 1972) involved the case of Alberta Lessard, who was apprehended by two police officers in front of her Wisconsin home and involuntarily committed to a Milwaukee hospital on the basis of an alleged diagnosis of schizophrenia. The nature of Lessard's ordeal is captured in the list of due process violations alleged in her subsequent class action lawsuit, wherein the Wisconsin commitment statute was found wanting for the following reasons:

> [I]n permitting involuntary detention for a possible maximum period of 145 days without benefit of hearing on the necessity of detention; in failing to make adequate notice of all hearings mandatory; in failing to give adequate and timely notice where notice is given; in failing to provide for mandatory notice of right to trial by jury; in failing to give a right to counsel or appointment of counsel at a meaningful time; in failing to permit counsel to be present at psychiatric interviews; in failing to provide for exclusion of hearsay evidence and for the privilege against self-incrimination; in failing to provide access to an independent psychiatric examination by a physician of the mentally ill person's choice; in permitting commitment of a person without a determination that the person is in need of commitment beyond a reasonable doubt; and in failing to describe the standard for commitment so that persons may be able to ascertain the standard of conduct under which they may be detained with reasonable certainty. (p. 1082)

Lessard was not heard or decided by the U.S. Supreme Court; in fact, this case was conducted at the lowest level of the federal trial system. Nonetheless, this decision was highly influential and lives on, in some fashion or another, in the statutory requirements of nearly every state jurisdiction in the country (Bloom 2004; Werth 2001). As a result, respondents facing commitment for mental health issues allegedly relevant to potential gun violence or for any other reason are typically afforded—among other codified rights—legal counsel, monitoring of any potentially adverse psychiatric examination, and the right to procure a psychiatric examination of their own.

Least Restrictive Alternative

In addition to specifying the nature of due process in an involuntary commitment procedure, the *Lessard* court specified that the imposition of some form of treatment was not a binary determination, consisting of either being consigned to a psychiatric facility or being discharged to the community scot-free:

> [P]ersons suffering from the condition of being mentally ill, but who are not alleged to have committed any crime, cannot be totally deprived of their liberty if there are less drastic means for achieving the same goal.... We believe that the person recommending full-time involuntary hospitalization must bear the burden of proving (1) what alternatives are available; (2) what alternatives were investigated; and (3) why the investigated alternatives were not deemed suitable. These alternatives included voluntary or court-ordered outpatient treatment, day treatment in a hospital, night treatment in a hospital, placement in the custody of a friend or relative, placement in a nursing home, referral to a community mental health clinic, and home health aide service. (p. 1096)

Under this scheme, depending on state firearm prohibition statutes and the compelled treatment option ultimately chosen, a respondent with serious mental illness for whom gun violence is alleged to be an issue could well enjoy continued access to firearms. Unless state law expressly prohibits firearm purchase or possession for persons involuntarily committed to outpatient treatment, otherwise known as assisted outpatient treatment, individuals under such orders may not be legally barred from access to firearms. For example, as has been widely publicized, the shooter in the 2007 Virginia Tech incident had been placed under an outpatient commitment order but was still able to legally purchase the firearms with which he committed the mass shootings that killed 32 people and wounded 17 more before he committed suicide (Bonnie et al. 2009). The growing emphasis among mental health service providers on outpatient commitment and community-based deterrents to gun violence (Farberman 2014; Miller 2014) does not address the fact that state law and outpatient treatment may not include a primary focus on even temporarily limiting access to firearms.

The Burden and Standard of Proof

The petitioner bears the burden of proof in commitment hearings. Depending on the state, the petitioner may be a prosecutor or a representative of the state mental health authority or other state agency. The petitioner must demonstrate that the temporarily detained individual suffers from a mental illness and as a result of that mental illness is dangerous to self or others. Some states' involuntary commitment statutes also include a criterion for mental illness and "grave disability," or a similar term. This criterion is generally interpreted to mean that as a result of mental illness, the individual may be in danger of dying due to inability to provide for basic necessities. An example might be a homeless person with mental illness who refuses to use a shelter and is in danger of dying from hypothermia.

A standard of "clear and convincing" evidence is typically required for an order of involuntary civil commitment. In *Addington v. Texas* (441 U.S. 584, 1979), pursuant to a petition by his mother, Frank Addington was confined to a state mental hospital after trial court jury members were told that they must base such a decision on "clear, unequivocal, and convincing evidence" (p. 418). In the 6-day trial, evidence had surfaced that Addington had recently been arrested for assaulting his mother, already had a lengthy mental hospitalization history, and had been found in need of confinement by a county psychiatric examiner.

Over the course of numerous appeals, Addington's attorneys had argued that a jury in such cases should be convinced "beyond a reasonable doubt" of the appropriateness of forced hospitalization. Ultimately, the U.S. Supreme Court held that "'a clear and convincing' standard of proof is required by the Fourteenth Amendment in a civil proceeding brought under state law to commit an individual involuntarily for an indefinite period to a state mental hospital." The Court held that "the reasonable-doubt standard is inappropriate in civil commitment proceedings because, given the uncertainties of psychiatric diagnosis, it may impose a burden the state cannot meet and thereby erect an unreasonable barrier to needed medical treatment" (p. 418). More recently, in *United States v. Comstock* (560 U.S. 126, 2010), the Supreme Court opined that the "clear and convincing standard" was sufficient for *federal* court involuntary civil commitment matters as well.

Although not as high a burden of proof as the "beyond a reasonable doubt" standard, the "clear and convincing" standard, where applicable, is still considerably more daunting than the "preponderance of the evidence" standard utilized in nearly every other form of civil proceeding (Taruffo 2003). If the judge finds that the individual meets the state's commitment criteria, the detained individual is then admitted involuntarily to a state psychiatric hospital or, much less frequently, placed under an outpatient treatment commitment order. If the judge finds that the individual does not meet the state's involuntary commitment criteria, the individual is free to leave the hearing without further intervention.

Intellectual Disability and Involuntary Commitment

The U.S. Supreme Court has also opined on the nature of specialized involuntary commitment standards for persons with "intellectual disability," formerly referred to as "mental retardation" (American Psychiatric Association 2013; Lifshitz-Vahav and Vakil 2014; Sappok et al. 2014). Paired concerns of gun violence and intellectual disability, as opposed to more typically cited diagnoses such as bipolar disorder or schizophrenia, may arise more often than many might think. Persons diagnosed with an intellectual disability make up "2% to 3% of the general population" but account for "4% to 10% of the prison population" (Petersilia 2000, p. 8). American studies from the late 1980s had previously suggested a prison population prevalence between 1% and 2% (Fazel et al. 2008).

Increasingly, mandatory reporting requirements for mental health professionals in cases of alleged patient or client dangerousness specifically include persons with intellectual or developmental disabilities who are believed to possess firearms (e.g., the Illinois Firearms Ownership Identification Card Act of 2013, 430 ILCS 65/1). McCreary (2011) advocated that with respect to gun violence regulation concerning persons with psychosis and other forms of major mental illness, "we should have the same laws regarding persons with intellectual disabilities" (p. 302).

Heller v. Doe (509 U.S. 312, 1993) resulted from a class action suit brought on behalf of intellectually disabled citizens of the Commonwealth of Kentucky who were involuntarily civilly committed. In 1990, Kentucky's revised involuntary commitment statutes specified that for persons with mental illness, the standard of proof was "beyond a reasonable doubt," but for persons with intellectual disability, the standard was "clear and convincing evidence." The class action argued, inter alia, that "the differences in treatment between the mentally retarded and the mentally ill—the different standards of proof and the right of immediate family members and guardians to participate as parties in commitment proceedings for the mentally retarded but not the mentally ill—violated the Equal Protection Clause's prohibition of distinctions that lack a rational basis, and that participation by family members and guardians violated the Due Process Clause" (p. 318).

The emphasis in this case on "family" certainly comports with the prevailing clinical understanding that "the family context is an important influence on the development and continuing" of aggressive behaviors and behavioral propensities that specifically include "risk for gun violence" in general (Williamson et al. 2014, p. 90). When in *Heller* the District Court for the Western District of Kentucky granted summary judgment in favor of these arguments, the U.S. Supreme Court agreed to hear the case in response to the Commonwealth of Kentucky's petition for certiorari. Reversing the lower court's decision, the Supreme Court, per Justice Kennedy, noted:

> Kentucky argues that a lower standard of proof in commitments for mental retardation follows from the fact that mental retardation is easier to diagnose than is mental illness. That general proposition should cause little surprise, for mental retardation is a developmental disability that becomes apparent before adulthood. . . . Mental illness, on the other hand, may be sudden and may not occur, or at least manifest itself, until adulthood.... If diagnosis is more difficult in cases of mental illness than in instances of mental retardation, a higher burden of proof for the former tends to equalize the risks of an erroneous determination that the subject of a commitment proceeding has the condition in question. (pp. 321–322)

The primary impact of this decision is that in those states that exceed the minimal *Addington* burden of proof requirement by mandating a "beyond a reasonable doubt" standard for involuntary civil commitments in general, it is nonetheless permissible for those jurisdictions to institute a lower standard of "clear and convincing evidence" in those proceedings in which the focus is intellectual disability instead of mental illness.

Commitment Criteria

In addition to establishing the requirements for due process and defining the standard of proof for civil commitment, courts have also defined the criteria that justify the involuntary deprivation of liberty for an individual with mental illness. In the case of *O'Connor v. Donaldson* (422 U.S. 563, 1975), Kenneth Donaldson, who was diagnosed with schizophrenia, had been committed to a state psychiatric hospital in Florida in 1957 after being told by a judge that he would be hospitalized for a few weeks. Donaldson was held for 15 years. He filed a lawsuit against the hospital, claiming that his constitutional rights had been violated because he had been confined against his will. Donaldson won his case (including monetary damages) in U.S. District Court as well as the appeals, and in 1975, the U.S. Supreme Court upheld the lower court rulings.

The Supreme Court unanimously held that a finding of "mental illness" alone cannot justify a state's indefinite involuntary commitment for provision of simple custodial confinement. The court ruled that although state law may have authorized confinement of the harmless mentally ill, mental illness alone does not itself establish a constitutionally adequate purpose for the confinement. Nor was it enough that Donaldson's original confinement was founded upon a constitutionally adequate basis, if in fact it was, because the court found no constitutional basis for confining such persons involuntarily if they are dangerous to no one and can live safely in freedom.

Justice Stewart, in writing the U.S. Supreme Court's decision, dispensed with any notion that a state might confine persons with mental illness based on "a finding of 'mental illness' alone," or "merely to ensure them a living standard superior to that they enjoy in the private community," or "solely to save its citizens from exposure to those whose ways are different" (p. 575). Justice Stewart concluded, "In short, a State cannot constitutionally confine without more a nondangerous individual who is capable of surviving safely in freedom by himself or with the help of willing and responsible family members or friends. Since the jury found, upon ample evidence, that O'Connor [the hospital superintendent], as an agent of the State, knowingly did so confine Donaldson, it properly concluded that O'Connor violated Donaldson's constitutional right to freedom" (p. 576).

Right to Treatment

Another issue relevant to an understanding of the challenges of involuntary civil commitment is that of "right to treatment." In the 1960s, Morton Birnbaum, a lawyer and a physician, first proposed that individuals involuntarily committed to psychiatric hospitals had a right to treatment (Birnbaum 1960, 1965). Although in *O'Connor v. Donaldson* (422 U.S. 563, 1975), the U.S. Supreme Court wound up steering clear of the issue, *Donaldson v. O'Connor* (493 F.2d 507, 5th Cir., 1974) had been argued and decided in the lower courts as a right-to-treatment case. A federal appellate court majority opinion commenced with the statement that "this case requires us to decide for the first time the far-reaching question whether the Fourteenth Amendment guarantees a right to treatment to persons involuntarily civilly committed to state mental hospitals" (*Donaldson v. O'Connor* 1974, p. 509).

As noted above, Donaldson was committed to and confined in a Florida state psychiatric hospital. At the time Donaldson was committed, in addition to being told he would be held for a matter of weeks, the judge also stated that Donaldson would be hospitalized in order to "take some of this new medication," with the understanding that he would be "all right" and would then "come back here [to court]" (*Donaldson v. O'Connor* 1974, p. 510). For the next 14.5 years, Donaldson remained in confinement but received virtually no psychiatric treatment during that time. It was alleged at trial that Donaldson had refused both medication and electroshock treatment on religious grounds, with the result that no subsequent therapy was offered. Donaldson's attorneys contended that he had a constitutional right either to affirmative treatment or to be released from the hospital.

In handing down its decision, the federal appellate court cited several key cases in justification of its ultimate holding that persons involuntarily committed to psychiatric facilities have a right to treatment that will provide a "reasonable opportunity" (*Donaldson v. O'Connor* 1974, p. 520) for cure or at least improvement of their mental conditions. These cases included *Wyatt v. Stickney* (325 F. Supp. 781, M.D. Ala., 1971), in support of treatment as a safeguard against the arbitrary exercise of state power; *Powell v. Texas* (392 U.S. 514, 1968), in support of treatment as a quid pro quo for confinement in the absence of specific offenses, sentence limitations, and procedures; and *Rouse v. Cameron* (373 F.2d 451 [D.C. Cir.], 1966), in support of requiring realization of any treatment goals alleged as the basis for confinement.

Commitment Criteria: Mentally Ill *and* Dangerous

Clinical Assessment of Statutory Criteria

Involuntary psychiatric commitment now requires both the presence of mental illness and a demonstration of dangerousness to self or others due to mental illness. Civil commitment in which psychiatric hospitalization is being pursued on the basis of mental illness *and* alleged dangerousness connected to potential for violence, including gun violence, is therefore not undertaken lightly or assured of success. Petitioners concerned that someone may commit gun violence due to mental illness are faced with complex and at times logically compromised statutory schemes. They must provide clear and convincing evidence that answers questions raised by individuals' rights and legal due process: What is the specific disease entity underlying the alleged dangerousness in question? Would treatment provide a reasonable opportunity to cure some mental condition that the court may recognize? How will mental health professionals undertake to provide that treatment, rather than simply confining and separating respondents from whatever weapons they may have in their possession?

Consider, for example, the current involuntary civil commitment scheme for New Hampshire. This law states that "a person shall be eligible for involuntary emergency admission if he is in such mental condition as a result of mental illness to pose a likelihood of danger to himself or others" (N.H. Rev. Stat. Ann. § 135-C:27, 1998). One might assume at first blush that establishing a mere "likelihood" of danger is an exceptionally straightforward and permissive standard and would be relatively simple to meet. However, the meaning of "eligible" in this context is unclear: is this a standard for determining who meets criteria for hospitalization or a standard for determining who might ultimately be *considered* for hospitalization?

Meeting this standard becomes even more complicated when the statute then undertakes to define what "danger to himself" means:

> (a) Within 40 days of the completion of the petition, the person has inflicted serious bodily injury on himself or has attempted suicide or serious self-injury and there is a likelihood the act or attempted act will recur if admission is not ordered;
> (b) Within 40 days of the completion of the petition, the person has threatened to inflict serious bodily injury on himself and there is likelihood that an act or attempt of serious self-injury will occur if admission is not ordered; or
> (c) The person's behavior demonstrates that he so lacks the capacity to care for his own welfare that there is a likelihood of death, serious bodily injury, or serious debilitation if admission is not ordered. (N.H. Rev. Stat. Ann. § 135-C:27, 1998)

Critical in the analysis of these additional requirements is the fact that "likelihood" is now piled upon "likelihood," a situation that can engender considerable confusion. Presumably, the "within 40 days" clause refers to the 40 days *preceding* the petition. Strange parallel structure issues aside (legislators, unlike authors, are not afforded professional editors), the bottom line is that within the context of a potential for violence, including gun-related violence, respondents would essentially need to try to harm themselves or overtly threaten to do so in order to fall within the purview of this statute.

The definition of "danger to self" under New Hampshire's statutes also requires such additional elements as a finding that the respondent fits all the following criteria:

- Has been "severely mentally disabled" for at least a year
- Has already been involuntarily hospitalized within the preceding 2 years
- Does not have a guardian
- Is not currently conditionally discharged from the hospital
- Has already refused treatment deemed necessary by a specifically approved mental health program
- Has been determined by a psychiatrist from a specifically approved mental health program "based upon the person's clinical history" to be subject to a "substantial probability" (distinct in some fashion, presumably from a "likelihood") that his or her "refusal to accept necessary treatment will lead to death, serious bodily injury, or serious debilitation if admission is not ordered"

Despite all of the high statutory drama surrounding "danger to self," the criterion for "danger to others" is established by demonstrating that "within 40 days of the completion of the petition, the person has inflicted, attempted to inflict, or threatened to inflict serious bodily harm on another" (N.H. Rev. Stat. Ann. § 135-C:27, 1998). In other words, unless the person suspected of becoming potentially violent toward other individuals, with or without a gun, actually tries to hurt someone or explicitly claims that he or she will do so, then involuntary civil commitment is simply not an option.

As a general matter, persons in any jurisdiction who are alleged to be "dangerous" based on stated suspicions of looming gun violence are unlikely to meet criteria for involuntary civil commitment without the establishment of a diagnosis that is both treatable and sufficiently salient to require, and not merely to merit, hospitalization. Nevertheless, in many commitment hearings, demonstrating acute and/or chronic mental illness is not the primary challenge. Many individuals with serious and chronic mental illnesses cycle in and out of state hospitals and local criminal detention centers, and are often well known to the presiding judges, magistrates, state petitioners, and hospital personnel.

Some states include a criterion of "gravely disabled," interpreted as the inability to care for oneself, but the interpretation of this phrase is so attenuated that it is typically little more than a nod to the concept of a need for treatment. This criterion is most typically applied to a respondent who, due to mental illness, is wandering on a highway and is likely to be hit by a car or who refuses shelter and is likely to die of hypothermia. Those petitioning for commitment would find it exceptionally difficult to bootstrap, for example, an individual with a nonacute and lifelong personality disorder into an argument that respondents suffer from such a major mental illness that confinement is necessary, and that services received on an involuntary inpatient basis would reverse a condition that reflects, as the label implies, long-standing character traits. This is not, of course, to suggest that personality disorders are not "treatable," as clinicians are well aware in light of ongoing advancements in the field (Gianoli et al. 2012; Muran et al. 2005; Strauss et al. 2006).

"Imminent Danger" and Clinical Determination of Dangerousness

Similarly, persons who have a psychiatric diagnosis and acute symptoms that might benefit from hospitalization are unlikely to meet involuntary commitment criteria without the establishment of an acute and elevated risk of "dangerousness" due to mental illness. In fact, the issue that most often prevents involuntary commitment of people with acute and severe mental illness, even in the face of evidence of need for treatment, is demonstrating that the individual is dangerous to self or others. Regardless of jurisdiction, the definition of *dangerousness* either is specified or is interpreted to be "imminent dangerousness." The New Hampshire statutes reviewed above specify a relatively brief time period for consideration of dangerousness. Other states' statutes may present a less specific time period, but typically include the word *imminent,* as in Colorado (Colorado Revised Statutes § 27-65-105, 2014); "in the near future," as in Virginia (Code of Virginia § 37.2-817, 2014); or other similar language. Translation of the concept of "imminent dangerousness" into clinical assessment presents a significant challenge.

The notion of "dangerousness" is omnipresent in all risk assessments, but what does it really mean? It surfaces in the case law and statutes that direct clinical practice (Slobogin 2007) but is rarely defined in operationalized terms for purposes of psychiatric and psychological assessment. *Black's Law Dictionary* (Garner 2014) defines *dangerous* as "likely to cause serious bodily harm," noting further that the concept is "relevant in several legal contexts," including the following: "For example, if a mental condition renders a person imminently dangerous to himself or others, he or she may be committed to a mental hospital" (p. 477). The circular and self-referential nature of such definitions does little to inform the civil forensic evaluator.

The *American Psychological Association Dictionary of Psychology* (VandenBos 2007) is somewhat more illuminating, defining *dangerousness* as "the state in which individuals become likely to do harm to either themselves or others, representing a threat to their own or other people's safety" (p. 255).

Dangerousness is not an indexed term in DSM-5 (American Psychiatric Association 2013), and no diagnostic entity identified by that reference is either inherently "dangerous" or solely defined in terms of "dangerousness." Antisocial personality disorder draws on a history of such behaviorally relevant notions as "aggressiveness, as indicated by repeated physical fights or assaults" and "reckless disregard for safety of self or others" (p. 659), but does not seek to establish that these negative attributes can be projected with any reliability into the future. McCallum (2001) and Meloy (1997) are among those who, nonetheless, have convincingly asserted significant ties between this diagnosis and the sorts of mass killings readily identified with gun violence.

Certain psychiatric diagnoses include behavior that could be dangerous. Schizophrenia is described in DSM-5 in terms of "grossly disorganized" behavior (p. 99) that could qualify as dangerous under certain circumstances. Bipolar disorder's diagnostic criteria include the potential for "excessive involvement in activities that have a high potential for dangerous consequences," but the examples provided are "engaging in unrestrained buying sprees," "sexual indiscretions," and "foolish business investments" (p. 124). The provocatively titled and at times controversial (Anand 2013; Coccaro 2012) diagnosis of intermittent explosive disorder is described in DSM-5 as one that may reflect "physical aggression toward property, animals, or other individuals, occurring twice weekly, on average, for a period of 3 months," but it is also noted that "this physical aggression does not result in damage or destruction of property and does not result in physical injury to animals or other individuals" (p. 466). Newly configured DSM-5 diagnoses within the broadly defined class of substance-related and addictive disorders are minimally informative with regard to manifestations of "dangerousness" per se, although social scientific research has long substantiated a well-recognized link between intoxication and interpersonal violence (Hill et al. 2009; Howard and Menkes 2007; Korcha et al. 2014).

Overall, the civil forensic evaluator will find it difficult to substantiate clinically the presence of "dangerousness" on the basis of having ascribed a particular psychiatric malady to the respondent suspected of susceptibility to violence in general and gun violence in particular. Even if "dangerousness" can be established to the satisfaction of the clinician, more than diagnostic labeling will be necessary to achieve compelled hospitalization. Rather than attempting to prove that a given individual is "dangerous," mental health professionals by and large have progressed to engaging in complex, often actuarially driven approaches to "risk assessment" (Buchanan 2013; Claussen-Schulz et al. 2004; Gold 2013; Harris and Rice 2013; Mills and Gray 2013; Mossman 2010; Singh et al. 2014), utilizing techniques described in other chapters in this volume.

However, core aspects of data collection in cases in which involuntary civil commitment is being considered can be broken down into the domains that research has identified as relevant to increasing levels of risk for suicide or perpetration of violence toward others (Mrad and Watson 2011; also see Chapters 2, 9, and 10):

1. Danger to self
    a. Mental disorders
    b. Demographic characteristics
    c. Previous attempts and current ideation
    d. Social support
    e. Other risk factors
2. Danger to others
    a. Base rates of suspected violence
    b. Personal characteristics
    c. Clinical factors
    d. Situational factors

Nevertheless, potentially lacking in the mental health clinician's collation, review, and synthesis of such data is a consideration of the concept of "imminent dangerousness." When first addressed in evidence-based depth in the clinical literature over three decades ago, this factor was described by Werner et al. (1983) as "central in evaluating patients for detention and release" but at the same time subject to considerable concerns with respect to "the reliability and accuracy of clinicians' predictions of imminent dangerousness" (p. 816). Despite the legal system's emphasis on the "imminent" nature of this construct for purposes of decision making in cases of involuntary psychiatric commitment, from a clinician's evaluation standpoint "more often what emerges throughout the process of conducting risk assessments is a more nuanced continuum of risk" (Helms and Prinstein 2014, p. 180). Indeed, it has been posited that where "imminent" danger is concerned, clinicians are being tethered by external demands to what is no less than "the illusion of short-term prediction" (Simon 2006, p. 296).

This clash between legal commitment requirements, their legal interpretations, and the acknowledged clinical "state of the art" means that even when the evaluator is increasingly convinced that an incident of any type of violence, including gun violence, is in the offing, it may be difficult or even impossible, based on the nature of available inpatient commitment statutes and the restrictiveness of a given jurisdiction's statutes, to satisfy both the "mental illness" and "imminent dangerousness" criteria for compelled psychiatric treatment. A central irony here is that although the police are both trained and enabled to act in a decisive fashion on their understanding that "in real-world law enforcement encounters, a seemingly docile situation can turn violent in a matter of seconds" and that "being able to identify the signs of imminent aggression" is the critical factor in the decision to employ force (Matsumoto and Hwang 2014, p. 118), clinicians armed with professional behavioral science backgrounds and afforded considerably more time to reach a measured conclusion face far more stringent restraints in providing a basis for needed mental health care.

Commitment Resources and Options

Federal and state governments do not provide an adequate number of beds for individuals with acute mental illness, even those who have been involuntarily committed. In addition, people who have been involuntarily committed often find it very difficult to continue accessing mental health services upon discharge. Thus, when a mental health evaluator attempts to seek compelled psychiatric care for a person suspected of dangerousness with respect to potential violence, one practical hurdle is the state's failure to provide sufficient resources for inpatient treatment (see Chapter 8).

According to research that was commissioned by the Treatment Advocacy Center (Torrey et al. 2014), 42 of the 50 states offer less than half of the minimum number of requisite public psychiatric beds. On average, only 17 beds per 100,000 population are available in the combined 50 states. This shortage has contributed to higher levels of homelessness, increases in the jailing of persons with mental illness, and emergency room overcrowding. More specifically, the Treatment Advocacy Center (2014) has cited a 14% decrease in state psychiatric beds between 2005 and 2010—resulting in a per capita state psychiatric bed population virtually identical to that in 1850.

In light of such chilling statistics, some have suggested that outpatient commitment be employed to fill the gaps created by this egregious lack of institutional support. According to Swartz and Swanson (2013),

> Involuntary outpatient commitment is a controversial policy that involves providing court-ordered community services to adults with severe mental illness who are nonadherent to treatment. Research has shown, with some exceptions, that sustained court-ordered outpatient treatment can improve a range of consumer outcomes.... Although most states permit outpatient commitment, many have not implemented it, possibly because officials believe that the program is too costly. However, improved consumer outcomes can result in reduced net costs over time. (p. 7)

Initial research at least suggests, albeit with minimal replication, that outpatient commitment is "associated with a sizeable reduction in the probability of arrest for both overall and violent offenses" (Link et al. 2011, p. 507). With respect to outpatient commitment laws in general, however, "there remains a paucity of definitive empirical date on their effectiveness," because "researchers have carried out only a small number of studies, the results of which seem inconclusive" (Kahan et al. 2010, p. 118). Nevertheless, the presence of such laws in upward of 42 states and in the District of Columbia (Segal and Burgess 2006) does provide substantial opportunity for further social scientific investigation.

For mental health clinicians seeking clinical assistance for patients with severe mental illnesses who may commit acts of violence, including gun violence, the challenges associated with outpatient commitment are twofold. The first of these is determining whether an unsupervised setting will be sufficient when access to firearms is a critical issue. The second is an entrenched perspective on the part of some courts, legal advocates, and clinicians that "after more than 20 years of mandates and programs, outpatient commitment remains a costly, coercive, and unproven approach" (Rowe 2013, p. 336).

Conclusion

An understanding of the legal context of involuntary commitment proceedings is important when reviewing how mental health clinicians actually conduct the evaluations that may or may not lead to compelled treatment for persons suspected of having a serious mental illness and dangerousness regarding guns. The labyrinthine requirements, varying standards, and restrictive mandates for involuntarily hospitalizing these potential patients from a legal perspective are made even more complicated by the daunting clinical practice issues in determining need and appropriateness for confinement. These turn upon risk assessment for dangerousness to self or others—that is, for suicide or aggression against other people.

Overall, the currently available evidence does *not* support the notion that involuntary civil commitment on either an inpatient or outpatient basis is the method of choice for combating the plague of gun-related violence that is threatening our citizens and periodically captivating the local and national news media. Even if involuntary commitment criteria were expanded, the process simplified, and more resources made available, most gun violence directed toward others is not committed by individuals with serious mental illness and therefore cannot be prevented by compelled hospitalization. In contrast, involuntary commitment can be an important intervention in regard to suicide and firearm-related suicide mortality.

Commitment standards, however, are narrowly and at times even contradictorily defined from a legal perspective. They place demands on the clinicians that the current state of the behavioral sciences, while still evolving, are often not yet in a position to meet. Moreover, should the clinician reach a medically supportable conclusion that comports with the legal system's notions of "dangerousness" or "risk," the necessary hospital-based or other treatment resources are often inadequate or simply unavailable. This results in denial of care and in short-term hospitalizations that do little more than attempt to stabilize briefly an individual who may then lack access to outpatient resources to maintain what stability the hospitalization may have provided. Simply put, by the time the system has employed, or ignored, its other options, a medically based solution involving compelled treatment or hospitalization may be too little, too late.

Suggested Interventions

To reduce to the extent possible the misconception that involuntary psychiatric commitment is a solution to the problem of gun violence directed toward others, policy makers and social science researchers should emphasize preventive measures such as the following:

- *Public service messages:* Citizens need to be educated about the dangers inherent in weapons that are unsecured, poorly maintained, and accessible by children or by persons with severe mental illness, significant mental disabilities, and/or substance abuse problems. These messages need to emphasize safety consistently and explicitly, to avoid rejection on the basis that they constitute a covert attack on constitutionally based guarantees with respect to gun ownership.
- *Public psychiatric beds:* Ongoing advocacy is necessary on the part of all mental health professional guilds to ensure that funding authorities uphold their responsibility to provide needed inpatient care resources for persons with mental illness. It may be helpful in this regard to stress the alarming rate of deterioration of treatment availability as well as the future implications of a lack of public psychiatric beds for a host of public health and safety issues, particularly suicide.
- *Outpatient commitment research:* Government agencies and research centers should increase research on the increasingly discussed legal intervention for compelled treatment. Surprisingly little evidence-based scholarship exists with respect to this mode of compelled psychiatric treatment, despite the long-standing presence of related laws on the books in the substantial majority of state jurisdictions. Arrest subsequent to commitment is a relatively easy research criterion to quantify and stands to make a sufficient impression on policy makers and law enforcement representatives alike.
- *Bases for commitment:* As noted above, notions of "dangerousness" and "risk" seem to engender as much confusion as clarity when the time comes for clinicians to make recommendations to the courts. Perhaps a broader criterion of the "need for treatment" would be more easily operationalized and more handily explainable to legal decision makers. Essentially, rather than having to establish that an examinee is going to "do something bad" within an artificially defined period of time, the evaluator would instead be tasked with explaining how the person in

question requires assistance, the by-product of which might or might not be the incidence of suicide or violence toward others, either of which could involve guns.

References

American Psychiatric Association: Diagnostic and Statistical Manual of Mental Disorders, 5th Edition. Washington, DC, American Psychiatric Association, 2013

American Psychological Association: Gun Violence: Prediction, Prevention, and Policy. Washington, DC, American Psychological Association, 2013. Available at: http://www.apa.org/pubs/info/reports/gun-violence-prevention.aspx. Accessed September 8, 2014.

Anand S: Intermittent explosive disorder and DSM-5: a flawed conceptualization of pathological anger. Aust N Z J Psychiatry 47(6):578–579, 2013 23719736

Appelbaum PS: Almost a Revolution: Mental Health Law and the Limits of Change. New York, Oxford University Press, 1994

Appelbaum PS, Gutheil TG: Clinical Handbook of Psychiatry and the Law, 4th Edition. Philadelphia, PA, Lippincott Williams & Wilkins, 2007

Birnbaum M: The right to treatment. Am Bar Assoc J 46:499–504, 1960

Birnbaum M: Some comments on "The right to treatment." Arch Gen Psychiatry 13(1):34–45, 1965 14306531

Bloom JD: Thirty-five years of working with civil commitment statutes. J Am Acad Psychiatry Law 32(4):430–439, 2004 15704628

Bonnie RJ, Reinhard JS, Hamilton P, et al: Mental health system transformation after the Virginia Tech tragedy. Health Aff (Millwood) 28(3):793–804, 2009 19414889

Brown RP, Imura M, Osterman LL: Gun culture: mapping a peculiar preference for firearms in the commission of suicide. Basic Appl Soc Psych 36(2):164–175, 2014

Buchanan A: Violence risk assessment in clinical settings: being sure about being sure. Behav Sci Law 31(1):74–80, 2013 23281104

Claussen-Schulz AM, Pearce MW, Schopp RF: Dangerousness, risk assessment, and capital sentencing. Psychol Public Policy Law 10(4):471–491, 2004

Coccaro EF: Intermittent explosive disorder as a disorder of impulsive aggression for DSM-5. Am J Psychiatry 169(6):577–588, 2012 22535310

Cooke CA, Puddifoot JE: Gun culture and symbolism among U.K. and U.S. women. J Soc Psychol 140(4):423–433, 2000 10981372

Dain N: Clifford W. Beers, Advocate for the Insane. Pittsburgh, PA, University of Pittsburgh Press, 1980

Draper E: Gun-rights groups opposed Colorado mental health bill. Denver Post, May 2, 2014. Available at: http://www.denverpost.com/news/ci_25680316/nra-others-see-colorado-mental-health-bill-gun. Accessed November 22, 2014.

Farberman R: What works to reduce gun violence? Monitor on Psychology 45(2):14–15, 2014

Fazel S, Xenitidis K, Powell J: The prevalence of intellectual disabilities among 12,000 prisoners—a systematic review. Int J Law Psychiatry 31(4):369–373, 2008 18644624

Frattaroli S, Vernick JS: Separating batterers and guns: a review and analysis of gun removal laws in 50 states. Eval Rev 30(3):296–312, 2006 16679498

Garner BA (ed): Black's Law Dictionary, 10th Edition. St Paul, MN, Thomson Reuters, 2014

Gianoli MO, Jane JS, O'Brien E, et al: Treatment for comorbid borderline personality disorder and alcohol use disorders: a review of the evidence and future recommendations. Exp Clin Psychopharmacol 20(4):333–344, 2012 22686496

Gold LH: Gun violence: psychiatry, risk assessment, and social policy. J Am Acad Psychiatry Law 41(3):337–343, 2013 24051585

Harris GT, Rice ME: Bayes and base rates: what is an informative prior for actuarial violence risk assessment? Behav Sci Law 31(1):103–124, 2013 23338935

Helms SW, Prinstein MJ: Risk assessment and decision making regarding imminent suicidality in pediatric settings. Clin Pract Pediatr Psychol 2(2):176–193, 2014

Hill TD, Nielsen AL, Angel RJ: Relationship violence and frequency of intoxication among low-income urban women. Subst Use Misuse 44(5):684–701, 2009 19306220

Howard RC, Menkes DB: Brief report: changes in brain function during acute cannabis intoxication: preliminary findings suggest a mechanism for cannabis-induced violence. Crim Behav Ment Health 17(2):113–117, 2007 17393553

Kahan DM, Braman D, Monahan J, et al: Cultural cognition and public policy: the case of outpatient commitment laws. Law Hum Behav 34(2):118–140, 2010 19169799

Korcha RA, Cherpitel CJ, Witbrodt J, et al: Violence-related injury and gender: the role of alcohol and alcohol combined with illicit drugs. Drug Alcohol Rev 33(1):43–50, 2014 24261437

Lamb HR: The 1978 APA conference on the chronic mental patient: a defining moment. 1978. Psychiatr Serv 51(7):874–878, 2000 10875950

Lifshitz-Vahav H, Vakil E: Taxonomy of moderators that govern explicit memory in individuals with intellectual disability: integrative research review. J Appl Res Mem Cogn 3(2):101–119, 2014

Link BG, Epperson MW, Perron BE, et al: Arrest outcomes associated with outpatient commitment in New York State. Psychiatr Serv 62(5):504–508, 2011 21532076

Matsumoto D, Hwang HC: Facial signs of imminent aggression. Journal of Threat Assessment and Management 1(2):118–128, 2014

McCallum D: Personality and Dangerousness: Genealogies of Antisocial Personality Disorder. New York, Cambridge University Press, 2001

McCreary JR: Falling between the Atkins and Heller cracks: intellectual disabilities and firearms. Chapman Law Review 15(2):271–305, 2011

Meloy JR: Predatory violence during mass murder. J Forensic Sci 42(2):326–329, 1997 9068195

Mental Illness Policy Organization: State-by-state standards for involuntary commitment (assisted treatment). New York, Mental Illness Policy Organization, 2011. Available at: http://mentalillnesspolicy.org/studies/state-standards-involuntary-treatment.html. Accessed September 9, 2014.

Metzner JL, Dvoskin JA: Correctional psychiatry, in The American Psychiatric Publishing Textbook of Forensic Psychiatry. Edited by Simon RI, Gold LH. Washington, DC, American Psychiatric Publishing, 2010, pp 395–411

Miller A: Stop gun violence. Monitor on Psychology 45(5):64–65, 2014

Mills JF, Gray AL: Two-Tiered Violence Risk Estimates: a validation study of an integrated-actuarial risk assessment instrument. Psychol Serv 10(4):361–371, 2013 23815361

Mossman D: Understanding risk assessment instruments, in The American Psychiatric Publishing Textbook of Forensic Psychiatry. Edited by Simon RI, Gold LH. Washington, DC, American Psychiatric Publishing, 2010, pp 563–586

Mrad DF, Nabors E: The role of the psychologist in civil commitment, in Forensic Psychology: Emerging Topics and Expanding Roles. Edited by Goldstein AM. Hoboken, NJ, Wiley, 2007, pp 232–259

Mrad DF, Watson C: Civil commitment, in Handbook of Forensic Assessment: Psychological and Psychiatric Perspectives. Edited by Drogin EY, Dattilio FM, Sadoff RL, et al. Hoboken, NJ, Wiley, 2011, pp 479–501

Muran JC, Safran JD, Samstag LW, et al: Evaluating an alliance-focused treatment for personality disorders. Psychotherapy: Theory, Research, Practice, Training 42(4):532–545, 2005

Nichols NJ: Eighth Circuit revisits restoration exception to domestic violence gun ban and says restore means restore. Miss Law Rev 71(1):267–284, 2006

Petersilia J: Doing Justice? Criminal Offenders With Developmental Disabilities. Berkeley, California Policy Research Center, 2000

Rowe M: Alternatives to outpatient commitment. J Am Acad Psychiatry Law 41(3):332–336, 2013 24051584

Samuel SE, Michals TJ: Competency restoration, in Handbook of Forensic Assessment: Psychological and Psychiatric Perspectives. Edited by Drogin EY, Dattilio FM, Sadoff RL, et al. Hoboken, NJ, Wiley, 2011, pp 79–96

Sappok T, Budczies J, Dziobek I, et al: The missing link: delayed emotional development predicts challenging behavior in adults with intellectual disability. J Autism Dev Disord 44(4):786–800, 2014 24002416

Schwartz HI, Mack DM, Zeman PM: Hospitalization: Voluntary and Involuntary. New York, Oxford University Press, 2003

Segal SP, Burgess PM: The utility of extended outpatient civil commitment. Int J Law Psychiatry 29(6):525–534, 2006 17070577

Simon RI: Imminent suicide: the illusion of short-term prediction. Suicide Life Threat Behav 36(3):296–301, 2006 16805657

Singh JP, Fazel S, Gueorguieva R, et al: Rates of violence in patients classified as high risk by structured risk assessment instruments. Br J Psychiatry 204(3):180–187, 2014 24590974

Slobogin C: Proving the Unprovable: The Role of Law, Science, and Speculation in Adjudicating Culpability and Dangerousness. New York, Oxford University Press, 2007

Strauss JL, Hayes AM, Johnson SL, et al: Early alliance, alliance ruptures, and symptom change in a nonrandomized trial of cognitive therapy for avoidant and obsessive-compulsive personality disorders. J Consult Clin Psychol 74(2):337–345, 2006 16649878

Swartz MS, Swanson JW: Economic grand rounds: can states implement involuntary outpatient commitment within existing state budgets? Psychiatr Serv 64(1):7–9, 2013 23280454

Taruffo M: Rethinking the standards of proof. Am J Comp Law 51(3):659–677, 2003

Torrey EF, Entsminger K, Geller J, et al: The Shortage of Public Hospital Beds for Mentally Ill Persons: A Report of the Treatment Advocacy Center. Arlington, VA, Treatment Advocacy Center, 2014. Available at: http://www.treatmentadvocacycenter.org/storage/documents/the_shortage_of_publichospital_beds.pdf. Accessed September 19, 2014

Treatment Advocacy Center: No Room at the Inn: Trends and Consequences of Closing Public Psychiatric Hospitals. Arlington, VA, Treatment Advocacy Center, 2014. Available at http://tacreports.org/bed-study. Accessed September 19, 2014.

VandenBos GR (ed): American Psychological Association Dictionary of Psychology. Washington, DC, American Psychological Association, 2007

Werner PD, Rose TL, Yesavage JA: Reliability, accuracy, and decision-making strategy in clinical predictions of imminent dangerousness. J Consult Clin Psychol 51(6):815–825, 1983 6655098

Werth JL Jr: U.S. involuntary mental health commitment statutes: requirements for persons perceived to be a potential harm to self. Suicide Life Threat Behav 31(3):348–357, 2001 11577919

Williamson AA, Guerra NG, Tynan WD: The role of health and mental health care providers in gun violence prevention. Clin Pract Pediatr Psychol 2(1):88–98, 2014

8

Accessing Mental Health Care

Robert L. Trestman, Ph.D., M.D.
Fred R. Volkmar, M.D.
Liza H. Gold, M.D.

Common Misperceptions

☒ Mental health treatment is readily available for people with serious mental illness.

☒ People with serious mental illness who are at high risk for committing mass shootings can be identified and treated, even against their wishes, before they become violent.

☒ Increased access to mental health treatment can prevent mass shootings by individuals with mental illness.

☒ People with serious mental illness are likely to be violent toward others, even if this violence does not involve use of firearms.

Evidence-Based Facts

☑ Accessing inpatient or outpatient treatment can be extremely difficult for individuals with serious mental illness, even if they are motivated to accept treatment.

☑ Mass shootings by individuals with serious mental illness are very rare events and therefore cannot be predicted. People who are at high risk for violence, with or without firearms, often cannot be identified and treated against their wishes before they become violent.

☑ Increased access to mental health treatment can reduce violent behavior in people with serious mental illness and can decrease the risk of suicide; however, available evidence does not support the belief that voluntary or involuntary mental health treatment can reduce or prevent mass shootings by individuals with or without mental illness.

☑ People with serious mental illness are more likely to be victims of violence than perpetrators of violence.

In the aftermath of highly publicized mass shootings, the media and the public immediately focus on the shooter's mental health. Why? Because the public widely assumes that mental disorders are good predictors of gun violence. The belief is that mental health clinicians could have or should have averted these acts of gun violence, even if this required involuntarily committing these individuals to a psychiatric hospital. In short, the implication is that if we mental health professionals were doing our jobs properly, fewer people would die from gun violence perpetrated by people with mental illness.

As reviewed in earlier chapters, mass shootings perpetrated by individuals with mental illness account for a disproportionately small percentage of firearm-associated morbidity and mortality. Only 3%–5% of individuals with mental illness perpetrate violence toward others, and only a small percentage of that violence involves firearms (Swanson and Gilbert 2011). Also, as discussed in Chapter 9, "Structured Violence Risk Assessment," despite the development of more than 200 violence risk assessment instruments, mental health professionals' assessments of violence risk are not predictive of specific acts of future violent behavior (Coid et al. 2011; Fazel et al. 2012; Singh et al. 2011).

For purposes of discussing access to mental health care, however, let us assume that the very small number of individuals who have serious mental illness (SMI) who commit murders of multiple strangers could be identified before they commit acts of violence. What then might mental health professionals do? What resources are available, and how can the people who need them access these resources? The answers to these questions reflect profound barriers to accessing mental health treatment in our fragmented mental health system.

The Mental Health System: One Family's Tragedy

On November 18, 2013, Austin "Gus" Deeds, the 24-year-old son of Virginia state senator Creigh Deeds, was in a dark place. According to Senator Deeds's public accounts, his son had been struggling for months with delusions, had expressed thoughts of suicide, and had recently referenced guns in his journal. Senator Deeds was so concerned that he removed from his house all guns but one and, to his knowledge, all the ammunition (Turner 2014). After unsuccessful efforts to get his son to voluntarily seek mental health services, Senator Deeds obtained an emergency custody order (ECO). The ECO allowed a sheriff's deputy to transport Gus involuntarily to a local hospital emergency department (ED) to be evaluated and, if needed, involuntarily hospitalized for further evaluation (Morehart 2014).

The evaluating clinician found that Gus Deeds met Virginia's statutory criteria for a temporary detention order (Morehart 2014), which require "a substantial likelihood that, as a result of mental illness, the person will, in the near future, cause serious physical harm to himself or others" (Virginia Code § 37.2-809). In Virginia, a person under a temporary detention order can be held involuntarily up to 48 hours pending a more complete evaluation and a hearing to determine whether the individual meets criteria for involuntary commitment. However, under the Virginia statute, a temporary detention order could not be executed unless the availability of an inpatient psychiatric bed could be confirmed.

Reportedly, no public or private psychiatric bed could be found before the ECO's statutory 6 hours expired. Gus refused voluntary treatment and refused to stay at the local hospital until a psychiatric bed was located. Under Virginia law, he could not be detained any longer. Gus and his father left the ED with an outpatient follow-up appointment scheduled for the next day (Morehart 2014). Thirteen hours after he was released, Gus stabbed his father multiple times, seriously wounding Senator Deeds. Within minutes of the attack on his father, Gus Deeds shot and killed himself (Morehart 2014). Senator Deeds stated he did not know where his son had found the ammunition (Turner 2014).

The Scope of the Mental Health Crisis

As a result of these events, Virginia's legislature amended state laws relating to civil commitment. Revisions in the law included, among other changes, increasing the amount of time individuals can be held on an ECO from 6 hours to 8 hours (with no extensions); requiring state hospitals to admit individuals on a temporary detention order if an ECO has expired and no other beds have been found; and requiring the Virginia Department of Behavioral Health and Developmental Services to maintain a Web-based statewide acute psychiatric bed registry to provide real-time information on acute bed availability in public and private inpatient psychiatric facilities to facilitate identification and designation of facilities for temporary detention of individuals who meet the TDO criteria (Code of Virginia, Chapter 8, §37.2-806 et seq.). These welcome changes in the Virginia Code were intended to reduce barriers to accessing mental health treatment.

Unfortunately, changes in the legal process such as these do not address the basic problems faced by Gus Deeds, his family, and thousands of others in attempting to access mental health care, even when patients meet the narrow criteria for involuntary commitment. Psychiatric inpatient bed shortages, increased use of emergency departments for acute psychiatric crises, and shortfalls in funding of community-based services have "led to a public health crisis for mentally ill people who have become homeless or who are incarcerated in the nation's jails and prisons" (Sharfstein and Dickerson 2009, p. 685; see also Salinsky and Loftis 2007). Patients, their families, and their mental health clinicians across the country struggle with this state of affairs on a daily basis (Grob 2000; Lamb 2000).

According to the Substance Abuse and Mental Health Services Administration (2013b), in 2012, an estimated 43.7 million adults (18.6% of all American adults age 18 or older) had any mental illness (AMI), defined as a diagnosed DSM-IV-TR (American Psychiatric Association 2000) disorder (other than developmental or substance use disorders), in the previous 12 months. Of these, 9.6 million (4.1% of all adults) had an SMI, defined as a DSM-IV-TR disorder that has resulted in serious functional impairment that substantially interferes with or limits one or more major life activities.

In the same year, 19.2% of adults with AMI (8.4 million adults) and 27.3% of adults with SMI (2.6 million) also had co-occurring substance use disorders, with associated increases in morbidity. In comparison, only 6.4% of adults who did not have mental illness in the previous year met criteria for a substance use disorder (Substance Abuse and Mental Health Services Administration 2013b).

Despite the hundreds of billions of dollars spent each year on mental health care, 59% of the adults with AMI and 37.1% of those with SMI did not receive any mental health treatment in 2012 (Substance Abuse and Mental Health Services Administration 2013b). Financial constraints to care, limited availability of treatment resources, and personal and institutionalized stigma associated with mental illness present tremendous barriers to mental health treatment. This is particularly the case for patients like Gus Deeds and others with SMI who need acute care.

Deinstitutionalization

Over the past 60 years, an unprecedented shift in mental health care from inpatient treatment to outpatient services has taken place. This process, commonly referred to as deinstitutionalization, was accompanied by changes in funding, social policy, and legal reform that have contributed to the current crisis. These changes reversed over 100 years of policy in which people with mental illnesses received centralized care in state-funded psychiatric hospitals.

In the nineteenth century, social activism for more humane and effective treatment of people with mental illness resulted in the construction of large asylums. By the mid-nineteenth century, virtually every state had established facilities for the care of individuals with mental illness. These asylums were "regarded as the symbol of an enlightened and progressive nation that no longer ignored or mistreated its insane citizens" (Grob and Goldman 2006, p. 4). By the mid-twentieth century, these asylums, now public psychiatric hospitals, housed patients in large numbers and often in deplorable conditions. In 1955, more than 550,000 people were patients in American psychiatric hospitals, fully 339 persons of every 100,000 in the population (Lamb and Weinberger 2005; Torrey 2014; Torrey et al. 2008).

The Community Mental Health Act of 1963 (Pub. L. No. 88-164, also known as the Community Mental Health Centers Construction Act) called for the creation of community mental health centers (CMHCs). The CMHCs were intended to provide a broad spectrum of services in lieu of long-term hospitalization (Frank and Glied 2006). The new CMHC services were to include linked and integrated outpatient care, aftercare programs, and continuous services to treat and support people in the community (Grob 2000; Grob and Goldman 2006). The Community Mental Health Act included the first direct federal funding commitment to mental health and provided seed grants to local communities (Frank and Glied 2006). In addition, new federal entitlement programs, such as Medicaid, were added to the Social Security Act, providing enhanced funding for outpatient treatment and services over those for inpatient services (Salinsky and Loftis 2007).

Prior to the 1960s, states were almost exclusively responsible for providing care for persons with mental illness. Funding changes associated with the Community Mental Health Act and new federal entitlement programs created an opportunity for the states to begin shifting costs for mental health care to the federal government, primarily by discharging patients in large numbers from public hospitals and closing beds (Frank and Glied 2006; Grob and Goldman 2006; Sharfstein and Dickerson 2009). Between 1955 and 1988, the number of patients in state and county mental hospitals decreased by more than 80% (Shorter 1997).

The reduction in inpatient psychiatric services was not balanced by the development of a comprehensive community-based system of medical care, psychiatric care, and social services (Salinsky and Loftis 2007). The implementation of the Community Mental Health Act was significantly underfunded, and states did not supply sufficient funds to meet the needs of the growing population of formerly institutionalized patients transitioning into their communities (Grob and Goldman 2006; Salinsky and Loftis 2007).

Despite shrinking resources, state hospitals remained the largest providers of total inpatient days of psychiatric care for patients with SMI (Grob 2000; Salinsky and Loftis 2007). In addition, although federal entitlement programs came to provide the greatest proportion of funding for individuals with SMI, accessing these funds was complicated, and the different entitlement programs were not linked in any meaningful or practical way with mental health care systems (Frank and Glied 2006; Grob and Goldman 2006).

The Courts Step In: Legal Rights of Individuals With Mental Illness

Until the mid-1960s, most states required only the presence of mental illness and a need for treatment to involuntarily commit a patient to a state mental hospital. The legal process of involuntary commitment, when present, was typically guided by the opinions of examining doctors or concerned family members, a process that many noted could be easily abused (Appelbaum 1994; Stone 1976). In the wake of the civil rights movement of the 1960s and 1970s, a series of judicial decisions and legislative changes supported and further incentivized deinstitutionalization of patients with mental illness by restricting the scope of commitment laws (Appelbaum 1994; Lamb 2000).

In the influential landmark case of *Lessard v. Schmidt* (349 F. Supp. 1078, [E.D. Wis.], 1972), a Wisconsin federal district court held that involuntary commitment required proof that a person was both mentally ill and dangerous to self or others; that a finding of dangerousness had to be based on an overt act, attempt, or threat to inflict substantial harm within 30 days preceding commitment; and that commitment hearings must follow strict legal procedures. *Lessard* shifted involuntary commitment from a medical model, in which need for treatment was the central criterion for involuntary commitment, to a legal model, based on liberty interests and due process (Appelbaum 1994; Stone 1976). Alan Stone predicted that "*Lessard* would invalidate the provisions of commitment laws in virtually all States, and would if followed exactly, put a virtual end to involuntary confinement" (Stone 1976, p. 52).

Although *Lessard* did not end involuntary civil commitment, it created a paradigm shift in the legal bases and procedures associated with involuntary commitment. Within a few years, nearly all states had revised their civil commitment laws to comply with the *Lessard* standards. By the end of the 1970s, individuals with mental illness could not be involuntarily committed to a psychiatric hospital in any state absent a judicial or semi-judicial hearing in which they were found to be both mentally ill and dangerous to themselves or others. The need for treatment as a rationale for involuntary commitment did not entirely disappear but became more narrowly and strictly applied (Appelbaum 1994; Frank and Glied 2006).

Other issues regarding the civil rights of people with mental illness and involuntary civil commitment became the subject of legal debate and judicial concern. These included a right to treatment and minimum standards for that treatment and care of individuals involuntarily committed to psychiatric hospitals (*Wyatt v.*

Stickney, 325 F. Supp. 781, M.D. Ala., 1971). Furthermore, the courts clearly articulated committed patients' rights to be treated in the least restrictive setting appropriate to the individual's condition (*Lake v. Cameron,* 364 F.2d 657, D.C. Cir., 1966; see also Appelbaum 1994; Frank and Glied 2006; Parks et al. 2014).

Many psychiatrists welcomed the increased autonomy and dignity these changes brought to their patients and the decrease in abuses associated with involuntary hospitalization. Nevertheless, the strict legal limitations on the involuntary commitment of individuals with SMI have been a mixed blessing for those with such disorders. On the one hand, their civil liberties are unquestionably better protected. On the other hand, these limits have increased the difficulty of accessing mental health treatment for individuals who may desperately need it. Many clinicians have concurred with the observation, first expressed in 1974, that their patients are "dying with their rights on" (see Appelbaum 1994, p. 30). This observation certainly comes to mind in regard to the death of Gus Deeds.

Consequences of Deinstitutionalization

For some chronically hospitalized patients, deinstitutionalization provided opportunities for an improved quality of life (Grob 2000; Torrey 2014). In addition, historically disempowered individuals found voices as consumers of mental health services. The social justice service-recipient movement resulted in organized advocacy, peer services, and visible and meaningful roles and services within state and federal initiatives (Frank and Glied 2006; Parks et al. 2014).

Nevertheless, the changes brought about by deinstitutionalization, in funding sources, and by an increased emphasis on legal rights and due process have had the serious and unintended negative consequences of creating multiple barriers to treatment. Although utilization of behavioral health services and mental health spending have increased over time, the 2012 National Survey on Drug and Health Use found that of the 43.7 million adults with AMI, almost 60% received no treatment; of the 9.6 million adults with SMI, almost 40% received no mental health treatment (Substance Abuse and Mental Health Services Administration 2013b).

Barriers to Accessing Mental Health Treatment: Finances, Availability, and Stigma

Paying for Mental Health Treatment

Cost is by far the largest barrier to care (Council 2004; Garfield 2011). In 2012, almost 60% of respondents in the National Survey on Drug and Health Use reported not receiving mental health care for financial reasons: inability to afford the cost of care (45.7%), health insurance that did not adequately cover the cost of treatment (7.9%), or health insurance that did not cover any mental health treatment (5.5%) (Substance Abuse and Mental Health Services Administration 2013b).

The biggest change in the financing of mental health care in past decades has been the shift from a centralized system of state dollars to a mix of public (largely federal) and private funding administered through multiple programs in various settings (Garfield 2011). Public payers account for the majority of funding for mental health, more so than for medical and surgical health care. For example, in 2009, public payers accounted for 60%, or $88 billion, of the $147 billion spent on mental health treatment (Garfield 2011; Substance Abuse and Mental Health Services Administration 2013a). In the same year, public funding accounted for only 49% of total health care spending. Private payers, including private insurance, out-of-pocket spending, and other private sources, pay less of the total of mental health spending (40% in 2009) compared to the total medical and surgical health care spending (51% in 2009) (Substance Abuse and Mental Health Services Administration 2013a).

A full description of all current funding sources for mental health care is beyond the scope of this discussion. The following subsections briefly review major sources of funding for mental health care and implications for accessing care. These sources include Medicaid (27% of mental health spending in 2009), private insurance (26%), state and local spending (other than state Medicaid; 15%), and out-of-pocket costs (11%) (Substance Abuse and Mental Health Services Administration 2013a).

Medicaid

Medicaid is the payment source for the majority of individuals served by state mental health agencies (Garfield 2011). Because eligibility for Medicaid coverage is based on income level or disability, Medicaid provides health insurance to the most economically vulnerable populations. Medicaid is often the only source of health care coverage available for low-income individuals with mental illness (Shirk 2008). In 2012, Medicaid provided health care assistance for approximately 16% of the entire U.S. population (about 50 million people) (DeNavas-Walt et al. 2013; Truffer et al. 2013).

The increase in Medicaid expenditures for mental health over the past 20–30 years is one of the major funding changes in the provision of mental health care. Medicaid was established as a joint federal-state public insurance program, with states eligible to receive funds from the federal government on the basis of per capita income. Its financing structure allows states to expand services with federal assistance and relatively fewer state dollars (Garfield 2011; Pinals 2014).

Medicaid spending grew so rapidly between 1986 and 2009 that it "became one of the most important drivers of overall mental health spending increases" (Substance Abuse and Mental Health Services Administration 2013a, p. 20). In

2009, Medicaid accounted for the largest component of mental health spending at 27%. Medicaid also accounted for the largest share of the increase in mental health spending at 29% between 1986 and 2009. Although reimbursement for any given service under Medicaid is relatively limited, Medicaid covers more of the services typically needed by individuals with SMI than does private insurance. For example, Medicaid often covers community-based services such as assertive community treatment, case management, clubhouses and drop-in centers, and some home and rehabilitation services (Garfield 2011; Shirk 2008).

Nevertheless, the limitations of Medicaid coverage, especially the institution for mental disease (IMD) exclusion, have had widespread effects on the availability of mental health services, especially for people with SMI. Medicaid does not cover hospital services for adults ages 22–64 in an IMD, defined as an institution in which more than 50% of the beds are occupied by primary mental health service recipients (Garfield 2011; Parks et al. 2014). Medicaid's exclusion of state psychiatric hospital coverage gave states a significant financial incentive to shift care to treatment facilities not subject to the IMD exclusion, such as smaller psychiatric units in larger general hospitals, CMHCs, and other community treatment options (Pinals 2014). This change resulted in substantial state savings in deinstitutionalizing patients, at the cost of a significant loss of inpatient care capacity (Garfield 2011; Shirk 2008).

In addition, Medicaid coverage is designed primarily to provide medically related treatment and support services. Individuals with SMI often need access to public housing, job training, and income support, each financed by its own government agency. This complex and bureaucratic system of benefits is challenging for consumers as well as mental health and social service professionals to navigate. However, without access to these necessary social supports, many individuals with SMI are unable to continue participating in mental health treatment (Garfield 2011; Shirk 2008).

Finally, many individuals with SMI and low income who would benefit from Medicaid coverage are not covered. Approximately one-third of people with mental illness, substance use disorders, or both have incomes under the federal poverty level and are uninsured (Honberg et al. 2011a; Shirk 2008). In 2012, just over 6% of adults with SMI had no health insurance, although many of these uninsured people were likely to be eligible for Medicaid coverage (Substance Abuse and Mental Health Services Administration 2012, 2013b).

Barriers to accessing Medicaid for those who might be eligible can include homelessness or psychiatric impairments that interfere with completing the Medicaid enrollment process (Garfield 2011; Honberg et al. 2011a; Shirk 2008). In addition, individual patients' eligibility for Medicaid is extinguished or suspended while they are inpatients in an IMD, such as a state psychiatric hospital, or if they become incarcerated. Once discharged, those who qualify for Medicaid coverage and other social benefits have to enroll, reenroll, or reactivate suspended coverage, a task many cannot accomplish without assistance. Failure to reenroll, which commonly occurs, often results in loss of Medicaid coverage and other social benefits, which in turn results in lack of treatment continuity or engagement (Davis et al. 2014; Slade et al. 2014; Smith et al. 2014).

The Affordable Care Act (ACA) of 2010 (PL 118-148) was intended to reduce the number of people who are uninsured. The ACA addressed reform in the public sector through expansion of Medicaid eligibility and is expected to result in new populations accessing mental health services through Medicaid as well as private health insurance plans (Beronio et al. 2013; Garfield et al. 2010; Kaiser Commission on Medicaid and the Uninsured 2014). Prior to the ACA, 1.9 million individuals received behavioral health treatment through Medicaid. Under the ACA, an estimated 16.3 million people are eligible for insurance coverage under Medicaid expansion; utilization of mental health services based on 100% state participation could increase by as much as 72% (Ali et al. 2014). Nationally, the rate of individuals without health insurance had fallen from 17.3% in 2013, when the ACA went into effect, to 11.7% through the first half of 2015 (Witters 2014). Limited evidence on the early effects of ACA coverage suggests that patients are facing fewer financial barriers to mental health care (Golberstein et al. 2015).

Nevertheless, the ACA may fall short in regard to increasing access to care for individuals with SMI eligible for Medicaid enrollment. In 2012, the Supreme Court ruled that states could choose to participate in the ACA's Medicaid expansion but could not be required to do so (*National Federation of Independent Business v. Sibelius,* 132 S.Ct. 1161, 2012). As of July 20, 2015, only 31 states and the District of Columbia have chosen to participate in the Medicaid expansion (Kaiser Family Foundation 2015). The ACA's Medicaid expansion also may not meet the needs of uninsured individuals with AMI as a result of some of the legislation's other provisions. For example, states that do participate in Medicaid eligibility expansion have the option of providing "benchmark" benefits, which are similar to those available through employer-based private coverage and are typically less than full Medicaid benefits. An analysis of the ACA's provisions indicates that even with federal parity requirements, some services needed by individuals with AMI, particularly those with SMI, may be excluded from coverage (Beronio et al. 2013; Garfield et al. 2010).

State General Funding

State general funding (which for purposes of this discussion includes non-Medicaid funding and local funding) of mental health care is the "safety net of last resort for children and adults living with serious mental illness" (Honberg et al. 2011a, p. 2). However, as states have increasingly relied on Medicaid to cover mental health treatment costs, significantly less state funding has been available to provide services for uninsured populations (Substance Abuse and Mental Health

Services Administration 2013a). In 1986, state non-Medicaid spending represented 27.4% of all mental health care expenditures; Medicaid represented 17%. In 2009, state funding had decreased to 15% of all mental health expenditures and Medicaid had increased to 27% (Substance Abuse and Mental Health Services Administration 2012, 2013a).

In addition, because state mental health spending is financed through general funds rather than a dedicated revenue source, these services are particularly sensitive to a state's budget conditions (Garfield 2011). States are able to save money when a patient is discharged from a state hospital to the community, and states save a lot of money when public psychiatric beds and hospitals are eliminated. People who rely on state mental health resources are in particular jeopardy because they often rely on additional state-funded services such as education or housing (Substance Abuse and Mental Health Services Administration 2012).

The economic recession that began in 2008 resulted in the largest reduction in state government revenues in 40 years and led to steep decreases in state funding for mental health services (Honberg et al. 2011a; Parks et al. 2014). From fiscal year 2010 through 2013, states cut mental health care funding by $4.4 billion. Relatively modest budget increases since 2012 did not reverse the effects of the decrease in spending in previous years, and many states have continued to decrease funding for mental health services (Honberg et al. 2011a, 2011b).

Private Insurance

Private health insurance is accessed primarily through employer-sponsored plans. In 2012, these private plans provided health coverage for over 60% of the U.S. population, a total of 198.8 million people (DeNavas-Walt et al. 2013). Nevertheless, in 2012, private health insurance covered only 15.4% of individuals with AMI and 2.7% of individuals with SMI (Substance Abuse and Mental Health Services Administration 2013b).

Despite covering fewer individuals with AMI, private health insurance in 2009 accounted for 26% of the total mental health spending in the United States, nearly equaling that of Medicaid at 27% (Substance Abuse and Mental Health Services Administration 2013a). Private insurance also accounted for 28% ($32 billion) of the increase in mental health spending between 1986 and 2009 (Substance Abuse and Mental Health Services Administration 2012, 2013a).

In attempts to control the spiraling increases in mental health care spending, private health insurance plans limit benefits. For example, private insurance commonly limits mental health coverage in ways not applied to medical and surgical benefits. These limits include higher cost sharing, lower dollar caps for services, and limits on the number of outpatient visits or inpatient days (Garfield 2011). In 2009, about 80% of all private insurance plans that offered mental health benefits had limits on those benefits and/or services (Substance Abuse and Mental Health Services Administration 2012). Nearly 20% had no coverage for mental health services, including outpatient therapy and inpatient crisis intervention and stabilization (Beronio et al. 2013).

State and federal government agencies have sponsored legislative attempts to create parity since the early 1970s (Garfield 2011). The 2008 Paul Wellstone and Pete Domenici Mental Health Parity and Addiction Equity Act was intended to stop most group health plans from imposing stricter treatment limits and financial requirements on mental health benefits than those for medical and surgical benefits (Garfield 2011). The ACA also addressed insurance reform and parity in the private sector through the creation of the state health insurance marketplaces ("exchanges") where private insurers compete for business.

The implementation of the ACA and parity enforcement (see, e.g., Moran 2014a, 2014b) under the Mental Health Parity and Addiction Equity Act of 2008 may eliminate some of the differences in costs and utilization rates. Nevertheless, evidence on parity to date indicates that parity laws may not substantially increase private payers' spending on mental health services, largely because of a concomitant reliance on intense case management through managed behavioral health organizations. In addition, under the ACA, group health plans in existence before March 23, 2010, are exempt from many of the ACA's provisions, and may still exclude or limit coverage of mental health services (Garfield 2011).

Out-of-Pocket Costs

Out-of-pocket payments for mental health services include copayments for services covered by insurance, payment for services excluded from insurance plans, and direct payment for all services by individuals with no insurance coverage. Publicly funded insurance programs do not pick up all those who do not have private coverage, and uninsured rates among those with mental illnesses are higher than among those without (Garfield 2011). Out-of-pocket payments for behavioral health care have actually been relatively stable since the early 1990s (Substance Abuse and Mental Health Services Administration 2013a).

However, out-of-pocket payment for behavioral health services varies depending on a person's insurance coverage and level of utilization of services. Under private insurance plans, patients' shares of costs increase as they use more behavioral health services and hit limits. In contrast, out-of-pocket costs decrease as individuals use general medical care services and meet deductibles. As a result of these policies, in 2009, those with private coverage paid about 25% of their total mental health expenditures out of pocket, a significantly higher amount than did those with Medicaid coverage, who paid only 6% of total out-of-pocket costs (Garfield 2011). The implementation of parity through the ACA and the 2008 Mental Health Parity and Addiction Equity Act may lead to similar levels and patterns of cost sharing across service types (Garfield 2011).

Summary

The various mental health care funding sources, including those discussed in this section as well as others, form a complex system of benefits and programs, each with its own particular eligibility, rules, and benefits package (Garfield 2011), and each having had different impact on availability of and access to mental health treatment. Although many funding programs interact closely, they were not designed as a coordinated system of care, and at times they appear to be more like a maze than a health care system (Garfield 2011). As a result, the nature of funding and the ability to pay for mental health treatment are formidable barriers to accessing treatment for those with SMI.

Availability of Mental Health Services

A critical shortage of treatment resources and capacity presents another significant barrier to accessing mental health services. In 2012, of individuals who identified a need for mental health services but did not receive services, almost one-fourth of respondents (22.8%) reported that they did not receive treatment because they "did not know where to go for services" (Substance Abuse and Mental Health Services Administration 2013b).

Mental Health Providers

Although states have worked to build community-based treatment and recovery support systems, this growth has often been insufficient to accommodate the level of community services needed (Parks et al. 2014). In 2006, thirty-three states had a 20%–30% shortage of mental health professionals (Substance Abuse and Mental Health Services Administration 2012). Communities report shortages of key outpatient staff, especially psychiatrists (Shirk 2008; Thomas et al. 2009). In 2009, of the 3,100 counties in the United States, 55% had no practicing psychiatrists, psychologists, or social workers (American Hospital Association 2012).

Facilities providing mental health care are also in short supply; in 2009, only 27% of community hospitals had an inpatient psychiatric unit (American Hospital Association 2012). The shortage of mental health professionals and barriers to access to mental health care are two factors in the increased utilization of nonspecialty mental health care, particularly in regard to prescription medication (Substance Abuse and Mental Health Services Administration 2013b).

Outpatient Psychiatric Care

Mental health care is most frequently delivered on an outpatient basis by primary care or mental health clinicians (American Hospital Association 2012; Frank and Glied 2006; Substance Abuse and Mental Health Services Administration 2012, 2013a). In 2012, the most common form of mental health treatment for individuals with AMI or SMI was prescription medication (12.4% or 29.0 million adults), followed by outpatient services (6.6% or 15.5 million adults), and then inpatient services (0.8% or 1.9 million adults) (Substance Abuse and Mental Health Services Administration 2013b).

As would be expected, utilization of all three types of mental health services is substantially higher among those with SMI (Garfield 2011; Substance Abuse and Mental Health Services Administration 2013b). Not surprisingly, in 2009, the uninsured paid the highest percentage of total out-of-pocket mental health expenditures (62%) (Substance Abuse and Mental Health Services Administration 2013b). In 2012, although 40.7% of adults held private health insurance, the percentage of adults using mental health services was higher among adults who were covered by Medicaid (21.4%) than among those with private health insurance (14.2%) (Substance Abuse and Mental Health Services Administration 2013b).

The disproportionate rates of payment relative to coverage may reflect another limitation common among private insurance health plans. Many private insurance plans require that individuals obtain treatment from "preferred" providers, who have independently agreed to provide services to a particular insurance or managed care plan at a reduced fee. This can significantly limit the range of providers available for patients covered by commercial insurance (Rosenberg et al. 2010). Many mental health providers are unwilling to spend increasing amounts of their time completing the paperwork required to receive direct reimbursement from managed care plans. Thus, prospective patients with private coverage often find psychiatrists reluctant to provide services through the patients' insurance (Bishop et al. 2014). Patients with managed care plans who access "out-of-network" mental health services may receive no reimbursement for out-of-pocket costs.

These limitations for patients with private insurance have been a major factor in loss of access to specialty care. Primary care physicians, whose services are not limited by the insurance restrictions on mental health care, are often the first point of contact for individuals seeking mental health treatment. General practitioners now write the majority of prescriptions for psychotropic medications, and many limit their treatment to pharmacology (Mark et al. 2011; Substance Abuse and Mental Health Services Administration 2013b).

In fact, acceptance rates for all types of insurance are significantly lower for psychiatrists than for physicians in other specialties (Bishop et al. 2014). For example, because of low reimbursement rates by Medicaid, many psychiatrists limit the number of Medicaid-covered outpatients they will take (Shirk 2008). A study using data from 2011 and 2012 found that over half of psychiatrists were not accepting new Medicaid outpatients (Decker 2013). Of adults in 2012 using outpatient services, only 10.1% were likely to use Medicaid to cover the costs of treatment, although 30.5% of adults with AMI and 8.5% of adults had Medicaid coverage (Substance Abuse and Mental Health Services Administration 2013b).

Anecdotal evidence in states that have opted for the ACA's Medicaid expansion provisions indicates that shortages of available services are now being encountered. Some states, such as Kentucky, are attempting to alleviate shortages of providers by allowing non-CMHC psychologists and social workers to be eligible for Medicaid reimbursement, thereby allowing these private mental health professionals to be able to accept Medicaid patients. Nevertheless, many private therapists also refuse to accept Medicaid because of low reimbursement rates, excessive paperwork, and the patients' clinical acuity. Those who are seeing Medicaid patients are reporting overwhelming caseloads, leading to long delays before an appointment can be made (Goodnough 2014).

Finally, outpatient services alone typically are not sufficient to treat individuals with SMI. Reasons may include individuals' lack of insight into need for treatment and high rates of treatment discontinuation. An extensive clinical literature documents a significant association between illness insight and treatment acceptance (Davis et al. 2014; Doyle et al. 2014; Slade et al. 2014; Smith et al. 2014). Increased risk of treatment dropout is associated with psychiatric comorbidity, absence of health insurance, average to low income, lack of family support and involvement, and substance use disorders (Davis et al. 2014). These factors are all more likely among individuals covered by Medicaid or those having no insurance coverage.

Inadequate follow-up is a strong predictor of inpatient readmission, homelessness, and incarceration (Smith et al. 2014). Homeless people with substance use and mental disorders are among those individuals who may have the most difficulty in accessing treatment, even if they have public health insurance (Council 2004; Kim et al. 2007). Lack of access to basic necessities such as housing or income support can exacerbate severe mental disorders and increase the need for inpatient treatment (Garfield 2011; Salinsky and Loftis 2007). For these individuals, psychiatric hospitals are a particularly important source of specialist care (Salinsky and Loftis 2007; Sharfstein and Dickerson 2009).

Inpatient Psychiatric Care

Inpatient mental health services are a critical part of the continuum of care for people with SMI. In 2009, most psychiatric admissions were due to an acute clinical crisis (Sharfstein and Dickerson 2009). Publicly funded psychiatric inpatient hospitals provide safety-net care to indigent patients and others who cannot access private sector care. People who are uninsured and severely ill, who meet involuntary commitment criteria, and who are found incompetent to stand trial or not guilty by reason of insanity are treated in state psychiatric hospitals.

Inpatient care is the most infrequently used but most expensive form of mental health care services. In 2009, less than 1% of all adults in the United States (3.1% of adults with AMI and 6.8% of adults with SMI) received inpatient services (Substance Abuse and Mental Health Services Administration 2012). Nevertheless, spending on psychiatric hospitalization in 2009 accounted for 26% of all mental health spending, approximately the same amount spent on prescription medications (28%), the most common form of mental health treatment (Substance Abuse and Mental Health Services Administration 2013a).

With a few exceptions, states and private sources rather than the federal government fund most psychiatric hospitals (Substance Abuse and Mental Health Services Administration 2012). Because of the high cost of maintaining inpatient hospitals and related services, Medicaid's IMD exclusion, and the emphasis on community mental health treatment, psychiatric hospitals and inpatient beds are often the first mental health services to be cut when states come under increasing budget pressures (Shumway et al. 2012; Substance Abuse and Mental Health Services Administration 2012).

Inpatient psychiatric beds have become increasingly difficult to access, regardless of insurance status or motivation for treatment. Deinstitutionalization, massive state mental health budget cuts, and lack of federal funding or reimbursement have resulted in a draconian reduction in the number of available inpatient beds. Between 1950 and 2012, the number of state psychiatric hospitals decreased by 36%, from 322 to 207; however, the number of patients in state psychiatric hospitals declined by 92% (Parks et al. 2014). Between 1955 and 2007, approximately 500,000 of the nation's 550,000 public psychiatric beds were shut down (Torrey 2014). In 2006, more than 80% of states were reporting a shortage of psychiatric acute care beds (Bloom et al. 2008; Sharfstein and Dickerson 2009).

The 2008 recession led to even more public psychiatric bed and hospital closures. Between 2005 and 2010, the number of state psychiatric beds decreased 14%, from just over 50,000 beds to just over 43,000 (Parks et al. 2014; Substance Abuse and Mental Health Services Administration 2012). By 2010, the number of public state psychiatric beds available had decreased to 14.1 per 100,000 of the U.S. population, the same number (14 beds per 100,000) as were available in 1850 (Torrey et al. 2012), when social advocacy to provide more humane care to those with mental illness first led to the construction of public hospitals.

The increasing share of beds occupied by forensic patients further limits the availability of inpatient beds (Pinals 2014). In 2010, approximately 33% of all public psychiatric beds (although this varied greatly by state) were occupied by individuals with mental illness hospitalized pending an evaluation of their competency to stand trial or criminal responsibility (or insanity), or after a legal finding of not guilty by reason of insanity (Treatment Advocacy Center 2013b). Costs associated with justice-involved inpatients have also come to represent increasing percentages of increasingly limited state hospital expenditures, rising from 7.3% in 1983 to 36% in 2012 (Parks et al. 2014; Pinals 2014). In a few states, over 90% of the state psychiatric hospital expenditures are devoted to the treatment of persons under forensic commitment (Parks et al. 2014).

Moreover, state psychiatric hospitals have no control over the admissions or discharges of forensic patients. Lengths of inpatient stays for forensic service recipients are not determined by treatment needs or medical necessity but by the judicial system (Parks et al. 2014; Pinals 2014). In one study, the average length of an inpatient stay for nonforensic patients with SMI was 10 days, plus or minus 3 days (Lee et al. 2012). In contrast, in many states, courts refuse to discharge individuals who have been clinically stable after months or years of treatment. In spite of the lack of control over forensic admissions and discharges, state psychiatric hospitals cannot exceed their licensed and staffed bed capacity or they risk losing Centers for Medicaid & Medicare Services certification, Joint Commission accreditation, and federal funding (Pinals 2014; Parks et al. 2014).

Finally, as discussed below (see "Consequences of Barriers to Accessing Mental Health Care"), admission to the state hospitals can trigger termination of public insurance and other social benefits. Justice-involved individuals with mental illness are at risk for a host of social and occupational challenges, including unemployment, homelessness, and rearrest, due to repeated interruptions in health care and other public benefits. Individuals with both mental health and criminal justice involvement therefore have an increased risk of significantly fractured care, resulting in a high risk of mortality and poor outcomes (Pinals 2014).

Mental Illness and Stigma

In a 2012 study, individuals who did not receive mental health services but who acknowledged they might have needed such services gave reasons for avoiding treatment that reflect the stigma associated with mental illness (Substance Abuse and Mental Health Services Administration 2013b). A review of social policies and the stigma associated with mental illness found "extensive changes in social policies, court decisions, treatments, and living conditions" but "surprisingly little evidence of significant shifts in public perceptions about mental illness" (Frank and Glied 2006, p. 133). A full discussion of the effects of stigma associated with mental illness is beyond the scope of this chapter. In brief, ignorance and misinformation about mental illness and prejudicial attitudes and discriminatory behavior toward individuals with mental illness create additional barriers to availability of, and access to, care.

Studies repeatedly confirm that self-stigma and fear of public stigma are powerful influences on decisions to seek treatment (e.g., Drapalski et al. 2013; Mojtabai et al. 2011; Substance Abuse and Mental Health Services Administration 2013b). In one recent study, 58% of individuals with a first episode of psychosis felt the need to conceal their diagnosis (Lasalvia et al. 2014); nondisclosure can interfere with help-seeking behavior, creating a major obstacle to receiving effective treatment (Frank and Glied 2006; Lasalvia et al. 2014). In addition, institutionalized stigma—that is, pervasive and unquestioned negative stereotypes and assumptions so widely held among legislative and corporate decision makers that they become incorporated into legal, social, and business policies—perpetuates unequal and inadequate funding of mental health care (Corrigan et al. 2011; Golberstein et al. 2008; Lasalvia et al. 2014).

Consequences of Barriers to Accessing Mental Health Care

The many barriers to accessing mental health treatment, particularly for those with SMI, have resulted in a public health crisis of epidemic proportions. Those who seek treatment voluntarily find their options limited by lack of mental health resources as well as by financial costs. Those who may be involuntarily committed find that their access to government entitlements and benefits, including housing, has been disrupted. Upon discharge, they are often unable to maintain therapeutic gains provided by acute treatment, with profound social and mental health consequences.

Homelessness

The incidence of homelessness among those with SMI has increased dramatically since the 1960s. Persons with SMI are 10–20 times more likely than the general population to be at risk for homelessness (Frank and Glied 2006; Khadduri et al. 2008; Parks et al. 2014). One large study found a 15% prevalence rate of homelessness among those with SMI (Folsom et al. 2005). Homelessness increases risk of victimization as well as substance use, involvement in the criminal justice system, and morbidity (Roy et al. 2014).

Victimization

Persons with SMI are more likely to be the victims than the perpetrators of crime. The stereotypical association of violence with SMI is so pervasive that publications that focus on the link between mental illness and the perpetration of violence number significantly more than the publications regarding victimization of individuals with mental illness (Choe et al. 2008; Roy et al. 2014). Nevertheless, studies report that crime victimization rates for those with mental illness, even after relevant demographic factors were controlled for, are between 2.4 and 11 times greater than those for the general population (Desmarais et al. 2014; Pandiani et al. 2000; Teplin et al. 2005). Homeless individuals with SMI are at higher risk of victimization than homeless individuals without SMI (45% vs. 26%), and homeless women with mental illnesses in particular experience extreme levels of victimization (Roy et al. 2014).

Law Enforcement Contacts

Unfortunately, the police are now all too often the first point of contact with severely mentally ill individuals in crisis, and often with dire consequences. When individuals with SMI are homeless and thus visible in public spaces, they are more likely to draw law enforcement's attention (Roy et al. 2014). In 2015, a *Washington Post* team of investigative reporters began tracking the national number of police shootings that involved people with mental illness. They report that individuals in crisis who were either explicitly suicidal or had a history of mental health problems accounted for 25% of all the people shot and killed by police across the United States in the first 6 months of 2015 (Lowery et al. 2015). The *Post*'s analysts also state that the 25% figure is likely to be an underestimate. Other organizations indicate substantially higher percentages. A joint report by the Treatment Advocacy Center and the National Sheriffs' Association asserts that approximately half the people shot and killed by the police each year have mental health problems (Treatment Advocacy Center 2013a). In Albuquerque, New Mexico, according to a report by the New Mexico Public Defender Department, nearly 75% of people shot by police in 2010 and 2011 had mental illness (Santos and Goode 2014).

Marginalized individuals with SMI who come in contact with law enforcement are more often arrested, resulting in a substantial increase in the number of incarcerated individuals with mental illness. Although the increase in the number of justice-involved persons with mental illness has multiple causes (Pinals 2014), the higher likelihood of arrest during police interventions involving individuals with mental illness is well established (Fisher et al. 2006; Teplin 2000). In studies of clients from a state mental health agency (Fisher et al. 2006) and of Medicaid beneficiaries (Cuellar et al. 2007), rates of arrest have been found to be between 25% and 28% over a 10-year period.

Incarceration

Given the rates of homelessness and arrest among people with SMI, the finding that correctional facilities now house a disproportionate number of individuals with SMI is not surprising (Hawthorne et al. 2012; Prins 2014; Steadman et al. 2009). The widespread and national phenomenon of increased incarceration of those with mental illness as a result of deinstitutionalization has led to increased use of the term *transinstitutionalization* (i.e., incarceration in lieu of hospitalization) to refer to the changes in the delivery of mental health care in past decades.

The current and lifetime prevalence of numerous mental illnesses is higher among incarcerated populations than among nonincarcerated populations, sometimes by wide margins (Hawthorne et al. 2012; Prins 2014). Although the exact number of individuals with SMI currently in jails and prisons is not known (Prins 2014), more than 2.1 million people with SMI were estimated to be booked into jails in 2007 (Steadman et al. 2009). A Bureau of Justice assessment of correctional inmates and mental health in 2005 (James and Glaze 2006) indicated that 56% of state prisoners, 45% of federal prisoners, and 64% of jail inmates had symptoms of mental illness in the 12 months prior to the interview. The country's three biggest jail systems (Cook County in Illinois; Los Angeles County; and Riker's Island in New York City) are widely reported to be the largest mental health treatment facilities in the country (Fields and Phillips 2013; NPR Staff 2011).

For the socially vulnerable population of individuals with SMI, contact with the criminal justice system exacerbates their marginalization and disrupts treatment and linkage to service systems beyond the degree associated with the effects of mental illness (Fisher et al. 2011; Prins 2014). Predictably, interruption of benefits leads to lack of treatment, lack of social services, homelessness, and increased rates of rearrest and incarceration (James and Glaze 2006; Hawthorne et al. 2012; Luciano et al. 2014). One literature review found that among homeless individuals, lifetime rates of incarceration were 48%–67%; the rate in the general population is estimated to be about 15% (Roy et al. 2014).

Legal and justice system involvement of people with mental illness also comes with significant economic costs. Administrative records for 25,133 Connecticut adults with a diagnosis of schizophrenia or bipolar disorder were matched across judicial, correctional, and Medicaid databases over a 2-year time span. The group who became involved with the justice system (about 25% of the sample) cost state and federal agencies approximately twice as much, per person, as the group with no justice involvement ($48,980 vs. $24,728) (Swanson et al. 2013).

Nevertheless, officers who encounter an irrational person creating a disturbance have three choices: transport that person to a hospital, arrest the person, or resolve the matter informally (Teplin 2000). When police become involved in a situation with individuals who have SMI or who are in acute psychiatric crisis, an informal resolution is less likely than an arrest or transport to a hospital ED. Thus, the two primary venues of acute psychiatric care in the United States for those with SMI are psychiatric inpatient hospitals and EDs of general medical hospitals (Salinsky and Loftis 2007), and both are overwhelmed.

Options for Accessing Mental Health Care in the Early Twenty-First Century

Emergency Departments

Hospital EDs across the United States serve as de facto primary care and treatment sites for many uninsured or indigent individuals. This population specifically includes those with SMI, who are overrepresented among this disadvantaged population (Nicks and Manthey 2012; Substance Abuse and Mental Health Services Administration 2012). From 2010 through 2013, as a result of cuts in state budgets for mental health services and continuing elimination of inpatient psychiatric beds, ED use by individuals with a primary diagnosis of a mental illness or substance use disorder increased 28% (Parks et al. 2014).

Compared with patients without psychiatric disorders, individuals with psychiatric illnesses have higher rates of ED use and are more likely to use the ED on multiple occasions (Baillargeon et al. 2008). Many of the psychiatric patients seen in EDs require hospitalization; not infrequently, they require involuntary hospitalization, adding another level of complexity to evaluation and management. According to one federal estimate, spending by general hospitals to provide ED care for psychiatric patients was expected to nearly double, from $20.3 billion in 2003 to $38.5 billion in 2014 (Creswell 2013).

The nonfinancial burden of treating people with mental disorders in EDs is also well established. Increased psychiatric utilization and overuse of EDs negatively affect access to emergency care for all patients by compromising the care and safety of all ED patients and diminishing the available pool of ED staff (Coffey et al. 2010; Nicks and Manthey 2012; Parks et al. 2014; Salinsky and Loftis 2007). Once a decision to admit has been made, ED staff spend twice as much time looking for beds for psychiatric patients as they do finding beds for nonpsychiatric patients (Salinsky and Loftis 2007). Psychiatric patients remain in hospital EDs 2–3.5 times as long as nonpsychiatric patients (Nicks and Manthey 2012; Salinsky and Loftis 2007), with 42% of primary psychiatric patients spending 9 or more hours in the ED (Nicks and Manthey 2012). The extended length of stay for each psychiatric patient translates into a capacity reduction in the ED of 2.2 fewer patients (Nicks and Manthey 2012; Parks et al. 2014).

The increased utilization of EDs by acute psychiatric patients, the shortage of inpatient beds, and the inordinate amount of time patients must wait for a bed to be found after a decision to admit has been made have led to a practice known as *boarding.* This term is used to describe a patient's status when held in the ED, often for excessive amounts of time, due to a delay in transfer to a psychiatric hospital because no inpatient beds are available. Boarding of psychiatric patients in EDs occurs regardless of whether the patient is consenting voluntarily to admission or requires involuntary admission (Bloom 2015).

Psychiatric boarding is practiced in differing degrees across the United States but is a commonplace occurrence, caused by the shortage of beds for psychiatric patients in general hospital psychiatric units, private psychiatric hospitals, and state hospitals (Bloom 2015). Boarding psychiatric patients in EDs is a trend that is increasing (American Hospital Association 2012). About 80% of ED medical directors have reported that their hospitals board psychiatric patients (American Hospital Association 2012). The most common reasons cited in one survey for extended ED length of stay were lack of an accepting facility (19.9%), inability to transfer to an accepting facility (19.9%), and lack of in-house psychiatric beds (16.5%) (American College of Emergency Physicians 2008).

Boarding can adversely affect ED psychiatric and nonpsychiatric patients alike. The external stimuli associated with the busy ED environment can increase patient anxiety and agitation, leading to increased risk of symptom exacerbation or patient elopement, posing dangers to the patient and to staff (American Hospital Association 2012). Patients may be given medication, but other types of treatment are rarely provided, and the use of physical restraints is common (Bender et al. 2009).

In a precedent-setting decision, the Washington State Supreme Court unanimously ruled in August 2014 that boarding involuntarily held psychiatric patients temporarily in hospital emergency rooms because no beds are available at psychiatric treatment facilities is unlawful and violates the state's Involuntary Treatment Act. The court said in its ruling that "patients may not be warehoused without treatment because of lack of funds" nor can lack of funds justify the state's failure to provide the treatment necessary for recovery (*Detention of D. W. v. Department of Social and Health Services,* 181 Wash. 2d 201, 2014).

The cost of creating more public treatment options to comply with the ruling was estimated to run to the "tens of millions of dollars" (Mannix 2014). However, if Washington State does not provide the resources in response to this court decision to meet the needs of those with serious mental illness brought to EDs, "we can hypothesize a situation in which the bar for continued hospitalization will be raised and premature discharge of patients becomes a new norm of this beleaguered system" (Bloom 2015, p. 221).

Acute Inpatient Care

Thus, we come full circle back to the state of affairs that contributed to the tragic death of Gus Deeds: the lack of available inpatient beds for individuals with SMI in crisis, regardless of voluntary or involuntary status. As many families can attest, involuntary civil commitment criteria are now so narrowly defined and interpreted that they present a major barrier to accessing care for individuals with SMI. These individuals may lack insight into the nature of their illness but desperately need mental health treatment before they become dangerous to themselves or others.

The events leading to Gus Deeds' death brought the practice of "streeting"—that is, releasing an individual who needs voluntary or involuntary acute inpatient treatment from an emergency room back to the community—into the national spotlight. A report released in June 2015 indicates that the number of civil commitments in Virginia has increased since the changes enacted in Virginia's laws in 2014 following the death of Gus Deeds (Allen and Bonnie 2015). Nevertheless, reform of involuntary commitment laws or laws regarding holding psychiatric patients in appropriate facilities will do little to increase the availability of acute inpatient services unless such reform is accompanied by increased state funding.

Just as boarding has been occurring across the country for years and is not unique to Washington State, streeting psychiatric patients is not unique to Virginia and did not begin in 2013 with the death of Gus Deeds (see Bevelacqua 2011). The lack of acute treatment inpatient beds is a systemic crisis across the United States and underlies the unfortunate practices of both boarding and streeting. Although Bloom referred only to boarding, the fact is that both the practices of boarding and streeting have "existed for many years in the shadows of mental health care" (Bloom 2015, p. 220). Regardless of where either practice occurs, both practices reflect a failure of the mental health system that affects the most vulnerable of our citizens and places patients, their families, and at times the public at risk (Bevelacqua 2011).

Fragmentation and Transformation of Mental Health Care

In 2002, President George W. Bush's Commission on Mental Health reported that the fragmentation of services for those with mental illness was such that the nation's mental health services were incapable of efficiently delivering and financing effective mental health treatment (President's New Freedom Commission on Mental Health 2003). For many patients, access to outpatient services, including social support services, effectively prevents the need for inpatient treatment. However, when in crisis and/or when dangerous to themselves or others, individuals with SMI need access to competent inpatient care.

The lack of availability of mental health treatment services, lack of funding of services, inability to pay for services, and both personal and institutionalized stigma have created barriers to accessing voluntary and even involuntary treatment. As the death of Gus Deeds demonstrates, these barriers to treatment, especially when combined with access to firearms, can have fatal consequences. Judicial or legislative mandates banning practices such as "boarding" or "streeting" will not improve access to mental health care if such mandates are not funded and services are not coordinated.

Increased integration and coordination of services is arguably the most critical need in decreasing barriers to mental health treatment (American Hospital Association 2012). Without such integration, increased funding and services will not reach the populations who most need them. For example, achieving continuity of Medicaid coverage across inpatient admissions requires a system that bridges inpatient and outpatient mental health care as well as social services. Similarly, individuals with mental illness transitioning from jail or prison to the community often experience homelessness and recidivism.

Changes in public policies and funding, when informed by evidence-based research that identifies problems, needs, and effective interventions, can improve access to mental health treatment. Correctional prerelease access to benefits such as Medicaid and Supplemental Security Income improves access to housing and reduces recidivism (Dennis et al. 2014). The restructuring of California's public mental health system promoted access to treatment by patients with SMI (Snowden et al. 2002). Homeless persons with mental illnesses who receive coordinated and intensive mental health and support services have been discharged from inpatient treatment to community support services without deterioration of mental or social functioning (Rosenheck and Dennis 2001; Shumway et al. 2012).

A promising attempt to integrate care was included in the ACA, which in 2010 funded a 3-year demonstration project through the Centers for Medicare & Medicaid Services. In this project, selected nongovernment inpatient psychiatric hospitals could be exempted from the IMD exclusion for psychiatric emergencies provided to Medicaid enrollees ages 21–64 who had an acute need for treatment. Although the 2013 evaluation of this pilot program did not draw definitive conclusions, evaluators recommended that the project continue for another 2 years to allow a more thorough evaluation of its effects (Parks et al. 2014).

Increased funding of mental health services is desperately needed and always welcome. Unfortunately, the needs of the current mental health system go beyond more beds and more dollars. As called for by the President's New Freedom Commission on Mental Health (2003), the National Association of State Mental Health Program Directors (Miller et al. 2014), and the Substance Abuse and Mental Health Services Administration (Salinsky and Loftis 2007), the entire mental health system in the United States needs system transformation. Mental health care treatment and delivery systems need to become recovery oriented, person centered, and family driven, and to emphasize autonomy, freedom of choice, and hope (Parks et al. 2014; Pinals 2014).

To be effective, transformation of the current fragmented and underfunded mental health systems should involve shifting the provision of mental health care to a public health care model that utilizes a full range of evidence-based preventive and intervention strategies to decrease the personal, community, and social costs of mental illness. A public health care approach to mental health that focuses on health promotion, disease prevention, and service integration would also include strategies for continued examination of fragmentation of services and gaps in care (Levin et al. 2010; Salkever et al. 2014).

To that end, more data are needed. The United States lacks a robust mental health surveillance system that collects and analyzes national and state data. Such data guide policy and expenditure of resources, as well as help in tracking overall mental health status; capacity of, access to, and receipt of treatment; and the degree to which the need for treatment is met. Public health surveillance systems that exist for other diseases, such as HIV/AIDS, serve as examples. Surveillance data, including data regarding gaps in treatment capacity, are particularly needed for people in vulnerable subpopulations, such as homeless or incarcerated populations, because many of these people have higher rates of mental illness (Salinsky and Loftis 2007; Substance Abuse and Mental Health Services Administration 2012).

Access to Mental Health Treatment and Gun Violence

Studies consistently demonstrate that ongoing treatment reduces the risk of violence, including suicide, among individuals with SMI (Golenkov et al. 2014; Keers et al. 2014; Langeveld et al. 2014; Lawlor et al. 2007; Swanson et al. 2003; Witt et al. 2013). That said, the explicit connection of calls for increased funding for mental health services as a means of decreasing the incidence of gun violence, particularly mass shootings, are misguided. No evidence of any kind supports the common misperception that increased mental health funding or services will decrease or prevent mass shootings by individuals with or without mental illness (see Chapter 1, "Gun Violence and Serious Mental Illness," and Chapter 4, "Mass Shootings and Mental Illness").

In contrast, the increased provision of mental health services, particularly "upstream" services that promote treatment engagement and adherence and decrease stigma, can potentially decrease high rates of firearm suicide (see Chapter 2, "Firearms and Suicide in the United States," and Chapter 10, "Decreasing Suicide Mortality"). Incidents of gun violence, especially mass shootings, committed by individuals with SMI are relatively rare. Nevertheless, casting a wider net by decreasing barriers to accessing mental health care through increasing resources and integrating mental health and social services is much likelier to help someone who might be inclined toward violence, before a tragedy occurs.

Conclusion

The lack of access to a reasonably well functioning mental health care system is a public health crisis in the United States that calls for transformation. The financial and social costs of the barriers to effective mental health treatment, especially for those with SMI, are obvious and significant. The Deeds family is only one of the many families that can attest to the personal and community tragedies that result from a system that routinely denies care to those who most need it. However, regardless of whether boarding or streeting those with acute mental illness is unconstitutional or illegal, judicial and legislative decisions will do little to improve the current state of affairs without allocation of more resources.

With adequate resources, use of public health models, and proven effective practices, the mental health system in the United States could become more effective and accessible. This transformation requires coordinating mental health and social services and funding, implementing evidence-based mental health treatment across the spectrum of need, decreasing stigma, and collecting data to guide these efforts. Efforts to engage individuals before violence or suicide takes place, by improving treatment adherence and alleviating the symptoms of SMI, may also decrease the small portion of community violence associated with serious psychiatric disorders.

Suggested Interventions

- Resources need to be allocated so as to allow implementation of evidence-based programs that provide a continuum of care. At one end of the spectrum, individuals with SMI may at times need inpatient treatment or hospitalization, requiring increased availability of inpatient resources. At the other end of the spectrum, community and outpatient treatment can be highly effective and decrease the need for inpatient hospitalization.
- Dedicated case management services need to be created, with an emphasis on community outreach, to assist individuals with integrating mental health services with social, job placement, housing, and financial needs.
- An increase is needed in the funding and coordination of specialized justice-related interventions for individuals with mental illness. Such services include police and jail diversion, mental health courts, specialized probation, and forensic assertive community treatment. For those incarcerated, release planning includes social services, safe and supportive housing, job training, and health insurance reenrollment, as well as mental health and social services that support recovery and minimize risks of reincarceration.
- The federal government and each state should appoint a commission to review available mental health resources and their efficacy, and to recommend changes to decrease barriers to accessing mental health care and increase integration of existing resources.

References

Allen AA, Bonnie JK: Annual Statistical Report, Operation of the Civil Commitment Process in FY 2013–FY 2014. Available at: http://cacsprd.web.virginia.edu/ILPPP/PublicationsAndPolicy/DownloadPDF/75. Accessed August 21, 2015.

Ali MM, Teich J, Woodward A, Han B: The implications of the Affordable Care Act for behavioral health services utilization. Adm Policy Mental Health, November 19, 2014. DOI 10.1007/s10488-014-0615-8. Accessed August 9, 2015.

American College of Emergency Physicians: ACEP Psychiatric and Substance Abuse Survey 2008. Washington, DC, American College of Emergency Physicians, 2008. Available at: http://newsroom.acep.org/download/ACEP+Psychiatric+and+Substance+Abuse+Survey+-+April+2008.pdf. Accessed August 4, 2015.

American Hospital Association: Bringing behavioral health into the care continuum: opportunities to improve quality, costs, and outcomes. Trendwatch, January 2012. Available at: http://www.aha.org/research/reports/tw/12jan-tw-behavhealth.pdf. Accessed August 4, 2015.

American Psychiatric Association: Diagnostic and Statistical Manual of Mental Disorders, 4th Edition, Text Revision. Washington, DC, American Psychiatric Association, 2000

Appelbaum PS: Almost a Revolution: Mental Health Law and the Limits of Change. New York, Oxford University Press, 1994

Baillargeon J, Thomas CR, Williams B, et al: Medical emergency department utilization patterns among uninsured patients with psychiatric disorders. Psychiatr Serv 59(7):808–811, 2008 18587001

Bender D, Pande N, Ludwig M: Psychiatric Boarding Interview Summary. Washington, DC, U.S. Department of Health and Human Services, Assistant Secretary for Planning and Evaluation, Office of Disability, Aging and Long-Term Care Policy, 2009

Beronio K, Po R, Skopec L, Glied S: Affordable Care Act Will Expand Mental Health and Substance Use Disorder Benefits and Parity Protections for 62 Million Americans (research brief). Washington, DC, U.S. Department of Health and Human Services, Office of the Assistant Secretary for Planning and Evaluation, February 2013

Bevelacqua GD: Semi-annual Report In-Brief, Office of the Inspector General, Behavioral Health and Developmental Services. Richmond, VA, Commonwealth of Virginia, 2011

Bishop TF, Press MJ, Keyhani S, et al: Acceptance of insurance by psychiatrists and the implications for access to mental health care. JAMA Psychiatry 71(2):176–181, 2014 24337499

Bloom JD: Psychiatric boarding in Washington State and the inadequacy of mental health resources. J Am Acad Psychiatry Law 43:218–222, 2015 26071512

Bloom JD, Krishnan B, Lockey C: The majority of inpatient psychiatric beds should not be appropriated by the forensic system. J Am Acad Psychiatry Law 36(4):438–442, 2008 19092059

Choe JY, Teplin LA, Abram KM: Perpetration of violence, violent victimization, and severe mental illness: balancing public health concerns. Psychiatr Serv 59(2):153–164, 2008 18245157

Coffey R, Houchens R, Chu BC, et al: Emergency Department Use for Mental and Substance Use Disorders: Agency for Healthcare Research and Quality. Rockville, MD, U.S. Agency for Healthcare Research and Quality, August 23, 2010. Available at: https://www.hcup-us.ahrq.gov/reports/ED_Multivar_Rpt_Revision_Final072010.pdf. Accessed August 4, 2015.

Coid JW, Yang M, Ullrich S, et al: Most items in structured risk assessment instruments do not predict violence. J Forens Psychiatry Psychol 22(1):3–21, 2011

Corrigan PW, Roe D, Tsang HWH: Challenging the Stigma of Mental Illness: Lessons for Therapists and Advocates. New York, Wiley, 2011

Council CL (ed): Health Services Utilization by Individuals With Substance Abuse and Mental Disorders. Rockville, MD, Substance Abuse and Mental Health Services Administration, Office of Applied Studies, 2004

Creswell J: E.R. costs for mentally ill soar, and hospitals seek better way. New York Times, December 25, 2013, p A1

Cuellar AE, Snowden LM, Ewing T: Criminal records of persons served in the public mental health system. Psychiatr Serv 58(1):114–120, 2007 17215421

Davis M, Abrams MT, Wissow LS, et al: Identifying young adults at risk of Medicaid enrollment lapses after inpatient mental health treatment. Psychiatr Serv 65(4):461–468, 2014 24382689

Decker SL: Two-thirds of primary care physicians accepted new Medicaid patients in 2011–12: a baseline to measure future acceptance rates. Health Aff (Millwood) 32(7):1183–1187, 2013 23836732

DeNavas-Walt C, Proctor BD, Smith JC: Income, Poverty, and Health Insurance Coverage in the United States: 2012. Washington, DC, U.S. Government Printing Office, 2013

Dennis D, Ware D, Steadman HJ: Best practices for increasing access to SSI and SSDI on exit from criminal justice settings. Psychiatr Serv 65(9):1081–1083, 2014 24981962

Desmarais SL, Van Dorn RA, Johnson KL, et al: Community violence perpetration and victimization among adults with mental illnesses. Am J Public Health 104(12):2342–2349, 2014 24524530

Doyle R, Turner N, Fanning F, et al: First-episode psychosis and disengagement from treatment: a systematic review. Psychiatr Serv 65(5):603–611, 2014 24535333

Drapalski AL, Lucksted A, Perrin PB, et al: A model of internalized stigma and its effects on people with mental illness. Psychiatr Serv 64(3):264–269, 2013 23573532

Fazel S, Singh JP, Doll H, et al: Use of risk assessment instruments to predict violence and antisocial behaviour in 73 samples involving 24 827 people: systematic review and meta-analysis. BMJ 345(7868):e4692, 2012 22833604

Fields G, Phillips EE: The new asylums: jails swell with mentally ill. Wall Street Journal, September 26, 2013, p A1

Fisher WH, Roy-Bujnowski KM, Grudzinskas AJ Jr, et al: Patterns and prevalence of arrest in a statewide cohort of mental health care consumers. Psychiatr Serv 57(11):1623–1628, 2006 17085611

Fisher WH, Simon L, Roy-Bujnowski K, et al: Risk of arrest among public mental health services recipients and the general public. Psychiatr Serv 62(1):67–72, 2011 21209302

Folsom DP, Hawthorne W, Lindamer L, et al: Prevalence and risk factors for homelessness and utilization of mental health services among 10,340 patients with serious mental illness in a large public mental health system. Am J Psychiatry 162(2):370–376, 2005 15677603

Frank RG, Glied SA: Better but Not Well: Mental Health Policy in the United States Since 1950. Baltimore, MD, Johns Hopkins University Press, 2006

Garfield RL: Mental Health Financing in the United States: A Primer. Washington, DC, Kaiser Commission on Medicaid and the Uninsured, 2011

Garfield RL, Lave JR, Donohue JM: Health reform and the scope of benefits for mental health and substance use disorder services. Psychiatr Serv 61(11):1081–1086, 2010 21041345

Golberstein E, Eisenberg D, Gollust SE: Perceived stigma and mental health care seeking. Psychiatr Serv 59(4):392–399, 2008 18378838

Golberstein E, Busch SH, Zaha R, et al: Effect of the Affordable Care Act's young adult insurance expansions on hospital-based mental health care. Am J Psychiatry 172:182–189, 2015 25263817

Golenkov A, Nielssen O, Large M: Systematic review and meta-analysis of homicide recidivism and schizophrenia. BMC Psychiatry 14:46, 2014 24548381

Goodnough A: Expansion of mental health care hits obstacles (U.S. section). New York Times, August 28, 2014. Available at: http://www.nytimes.com/2014/08/28/us/expansion-of-mental-health-care-hits-obstacles.html?_r=0. Accessed August 4, 2015.

Grob GN: Mental health policy in the late twentieth century, in American Psychiatry Since World War II: 1944–1994. Edited by Menninger RW, Nemiah JC. Washington, DC, American Psychiatric Press, 2000, pp 232–258

Grob GN, Goldman HH: The Dilemma of Federal Mental Health Policy: Radical Reform or Incremental Change? Rutgers, NJ, Rutgers University Press, 2006

Hawthorne WB, Folsom DP, Sommerfeld DH, et al: Incarceration among adults who are in the public mental health system: rates, risk factors, and short-term outcomes. Psychiatr Serv 63(1):26–32, 2012 22227756

Honberg R, Diehl S, Kimball A, et al: State Mental Health Cuts: A National Crisis. Arlington, VA, National Alliance on Mental Illness, March 2011a. Available at: http://www.nami.org/Content/NavigationMenu/State_Advocacy/State_Budget_Cuts_Report/NAMIStateBudgetCrisis2011.pdf. Accessed August 4, 2015.

Honberg R, Kimball A, Diehl S, et al: State Mental Health Cuts: The Continuing Crisis. Arlington, VA, National Alliance on Mental Illness, 2011b

James DJ, Glaze LE: Bureau of Justice Statistics Special Report: Mental Health Problems of Prison and Jail Inmates. Washington, DC, U.S. Department of Justice, Office of Justice Programs, 2006. Available at: http://www.bjs.gov/content/pub/pdf/mhppji.pdf. Accessed August 4, 2015.

Kaiser Commission on Medicaid and the Uninsured: Key Facts About the Uninsured Population. Washington, DC, Kaiser Family Foundation, 2014. Available at: http://kff.org/uninsured/fact-sheet/key-facts-about-the-uninsured-population/. Accessed August 26, 2014.

Kaiser Family Foundation: Status of state action on the Medicaid expansion decision. Kaiser Family Foundation website, July 20, 2015. Available at: http://kff.org/health-reform/state-indicator/state-activity-around-expanding-medicaid-under-the-affordable-care-act/#table. Accessed August 9, 2015.

Keers R, Ullrich S, Destavola BL, et al: Association of violence with emergence of persecutory delusions in untreated schizophrenia. Am J Psychiatry 171(3):332–339, 2014 24220644

Khadduri J, Culhane DP, Buron L, et al: The Second Annual Homeless Assessment Report to Congress. Washington, DC, U.S. Department of Housing and Urban Development, 2008

Kim MM, Swanson JW, Swartz MS, et al: Healthcare barriers among severely mentally ill homeless adults: evidence from the Five-Site Health and Risk Study. Adm Policy Ment Health 34(4):363–375, 2007 17294124

Lamb HR: Deinstitutionalization and public policy, in American Psychiatry Since World War II: 1944–1994. Edited by Menninger RW, Nemiah JC. Washington, DC, American Psychiatric Press, 2000, pp 259–276

Lamb HR, Weinberger LE: The shift of psychiatric inpatient care from hospitals to jails and prisons. J Am Acad Psychiatry Law 33(4):529–534, 2005 16394231

Langeveld J, Bjørkly S, Auestad B, et al: Treatment and violent behavior in persons with first episode psychosis during a 10-year prospective follow-up study. Schizophr Res 156(2–3):272–276, 2014 24837683

Lasalvia A, Zoppei S, Bonetto C, et al: The role of experienced and anticipated discrimination in the lives of people with first-episode psychosis. Psychiatr Serv 65(8):1034–1040, 2014 24788167

Lawlor T, Grudzinskas AJ Jr, Geller JL, et al: A competency-based approach to managing violence with involuntary outpatient treatment. Adm Policy Ment Health 34(3):315–318, 2007 17115284

Lee S, Rothbard AB, Noll EL: Length of inpatient stay of persons with serious mental illness: effects of hospital and regional characteristics. Psychiatr Serv 63(9):889–895, 2012 22751995

Levin BL, Hanson A, Hennessey KD, et al: A public health approach to mental health services, in Mental Health Services: A Public Health Perspective, 3rd Edition. Edited by Levin BL, Hennessey KD, Petrila J. Oxford, UK, Oxford University Press, 2010, pp 5–11

Lowery W, Kindy K, Verma D: Distraught people, deadly results. The Washington Post, June 30, 2015. Available at: http://www.washingtonpost.com/sf/investigative/2015/06/30/distraught-people-deadly-results/. Accessed August 9, 2015.

Luciano A, Belstock J, Malmberg P, et al: Predictors of incarceration among urban adults with co-occurring severe mental illness and a substance use disorder. Psychiatr Serv 65(11):1325–1331, 2014 25022703

Mannix A: Court's psychiatric boarding ban will cost Washington tens of millions (The Today File). Seattle Times, August 14, 2014. Available at: http://blogs.seattletimes.com/today/2014/08/courts-psychiatric-boarding-ban-will-cost-washington-tens-of-millions. Accessed August 9, 2015.

Mark TL, Levit KR, Vandivort-Warren R, et al: Changes in U.S. spending on mental health and substance abuse treatment, 1986–2005, and implications for policy. Health Aff (Millwood) 30(2):284–292, 2011 21289350

Miller JE, Gordon SY, Shea P: Reducing the Burden of Mental Illness: The Role of Preventive Activities and Public Health Strategies. Alexandria, VA, National Association of State Mental Health Program Directors, 2014

Mojtabai R, Olfson M, Sampson NA, et al: Barriers to mental health treatment: results from the National Comorbidity Survey Replication. Psychol Med 41(8):1751–1761, 2011 21134315

Moran M: Patients score parity victories in two states: California. Psychiatric News, August 14, 2014a. Available at: http://psychnews.psychiatryonline.org/doi/full/10.1176/appi.pn.2014.8b6. Accessed August 9, 2015.

Moran M: Patients score parity victories in two states: New York. Psychiatric News, August 14, 2014b. Available at: http://psychnews.psychiatryonline.org/doi/full/10.1176/appi.pn.2014.8b11. Accessed August 9, 2015.

Morehart MFA: Office of the State Inspector General, Report to Governor McAuliffe and the General Assembly: Critical Incident Investigation, Bath County, Virginia, November 18, 2013. Richmond, VA, Office of the State Inspector General, 2014

Nicks BA, Manthey DM: The impact of psychiatric patient boarding in emergency departments. Emerg Med Int 2012:360308, 2012 22888437

NPR Staff: Nation's Jails Struggle With Mentally Ill Prisoners (audio report). Washington, DC, National Public Radio, September 4, 2011. Available at: http://www.npr.org/2011/09/04/140167676/nations-jails-struggle-with-mentally ill-prisoners. Accessed July 15, 2014.

Pandiani JA, Banks SM, Clements W, et al: Elevated risk of being charged with a crime for people with a severe and persistent mental illness. Justice Res Policy 2(2):19–36, 2000

Parks J, Radke AQ, Haupt MB: The Vital Role of State Psychiatric Hospitals. Alexandria, VA, National Association of State Mental Health Program Directors, Medical Directors Council, 2014

Pinals DA: Forensic services, public mental health policy, and financing: charting the course ahead. J Am Acad Psychiatry Law 42(1):7–19, 2014 24618515

President's New Freedom Commission on Mental Health: Achieving the Promise: Transforming Mental Health Care in America. Rockville, MD, Substance Abuse and Mental Health Services Administration, 2003

Prins SJ: Prevalence of mental illnesses in U.S. state prisons: a systematic review. Psychiatr Serv 65:862–872, 2014 24686574

Rosenberg RE, Mandell DS, Farmer JE, et al: Psychotropic medication use among children with autism spectrum disorders enrolled in a national registry, 2007–2008. J Autism Dev Disord 40(3):342–351, 2010 19806445

Rosenheck RA, Dennis D: Time-limited assertive community treatment for homeless persons with severe mental illness. Arch Gen Psychiatry 58(11):1073–1080, 2001 11695955

Roy L, Crocker AG, Nicholls TL, et al: Criminal behavior and victimization among homeless individuals with severe mental illness: a systematic review. Psychiatr Serv 65(6):739–750, 2014 24535245

Salinsky E, Loftis C: Shrinking Inpatient Psychiatric Capacity: Cause for Celebration or Concern? Washington, DC, National Health Policy Forum, George Washington University, 2007

Salkever D, Gibbons B, Ran X: Do comprehensive, coordinated, recovery-oriented services alter the pattern of use of treatment services? Mental health treatment study impacts on SSDI beneficiaries' use of inpatient, emergency, and crisis services. J Behav Health Serv Res 41(4):434–446, 2014 24481541

Santos F, Goode E: Police confront rising number of mentally ill suspects (U.S. section). New York Times, April 1, 2014. Available at: http://www.nytimes.com/2014/04/02/us/police-shootings-of-mentally-ill-suspects-are-on-the-upswing.html. Accessed August 4, 2015.

Sharfstein SS, Dickerson FB: Hospital psychiatry for the twenty-first century. Health Aff (Millwood) 28(3):685–688, 2009 19414876

Shirk C: Medicaid and Mental Health Services. Washington, DC, National Health Policy Forum, George Washington University, 2008

Shorter E: A History of Psychiatry: From the Era of the Asylum to the Age of Prozac. New York, Wiley, 1997

Shumway M, Alvidrez J, Leary M, et al: Impact of capacity reductions in acute public-sector inpatient psychiatric services. Psychiatr Serv 63(2):135–141, 2012 22302330

Singh JP, Grann M, Fazel S: A comparative study of violence risk assessment tools: a systematic review and metaregression analysis of 68 studies involving 25,980 participants. Clin Psychol Rev 31(3):499–513, 2011 21255891

Slade EP, Wissow LS, Davis M, et al: Medicaid lapses and low-income young adults' receipt of outpatient mental health care after an inpatient stay. Psychiatr Serv 65(4):454–460, 2014 24382558

Smith TE, Stein BD, Donahue SA, et al: Reengagement of high-need individuals with serious mental illness after discontinuation of services. Psychiatr Serv 65(11):1378–1380, 2014 25124372

Snowden L, Scheffler R, Zhang A: The impact of realignment on the client population in California's public mental health system. Adm Policy Ment Health 29(3):229–241, 2002 12033668

Steadman HJ, Osher FC, Robbins PC, et al: Prevalence of serious mental illness among jail inmates. Psychiatr Serv 60(6):761–765, 2009 19487344

Stone AA: Mental Health and Law: A System in Transition. New York, Jason Aronson, 1976

Substance Abuse and Mental Health Services Administration: Mental Health, United States, 2010. Rockville, MD, Substance Abuse and Mental Health Services Administration, 2012

Substance Abuse and Mental Health Services Administration: National Expenditures for Mental Health Services and Substance Abuse Treatment, 1986–2009. Rockville, MD, Substance Abuse and Mental Health Services Administration, 2013a

Substance Abuse and Mental Health Services Administration: Results from the 2012 National Survey on Drug Use and Health: Mental Health Findings. Rockville, MD, Substance Abuse and Mental Health Services Administration, 2013b

Swanson J, Gilbert AR: Mental illness and firearm violence. JAMA 306(9):930–931, author reply 931, 2011 21900130

Swanson JW, Swartz MS, Elbogen EB, et al: Effects of involuntary outpatient commitment on subjective quality of life in persons with severe mental illness. Behav Sci Law 21(4):473–491, 2003 12898503

Swanson JW, Frisman LK, Robertson AG, et al: Costs of criminal justice involvement among persons with serious mental illness in Connecticut. Psychiatr Serv 64:630–637, 2013 23494058

Teplin LA: Keeping the peace: police discretion and mentally ill persons. National Institute of Justice Journal (244):8–15, 2000

Teplin LA, McClelland GM, Abram KM, et al: Crime victimization in adults with severe mental illness: comparison with the National Crime Victimization Survey. Arch Gen Psychiatry 62(8):911–921, 2005 16061769

Thomas KC, Ellis AR, Konrad TR, et al: County-level estimates of mental health professional shortage in the United States. Psychiatr Serv 60(10):1323–1328, 2009 19797371

Torrey EF: American Psychosis: How the Federal Government Destroyed the Mental Illness Treatment System. New York, Oxford University Press, 2014

Torrey EF, Entsminger K, Geller JL, et al: The Shortage of Public Hospital Beds for Mentally Ill Persons. Arlington, VA, Treatment Advocacy Center, 2008

Torrey EF, Fuller DA, Geller MD, et al: No Room at the Inn: Trends and Consequences of Closing Public Psychiatric Hospitals, 2005–2010. Arlington, VA, Treatment Advocacy Center, 2012

Treatment Advocacy Center: Justifiable Homicides by Law Enforcement: What Is the Role of Mental Illness? A Joint Report by the Treatment Advocacy Center and National Sheriffs' Association. Arlington, VA, Treatment Advocacy Center, 2013a. Available at: http://tacreports.org/justifiable-homicides.

Treatment Advocacy Center: Trends in Hospital Bed Availability. Arlington, VA, Treatment Advocacy Center, 2013b

Truffer CJ, Klemm JD, Wolfe CJ, et al: 2013 Actuarial Report on the Financial Outlook for Medicaid. Washington, DC, Office of the Actuary, Centers for Medicare and Medicaid Services, U.S. Department of Health and Human Services, 2013

Turner T: Creigh Deeds: "No Reason to Believe There Would Be Any Violence." CNN.com, January 27, 2014. Available at: http://politicalticker.blogs.cnn.com/2014/01/27/creigh-deeds-no-reason-to-believe-there-would-be-any-violence/. Accessed August 18, 2014.

Witt K, van Dorn R, Fazel S: Risk factors for violence in psychosis: systematic review and meta-regression analysis of 110 studies. PLoS ONE 8(2):e55942, 2013 23418482

Witters D: Uninsured rate drops more in states embracing health law. Gallup Well-Being, August 16, 2014. Available at: http://www.gallup.com/poll/168539/uninsured-rates-drop-states-embracing-health-law.aspx. Accessed August 9, 2015.

PART II

Moving Forward

9

Structured Violence Risk Assessment

Implications for Preventing Gun Violence

Daniel C. Murrie, Ph.D.

Common Misperceptions

- ☒ People who will perpetrate gun violence can be identified through simple personality or behavioral "profiles."
- ☒ Competent mental health professionals have the ability to accurately predict acts of gun violence among people with mental illness.
- ☒ Structured violence risk assessment instruments are not useful in assessing the risk of gun violence in routine clinical practice.

Evidence-Based Facts

- ☑ No "profile," "checklist," or set of "warning signs" is necessary or sufficient to identify individuals, with or without mental illness, who are likely to commit acts of gun violence.
- ☑ No matter how competent, mental health professionals have no psychological tests or means to perfectly predict gun violence among people with or without mental illness.

☑ Standard, empirically supported, structured approaches to violence risk assessment are appropriate when considering the risk of violence, including gun violence, among people with or without mental illness.

Gun violence is a single outcome that results from innumerable causes and influences. As detailed throughout this text, these influences range from broad cultural, social, legal, and contextual factors to narrow situational, interpersonal, and individual factors. Mental illness plays only a small role in the broad public health problem of criminal violence, and when people with mental illness commit violence, they are not uniquely likely to use guns (Fazel and Grann 2006; Swanson 1994; Van Dorn et al. 2012).

Nevertheless, practicing mental health clinicians are often placed in positions where they must form an opinion about an individual's risk of violence, including gun violence. Concerns about violence can emerge over the course of treating a patient, or they may be the explicit focus of a referral, such as when clinicians are asked to make recommendations regarding hospitalization or civil commitment. In fact, state laws increasingly task mental health clinicians with various duties intended to reduce the likelihood of gun violence; these duties may include reporting a patient's gun possession to law enforcement or assessing the potential risk of a patient who is petitioning to have firearm ownership privileges restored after psychiatric hospitalization (Norris et al. 2006).

Perhaps because of highly publicized tragedies or a tendency to consider gun violence as distinct from other forms of violence, there is no shortage of misunderstandings and disagreements around assessing risk for gun violence. As the misperceptions about gun violence listed above (and in other chapters) demonstrate, the public appears understandably eager for clinicians to predict gun violence, perhaps on the basis of the "profile" of a prototypical gun violence perpetrator. In fact, however, no such profile exists, and *there is no violence risk assessment tool or strategy that is specific to gun violence.*

Fortunately, reducing gun violence, even the small proportion of gun violence that involves mental illness, does not depend on perfectly predicting gun violence. Nor does it require developing risk assessment approaches that are somehow unique to gun violence. Rather, mental health professionals attempting to assess and reduce the risk of gun violence among higher-risk individuals, with or without mental illness, can probably best do so by implementing the best practices from violence risk assessment and related fields.

A well-conducted violence risk assessment informs intervention, because the goal of violence risk assessment is *prevention,* not prediction. The best practices, and indeed the broad field of violence risk assessment, have advanced dramatically over the past several decades and have much to contribute to current efforts to reduce gun violence. Currently, these practices de-emphasize *prediction* of violence and instead emphasize the *assessment of violence risk.* The latter implies an ongoing process that considers the risks attributable to an individual, the environment, and their interaction, and recognizes that this risk will vary over time and across contexts.

Within the broad field of violence risk assessment, *structured approaches to violence risk assessment* may offer particularly practical contributions for identifying people, with or without mental illness, who are at higher risk for violence and for monitoring their risk over time. Structured violence risk assessment tools are often used by the justice system and by clinicians who perform violence risk assessments in correctional and forensic psychiatric contexts. These tools, however, are appropriate for clinicians in nearly all clinical contexts and for assessing risk in individuals whether or not they have symptoms of mental illness. Of course, even the best approaches to structured violence risk assessment will require individualized clinical judgment and case-specific practical interventions. To understand the contributions that structured violence risk assessment can—and cannot—make to gun violence prevention, it is worth considering some examples of these approaches and their history.

Violence Risk Assessment: A Brief History

Although violence risk assessment has assumed an increasingly important role in mental health and criminal justice contexts (Buchanan et al. 2012; Skeem and Monahan 2011), mental health clinicians have long been called on to perform violence risk assessments in a variety of contexts, ranging from routine clinical care to legal decisions about civil commitment or even death penalty sentencing (Shah 1975, 1981). Until at least the 1980s, clinicians typically answered questions about risk in a dichotomous fashion, just as the legal system requested (Heilbrun 2009). Clinicians categorized patients as either "dangerous" or "not dangerous," and the legal system responded accordingly. For example, individuals with mental illness identified as dangerous faced civil commitment, whereas those identified as not dangerous received no medical or legal interventions.

Clinicians providing these dangerousness assessments usually did so on the basis of unguided or unstructured clinical judgment, formulating opinions based on their training, experience, theories, or intuition (Monahan 2008). Perhaps not surprisingly, early research suggested that clinicians making these all-or-none dangerousness predictions tended to be wrong more often than not (Monahan 1981). Nevertheless, even as the limitations of popular approaches to "dangerousness prediction" became clear, the courts maintained that mental health clinicians could—and in some cases *must*—offer predictions regarding violence (*Barefoot v. Estelle* 463 U.S. 880, 1983; *Schall v. Martin* 467 U.S. 253, 1984; *Tarasoff v. Regents of the University of California* 17 Cal. 3d 425, 1976).

Faced with ongoing demands for violence risk assessment—alongside clear evidence of weaknesses in violence risk assessment practice—scholars began to work toward making violence predictions more empirically rigorous and ethically defensible (see Conroy and Murrie 2007 for a detailed history of the violence risk assessment field). As research progressed and violence was increasingly recognized as a public health concern (Douglas and Webster 1999; Mercy and O'Carroll 1988), scholars increasingly emphasized what is now commonly understood: that violence risk is not a fixed personal trait but rather the product of a complex interaction of personal and contextual factors that varies over time.

Researchers increasingly documented risk factors for violence, which included both characteristics of people (e.g., substance abuse, psychopathic personality) and characteristics of their context (e.g., high-crime neighborhoods). The paradigm began to shift from the dichotomous prediction of a violent act, or "dangerousness prediction," to an assessment of the degree of violence risk, or "risk assessment" (Heilbrun 2009). The latter acknowledged that clinicians could not perfectly predict or eliminate the possibility of future violence, although they could reasonably assess the degree of risk for future violence, to guide the degree of intervention applied. Thus, risk assessment generally implies an ongoing process and not simply a single, one-time definitive conclusion (as dangerousness prediction did).

Inasmuch as the mental health field has reached a generally accepted definition of *risk assessment,* it is probably best summarized by Kraemer et al. (1997) as "the process of using risk factors to estimate the likelihood (i.e., probability) of an outcome occurring in a population" (p. 340). Risk factors are those that precede a particular outcome, so they are related and potentially useful for assessing risk, although they do not necessarily *cause* the outcome.

Violence Risk Assessment: Efforts to Increase Structure

Unstructured Assessment Approaches

The primary professional approach to violence risk assessment has, at least historically, been unstructured clinical judgment. As Monahan (2008) explained,

> Unstructured risk assessment relies on the subjective judgment of professionally educated people who are experienced at making predictive judgments; in the case of violence, these typically include psychiatrists, psychologists, and social workers. In unstructured assessment, risk factors are selected and measured based on the mental health professional's theoretical orientation and prior clinical experience. What these risk factors are, or how they are measured, might vary from case to case depending on which seem most relevant to the professional doing the assessment. At the conclusion of the assessment, risk factors are

> combined in an intuitive or holistic manner to generate an overall professional opinion about a given individual's level of violence risk. (p. 19)

Although unstructured clinical judgment provides the flexibility to consider case-specific information, the process is not necessarily transparent, objective, accurate, or reliable across clinicians (Lidz et al. 1993; Monahan 1981, 2008). Indeed, unstructured approaches have appeared particularly ineffective when contrasted with the highly structured approach that has traditionally been called "actuarial" (also known as mechanical, statistical, or mathematical). Actuarial approaches define—in advance of any assessment—which data should be considered and what algorithm should be used to weigh and combine that data, leading to a fixed conclusion about risk (see Grove and Meehl 1996; Meehl 1954). Stated differently, an actuarial method is a formal approach that "uses an equation, a formula, a graph, or an actuarial table to arrive at a probability, or expected value, of some outcome" (Grove and Meehl 1996, p. 294). Perhaps the most familiar examples of actuarial approaches, for most people, are the algorithms insurance companies use to set insurance rates.

Following Paul Meehl's (1954) influential distinction between so-called clinical and actuarial models of prediction, researchers have repeatedly compared the unstructured-clinical-judgment approach to violence risk assessment with actuarial approaches and concluded that actuarial approaches are far superior (Dawes et al. 1989; Grove and Meehl 1996; Grove et al. 2000; Hanson and Morton-Bourgon 2009). For example, a comprehensive meta-analysis comparing clinical and actuarial prediction across many disciplines concluded that "one area in which the statistical method is most clearly superior to the clinical approach is the prediction of violence" (Ægisdóttir et al. 2006, p. 368).

Actuarial Assessment Approaches

Undoubtedly, actuarial approaches improve on the poor reliability and certain other problems that hamper unstructured clinical assessments. Most actuarial measures are easy-to-use tools, developed from a specific data set, that allow users to code—for a particular individual—certain clearly defined risk factors that were measured in the original data set and then examine the frequency of a particular outcome (e.g., violence) among individuals in the data set with the same risk factors or with the same number of identified risk factors. After using a strict actuarial method, a clinician offers a structured conclusion such as "Mr. Smith has X risk factors, making him similar to group Y in the instrument-development sample, of whom 27% went on to commit violence. Thus, Mr. Smith's risk for violence is approximately 27%." The perceived objectivity of actuarial approaches, along with the supportive research, has been sufficiently compelling that some scholars argue it is inappropriate to perform a violence risk assessment in any manner *other than* relying solely on an actuarial measure (e.g., Quinsey et al. 2006). Indeed, the strongest proponents of actuarial approaches have argued, "What we are advising is not the *addition* of actuarial methods to existing practice, but rather the *replacement* of existing practice with actuarial methods" (Quinsey et al. 2006, p. 197).

Most clinicians in routine practice appear reluctant, however, to adopt actuarial violence risk assessment instruments (Elbogen et al. 2002; Hilton et al. 2006; Monahan 2008; Tolman and Mullendore 2003), perhaps for understandable reasons. Some limitations of actuarial risk assessment measures, as summarized by Blanchard et al. (in press), include the following:

- Actuarial measures consider a small set of research-derived risk factors but do not allow the flexibility to consider the unique risk factors that may appear most salient in a particular case.
- The research-derived risk factors most relevant in an actuarial instrument development sample may not be as predictive in other contexts. In other words, the instrument may not generalize well.
- Although actuarial instruments may be excellent at addressing risk at the aggregate level, determining how to apply group estimates to individual cases is not always clear.
- Actuarial instruments tend to emphasize static variables rather than the dynamic variables that can be the focus of intervention.
- Because actuarial instruments are solely predictive, they have limited utility for guiding specific interventions or risk management strategies.

There may be more subtle reasons why clinicians have not adopted actuarial measures more widely; many advocates of actuarial instruments speculate that psychiatrists and psychologists "fear the loss of prestige in their clinical role" (Hilton et al. 2006, p. 406) if they rely completely on actuarial measures. However, many clinicians would counter that relying completely on actuarial measures would prove insufficient for certain risk-related questions, such as those requiring ongoing monitoring and intervention.

"Structured Professional Judgment" Approaches

Despite the historical emphasis on pitting clinical judgment against actuarial methods, this dichotomy does not accurately reflect the current range of violence risk assessment approaches available to clinicians (Monahan 2008). Rather, many modern violence risk assessment measures reflect an approach labeled *structured professional judgment* (SPJ; Blanchard et al., in press; Webster et al. 1997), intended to capture the strengths but minimize the weaknesses of both actuarial *and* clinical judgment approaches. Tools based on the SPJ model delineate research-identified risk factors (just as actuarial measures do) but rely on the clinician's judgment to gather, weigh, and combine these risk factors into a final risk formulation. Thus, like actuarial assessments, they tend to be more reliable, transparent, and accurate than unstructured assessment, but unlike actuarial measures, they also allow clinicians the flexibility to consider factors beyond the instrument and/or weigh some factors as more important than others (hence invoking clinical judgment).

Generally, SPJ instruments comprise 1) a list of historical (static and unchangeable) and dynamic (current, changing, and changeable) risk factors to consider and 2) a scheme for coding these factors (usually as absent, partially present, or present). SPJ instrument manuals usually provide recommendations for collecting information, determining final opinions, and communicating these opinions about violence risk. By listing predetermined, research-identified risk factors to consider in every case, SPJ approaches ensure some empirical basis. However, by encouraging users to incorporate additional case-specific risk factors and use their judgment to weigh each risk factor, SPJ approaches prioritize clinical judgment. Final opinions about risk are not determined solely by adding the risk factors; clinicians may conclude for qualitative reasons that actual risk is higher or lower than a simple tally of risk factors would suggest (Douglas et al. 2013; Webster et al. 1997). Likewise, final risk opinions are not communicated numerically but are more often conceptualized and communicated in a categorical manner (e.g., low, moderate, or high risk) to reflect the clinician's degree of concern about future violence (Blanchard et al., in press).

Continuum of Structure Among Violence Risk Assessment Approaches

Given the current breadth of approaches to violence risk assessment, particularly since the development of SPJ approaches, authorities have emphasized that violence risk assessment technology no longer involves a dichotomous choice between clinical or actuarial approaches (Monahan 2008; Monahan and Skeem 2014). Rather, "[t]he risk assessment process now exists on a *continuum of rule-based structure,* with completely unstructured (clinical) assessment occupying one pole of the continuum, completely structured (actuarial) assessment occupying the other pole, and several forms of partially structured assessment lying between the two" (Skeem and Monahan 2011, p. 39).

Current instruments can be categorized by the degree to which they structure four key components, or steps, of the risk assessment process: 1) identifying risk factors, 2) measuring or scoring the risk factors, 3) combining risk factors, and 4) producing a final risk estimate (Monahan 2008; Monahan and Skeem 2014; Skeem and Monahan 2011). Thus, purely unstructured approaches based on clinical intuition structure *none* of these components. A written list of research-identified risk factors, such as those often provided in medical textbooks, serves as a memory aid, which thereby adds structure to the first step but not to the subsequent ones. Popular SPJ approaches such as the Historical Clinical Risk Management–20 (HCR-20) structure two of these four components (i.e., identifying risk factors and scoring the risk factors). At the far end of the continuum, the highly structured, purely actuarial measures—of which the Violence Risk Appraisal Guide (VRAG; Quinsey et al. 1998, 2006) is probably the most popular example—structure all four components of the process: they identify risk factors, guide scoring, combine them mathematically, and produce a final numerical risk estimate.

Structured Violence Risk Assessments: Selected Instruments

Recent surveys reveal that violence risk assessments are quite common in the United States and internationally (Singh et al. 2014). Approximately half of these assessments are facilitated by a structured violence risk assessment instrument (Singh et al. 2014). Indeed, there appear to be at least 200 formal or published violence risk assessment tools in use internationally, as well as another 200 unpublished instruments that were developed by individuals or institutions (Singh et al. 2014). A review of every instrument is beyond the scope of this chapter, and not every instrument is appropriate for use. The assessments discussed in this section are illustrative examples of the most well-developed and well-researched instruments, arranged as they fall along the "continuum of rule-based structure" (Skeem and Monahan 2011).

Historical Clinical Risk Management–20

The HCR-20 (Webster et al. 1997), now in its third version (HCR-20V3; Douglas et al. 2013), is the most widely used and researched violence risk assessment approach using the SPJ model. Indeed, it is probably the most widely used violence risk assessment instrument of any sort (Hurducas et al. 2014; Singh et al. 2014); it has been translated into many languages and is used routinely in clinical, correctional, and forensic systems throughout the world (Douglas et al. 2013). The HCR-20 was developed for use with adult men or women—particularly civil psychiatric patients, forensic psychiatric patients, and criminal offenders—to assess risk of violence, defined in the most recent manual as the "actual, attempted, or threatened infliction of bodily harm on another person" (Douglas et al. 2013, p. 36).

The HCR-20 comprises 20 risk factors grouped according to three domains: Historical (past), Clinical (present state), and Risk Management (future planning). The Historical scale includes 10 historical risk factors addressing the individual's personality, adjustment, experiences, behavior, and mental disorder. The Clinical scale includes five dynamic risk factors related to current insight, ideation, symptoms, and stability. Finally, the Risk Management scale includes five dynamic risk factors related to future context, stress, support, and services. Clinicians rate each item as present, possibly/partially present, or absent.

A tremendous body of literature supports the utility of the HCR-20 as applied across numerous countries and clinical contexts; indeed, the HCR-20V3 manual mentions 200 studies from at least 35 countries (Douglas et al. 2013). These studies tend to support the instrument's reliability (across raters) and predictive validity (with respect to predicting violent outcomes). Regarding interrater reliability, most studies have found intraclass correlation coefficients (which represent rater agreement) in the good to excellent range for most HCR-20 scales (Douglas and Reeves 2010), although reliability tends to be stronger for the Historical and Clinical scales and weaker for the Risk Management scale and the final risk judgments. Thus, clinicians tend to reach similar but not identical conclusions using the instrument. Regarding predictive validity, the literature is too vast to review succinctly. Perhaps the strongest support comes from a comprehensive meta-analysis (Guy 2008) and several independent meta-analyses that compared various instruments (e.g., Campbell et al. 2009; Fazel et al. 2012; Singh et al. 2011) and concluded that the HCR-20 tended to perform as well as other risk assessment instruments.

Classification of Violence Risk

The Classification of Violence Risk (COVR; Monahan et al. 2005, 2006) is a structured risk assessment instrument developed with data from the seminal MacArthur Violence Risk Assessment Study (Monahan et al. 2001). This extensive study assessed more than 1,000 civil psychiatric patients, examined over 100 potential risk factors, and then followed the patients after hospital discharge for 20 weeks in the community, documenting their rates and types of violence. The study provided much of the field's best data regarding mental disorder and violence, and eventually led to the development of the COVR.

Unlike other instruments, the COVR is an interactive computer software program that guides the clinician through a chart review and brief patient interview necessary to measure 40 risk factors and calculate a risk estimate following an "iterative classification tree" methodology (Monahan 2010; Monahan et al. 2005). Examinees are asked initial questions (up to 27, depending on their responses) and directed to subsequent questions contingent on their answers. Thus, the COVR provides a structure for identifying, scoring, and combining risk factors (Monahan 2010). Finally, the COVR generates a report that places the examinee's violence risk into one of five categories based on the violence rates among subsamples of patients in the MacArthur study (e.g., a 1% rate of violence in the lowest-risk subsample and a 76% rate of violence in the highest-risk subsample).

Nevertheless, the authors emphasize that the clinician using the instrument, not the instrument itself, is responsible for the final risk estimate. Thus, the clinician should begin with the instrument-generated violence risk category but then also consider the possibility of any other factors (external to the instrument) that may raise or lower risk, before offering a final risk estimate and developing a risk management plan. In this regard, the COVR structures three stages of the risk assessment process—namely, identifying, measuring, and combining risk factors—but not the fourth step of producing the final risk estimate (Monahan 2008; Skeem and Monahan 2011).

The COVR may appear to have less empirical support than some other popular instruments, if *support* is defined solely by counting publications. However, the empirical foundations of the COVR are among the strongest of any risk assessment instrument. The development process, methodology, and analytic strategy were unusually sophisticated (see Monahan et al. 2005, 2006). As mentioned previously in this section, the measure was derived from the largest and best-designed study of violence and mental disorder to date, the MacArthur Violence Risk Assessment Study (Monahan et al. 2001; Steadman et al. 1998), and researchers then cross-validated the measure in a new sample (Monahan et al. 2005). In the first derivation sample, the predictive accuracy of the tool was remarkably strong (area under the curve [AUC] value=0.88), particularly compared with the predictive accuracies found in studies of other risk measures. As is typically the case when instruments are applied in new contexts, accuracy in the cross-validation sample was somewhat lower (AUCs of 0.63–0.70; Monahan et al. 2005). Nevertheless, the COVR appears as effective as other well-established violence risk assessment measures.

Violence Risk Appraisal Guide

The VRAG (Quinsey et al. 1998, 2006) is a 12-item actuarial instrument developed through an extensive program of research with mentally ill offenders in Canada. Researchers coded dozens of potential risk factors from the institutional files of a maximum-security forensic psychiatric hospital, then followed patient outcomes for an average of 7 years after release, documenting new criminal charges for violence (or return to the hospital for similarly violent behavior). The research resulted in an instrument that allows evaluators to code 12 risk factors, which are then statistically weighted and summed to produce an overall estimate of violence risk. This instrument-produced estimate *must* be the only final risk estimate; the instrument authors warn that "clinical judgment is too poor to risk contaminating" an objective actuarial estimate (Quinsey et al. 2006, p. 197; see also Rice and Harris 2005). In this regard, the VRAG structures all four stages of the risk assessment process—namely, identifying, measuring, and combining risk factors, then producing the final risk estimate (Skeem and Monahan 2011).

The VRAG has extensive research support, primarily (though not exclusively) from the instrument authors. Interrater reliability is strong (0.90), suggesting that different trained raters assign similar scores to the same examinee (Harris et al. 2002, 2003). Predictive validity has been fairly strong in replication samples that are similar to those on which the instrument was developed (with an average AUC value of 0.72 for the prediction of violence recidivism; Rice and Harris 2005), indicating that higher VRAG scores are associated with higher risk of future violence (Harris et al. 2002).

Caveat: Some Structured Violence Risk Assessment Instruments Lack Empirical Support

The three structured violence risk assessments just described are probably the most popular and well-researched violence risk assessment instruments, and each is an exemplar of instruments that structure fewer (i.e., the HCR-20), more (i.e., the COVR), or all (i.e., the VRAG) components of the risk assessment process. These are certainly not the only instruments in regular use, and a few others are similarly well designed and have emerging research support (for reviews see Blanchard et al., in press; Otto and Douglas 2010). However, it is important to emphasize that the discussion of structured violence risk assessment instruments in this chapter refers *only* to such measures that have been well designed and for which supporting research is easily accessible in peer-reviewed scientific literature.

This distinction between instruments with empirical support and those that lack such support is important. Since a series of widely publicized school shootings in the late 1990s, there has been no shortage of checklists, guidelines, or even computerized software that developers have marketed for purposes of assessing violence risk, particularly the risk of mass violence or gun violence. Like the more empirically supported instruments, these unsupported instruments fall along a continuum of structure, with some structuring fewer aspects of the assessment process and some structuring more.

At the least structured end of the continuum are popular lists of "warning signs" or "profiles" of individuals putatively likely to commit violence, based on characteristics shared by perpetrators of mass homicides. These profiles, often marketed as simple checklists, tend to include characteristics such as social isolation, depression, anger, recent stress, and similar common features. These characteristics may have been common among many (but not all) perpetrators of highly publicized homicides, and some may have some degree of empirical support. Nevertheless, these characteristics, even when grouped together, are commonplace in the general population and certainly are not specific to individuals at risk for gun violence. Therefore, such checklists are so broad as to be useless or even misleading. Indeed, the Federal Bureau of Investigation and other authorities tend to warn against using such checklists, profiles, and warning signs (O'Toole 1999).

At the other end of the spectrum are computer-based instruments or tools that appear highly structured, sophisticated, and specific to serious violence, but whose developers often treat the underlying data and algorithms as proprietary or confidential, and do not share research that can be examined by others. Thus, without an opportunity for public or peer review by qualified professionals other than the instrument developers, it becomes impossible to gauge the accuracy or utility of such instruments, despite claims of empirical rigor.

Thus, any discussion of empirically supported structured violence risk approaches (including the studies comparing risk approaches, as described in the following sections of this chapter) must exclude these unstudied approaches, whether they are simple popular checklists or ostensibly sophisticated computerized programs from private companies. Likewise, any discussion of structured violence risk assessment and gun violence must acknowledge that none of the best-developed instruments (and certainly none of the unstudied instruments) have any research base detailing the relationship between instrument scores and gun violence as distinct from other forms of violence.

Structured Violence Risk Assessment Tools in Practice: Key Considerations

Despite the caveats, structured assessment tools are among the most significant advances in violence risk assessment. Therefore, any discussion of violence risk assessment in practice, including discussions specific to gun violence, will need to consider the potential contributions of these tools to helping mental health professionals identify individuals at high risk of committing violence, including gun violence.

No Single Structured Violence Risk Assessment Is Always Best

No credible argument or data are available demonstrating that completely unstructured, unguided clinical judgment is better than more structured approaches. Research has consistently demonstrated that structured risk assessment approaches are more accurate than entirely unstructured approaches (Ægisdóttir et al. 2006; Grove et al. 2000; Hanson and Morton-Bourgon 2009). However, much room remains for reasonable disagreement about *which* structured approach (i.e., which instrument, tool, or type of tool) is most accurate.

Indeed, the literature is flush with such disagreement (Harris and Rice 2007; Hilton et al. 2006) as well as efforts to shed light on these disagreements with qualitative (e.g., Heilbrun et al. 2010) and quantitative (e.g., Singh et al. 2011) reviews.

Although a comprehensive review of such literature is beyond the scope of this chapter, a fair summary is that *no single structured violence risk assessment tool consistently outperforms all others.* One of the most compelling comparisons was a meta-analysis of 28 original studies that allowed for comparison of nine different risk assessment tools, including the popular HCR-20 and VRAG (Yang et al. 2010). After conducting careful analyses controlling for study features, the authors concluded, "All 9 tools and their subscales predicted violence at about the same moderate level of predictive accuracy.... If the intention is only to predict future violence, then the 9 tools are essentially interchangeable" (Yang et al. 2010, p. 740). Likewise, other independent meta-analyses that compared various instruments (e.g., Campbell et al. 2009; Fazel et al. 2012; Singh et al. 2011) failed to find substantial differences among popular violence risk assessment instruments developed for adults.

Why might such apparently different instruments perform so similarly? One innovative study compared four popular violence risk measures with four new "instruments" that were randomly generated from a pool of test items pulled from the four popular measures (Kroner et al. 2005). *None* of the four popular measures predicted criminal recidivism (including violence) significantly better than the four randomly generated instruments. The authors concluded that no instrument was sufficiently unique to outperform all others. Rather, most of the well-developed and well-validated measures assess similar common factors related to risk, and none of them do so in ways that are uniquely more accurate than others.

All Structured Violence Risk Assessment Approaches Have Limitations

On the one hand, using structured violence risk assessment tools appears to be an obvious evidence-based best practice. A variety of tools are available that perform demonstrably better than chance, and better than unstructured clinical judgment. As Heilbrun (2009) summarized, "The development of such specialized [violence risk assessment] tools has been one of the most important influences in promoting evidence-based practice in this area. Using such a specialized tool is clearly consistent with best practice" (p. 123). Indeed, a clinician may be hard-pressed to justify *not* using a structured instrument for violence risk assessment when assessing an examinee from a population and context for which such instruments have been developed; this would include most civil and forensic psychiatric patients.

On the other hand, *no* structured violence risk assessment instrument predicts violence with anywhere near perfect accuracy. Nearly all qualitative reviews conclude that predictive accuracy tends to be better than chance, but also far below perfect. Effect sizes (i.e., measures that describe the magnitude of a difference between groups, allowing researchers to quantify outcomes using a standard metric) for the prediction of violent outcomes tend to fall in the medium range (Campbell et al. 2009; Yang et al. 2010). These values are roughly similar to those for some widely used diagnostic and prognostic tools in medicine, but would still entail considerable prediction error in individual cases (Singh et al. 2011). Indeed, some scholars have argued that the margins of error (confidence intervals, in statistical prediction terms) surrounding individual risk assessments are so wide that risk instrument results for individuals are essentially meaningless (Cooke and Michie 2010; Hart et al. 2007). Although this extreme conclusion has faced vigorous rebuttal (e.g., Hanson and Howard 2010; Harris and Rice 2007; Mossman and Sellke 2007) and appears to reflect a minority viewpoint, it underscores the ongoing controversy regarding how risk instrument scores are best used (see Heilbrun et al. 2009).

Of course, risk assessment, by definition, involves drawing cautious inferences about an uncertain future, which will inevitably include unknowable contingencies. Violence is the outcome of many complex and interacting factors, differing across individuals and contexts, which can never be fully captured by any single instrument (or single clinical evaluation). For this reason, it seems unlikely that any significant advances will occur in the accuracy of structured violence risk measures that take them beyond this better-than-chance but far-from-perfect prediction. Indeed, many scholars suspect that there is a "sound barrier" (Menzies et al. 1985), "glass-ceiling effect" (Coid et al. 2011), or "ceiling on the accuracy that can be expected" (Buchanan 2008) from any future risk measures.

The Value of Structured Violence Risk Assessments Lies in Prevention, Not Prediction

If structured violence risk assessment tools are inevitably limited to better-than-chance but less-than-perfect accuracy, do they have a role in reducing gun violence? Absolutely. The research on structured violence risk assessment instruments has, for understandable and appropriate reasons, explored their utility almost exclusively in terms of predictive accuracy. Following study participants to gauge which ones went on to commit violence is probably the most straightforward way to examine the relationship between instrument scores and violence, and doing so provides a meaningful metric for a risk instrument's accuracy.

Most clinicians, however, are concerned more with violence *prevention* than with violence *prediction*. In other words, clinical duties rarely require a single-instance violence prediction, and more often require some sort of planning, monitoring, or intervention to prevent violence. Fortunately, "prevention does not require prediction of a specific individual's behavior" (American Psychological Association 2013, p. 5).

To be clear, clinicians do face a *few* tasks that appear to call for prediction. The most common scenarios involve civil commitment laws, in which the legal system considers whether an individual's risk of harming self or others is significant enough to warrant involuntary hospitalization as an intervention to protect the safety of the potential patient or others (see Chapter 7, "Mental Illness, Dangerousness, and Involuntary Commitment"). In this context, clinicians are usually asked to offer a single-point-in-time assessment of the patient's risk of violence in the near future, absent intervention (essentially a prediction). The court or other administrative body then decides whether that likelihood of violence is high enough to justify involuntary hospitalization. This is one of a few instances in which the legal context requires a violence risk assessment that is more similar to a single prediction than an ongoing risk management plan (Heilbrun 1997).

Nevertheless, most clinical roles do *not* require a clinician to *predict* that a particular patient will commit violence. Rather, most clinical roles require clinicians 1) to formulate an initial violence risk assessment of each individual so that clinicians can provide more risk management interventions to individuals at relatively higher risk of violence and fewer to those at lower risk and 2) to monitor an individual's risk, with plans to increase violence risk management strategies if and when an individual's risk appears to increase. Will every individual whom clinicians identify as being at high risk go on to commit gun violence? Certainly not. Only a small minority of any clinical population would progress to commit serious violence, although a greater proportion may commit minor violence or self-harm (Monahan et al. 2001; Steadman et al. 1998). However, by regularly assessing violence risk and then intervening in a manner proportional to risk, clinicians will probably have prevented some (unknown and unknowable) degree of violence that might have otherwise occurred. Just as importantly, clinicians will have helped, in more general ways, the most troubled individuals in their care.

Using Structured Violence Risk Assessment Tools to Inform Risk Status and Risk State

To describe the complexity of violence risk, Douglas and Skeem (2005) distinguished between risk status and risk state. Generally, *risk status* involves a person's risk of violent behavior relative to others in a particular population or context. Risk status is informed by the base rates of violence in the relevant population, and well-known, empirically supported risk factors drawn from epidemiological research. These risk factors tend to be more enduring (i.e., fixed, historical, unchanging) characteristics such as history of violence, early onset of violence, and history of substance abuse. In contrast, *risk state* refers to a person's current violence risk compared with his or her own risk at baseline or at another point in time. In other words, risk state involves an "individual's propensity to become involved in violence at a given time, based on particular changes in biological, psychological, and social variables in his or her life" (Douglas and Skeem 2005, p. 349; see also Skeem and Mulvey 2002).

Violence prevention often requires considering both risk status and risk state. The former is crucial to understanding an individual's risk relative to others, and the latter is crucial to understanding changes in risk over time. Either may be appropriately assessed using structured violence risk assessment tools. However, the purposes of the assessment will determine whether the clinician prioritizes risk status, risk state, or both. These priorities, as well as the context of the assessment, will determine which violence risk assessment measure is most appropriate.

Structured Violence Risk Assessment Tools Applied to Individuals Without Mental Illness

As emphasized throughout this text, gun violence is not uniquely or strongly associated with mental illness. Therefore, any reasonable approach to violence risk assessment must be developed to consider the vast majority of risk factors that do not relate to mental illness but that occur among the many potentially violent individuals who do not manifest mental illness. Furthermore, "a person with serious mental illness—*even one that bears a causal relationship to violence*—may have a high (or low) overall likelihood of violent recidivism for reasons independent of their illness" (Monahan and Steadman 2012, p. 247). Thus, structured violence risk assessment tools help clinicians—who, by training, are prone to focus primarily on psychiatric symptoms—avoid an overemphasis on psychiatric symptoms and additionally consider the much broader range of (nonpsychiatric) risk factors for violence. Well-developed violence risk assessment tools are applicable to individuals with and without mental illness.

Selecting and Using Structured Violence Risk Assessment Tools

Among the several well-researched and widely accessible violence risk assessment measures, there appears to be no single "best pick" in terms of consistently predicting violence more *accurately* than the others (Fazel et al. 2012; Yang et al. 2010). Thus, clinicians and systems should probably choose well-validated tools that best fit the practicalities of their context and clinical needs. Because clinicians assess violence risk in a variety of contexts, among a variety of examinees, for a variety of reasons, the best instrument for one violence risk assessment task may not be the best selection for another.

Delineating Groups for Differential Policies, Interventions, or Services

Harris (2006) emphasized that the relative superiority of any particular risk assessment method depends on the questions asked. He concluded that if the question involves the "aggregated long-term risk posed by a group of individuals [then] actuarial instruments almost certainly provide the most valid means of assessing such risk" (p. 39). Indeed, using actuarial approaches to subdivide groups into those at relatively higher or lower risk is one of the least controversial and most empirically supported applications of violence risk assessment tools (Heilbrun et al. 2009).

Many systems use actuarial tools in just this manner, to decide which groups of patients or offenders are likely to warrant the most intensive oversight. Correctional departments sometimes must decide which offenders should exit prison to more intensive versus less intensive parole conditions or supervision arrangements. For example, Virginia requires by statute that the state department of corrections screen all sex offenders on a popular actuarial risk measure specific to *sexual* violence in order to identify those who warrant further clinical evaluation for potential commitment under sex offender civil commitment laws (Virginia Code Ann. § 37.2-903). More specific to mental health services, large psychiatric facilities or community agencies may benefit, at certain stages, from using actuarial measures to screen patients into low-, medium-, or high-risk groups.

Most highly structured actuarial instruments have several advantages that make them ideal for these kinds of grouping or screening tasks. These tools tend to list straightforward items, which require less subjective clinical judgment to score. They can thus be scored more objectively, and scored by staff other than doctoral-level psychologists and psychiatrists. Screening with these measures is often more efficient, and may be perceived as less arbitrary, than more intensive clinical assessments. Indeed, these tools are used at many points in the criminal justice system, for offenders with or without mental illness, to inform risk-related decisions such as assigning a security or custody level, granting bail or bond, requiring supervision on release, and related issues.

Thus, the screening or group-delineation function of actuarial assessments may be appropriate for efficiently estimating risk status (i.e., an individual's general risk level compared to others) so as to separate groups of much-higher-risk or much-lower-risk individuals, who warrant greater or lesser services. Screening with actuarial instruments is particularly appropriate to inform single-point-in-time assessments for which the goal is optimal long-term accuracy, as opposed to risk assessments performed to provide ongoing monitoring of risk state (i.e., individual variation in risk over time). When ongoing assessment is necessary for some portion of the population, actuarial measures may help efficiently screen large groups of individuals to identify those who are likely to warrant more intensive assessment or monitoring. Conversely, actuarial measures of risk status may be useful to "screen out" those individuals who are at such low risk as to warrant no further assessment.

With respect to firearm policies in particular, actuarial measures may have a place in some of the wide-scale policies governing firearm access. States have increasingly passed laws that attempt to restrict those with mental illness (defined in various ways, depending on the jurisdiction and policy) from owning or purchasing handguns (Norris et al. 2006). These laws vary tremendously, and a review of them is well beyond the scope of this chapter (see Norris et al. 2006; Simpson 2007; Swanson et al. 2013), so it is not feasible to speak in general terms about their overall effectiveness. Nevertheless, some evidence suggests that strategies that prioritize identifying individuals who are genuinely at higher risk for violence, rather than strategies applying broad categorical exclusions, may indeed reduce gun violence (American Psychological Association 2013; Swanson et al. 2013).

For example, current federal and many state laws prohibit firearm ownership by individuals who have been involuntarily committed for psychiatric treatment. Rather than broad restrictions for a group for whom the risk of gun violence varies from high to none, a possible strategy is to screen individuals who are involuntarily committed in order to more accurately assess their risk of violence and to inform whether their gun rights should be suspended temporarily or permanently. To the extent that these firearm-ownership restrictions may require screening large groups to identify individuals with empirically supported risk factors for violence, brief structured methods may be the most fair and efficient approach. Depending on the context and resources, it may be appropriate to use an existing actuarial measure such as the VRAG or a more comprehensive structured measure such as the COVR. Structured screening tools may be used to screen out individuals who are at particularly low risk for violence (and would require no further consideration) from those who are at high enough risk to warrant a more comprehensive assessment. Theoretically, it may be feasible to develop an actuarial screening tool that is more specifically tailored to the population and purpose of firearm restriction laws; however, practically speaking, the field appears far from this development.

Assessing Baseline Risk and Designing Intervention

As detailed in the previous subsection, "Delineating Groups for Differential Policies, Interventions, or Services," some risk assessment tasks may require a single-point-in-time screening of risk status, yielding only an estimate of an individual's relative risk compared to that of other individuals. However, other risk assessment tasks will require a careful assessment of risk status that lays the groundwork for intervention and ongoing risk management.

A primary influence in modern violence risk assessment has been the influential model of offender assessment and rehabilitation approaches labeled "risk-needs-responsivity" (RNR; Andrews and Bonta 2006; Andrews and Dowden 2006; Andrews et al. 1990). As applied to violence risk assessment, the principles of the RNR model posit that individuals at greater *risk* for violent behavior require more intensive intervention or management efforts. Furthermore, these intervention efforts should be specifically targeted to each individual's unique criminogenic (or risk-relevant) *needs*—that is, the deficits, symptoms, or risk factors that are most related to the person's violence risk. Finally, *responsivity* refers to the anticipated likelihood that the individual will respond favorably to these violence-reduction interventions.

Forensic clinicians tasked with conducting comprehensive risk assessments often approach these assessments from an RNR perspective, and some describe the model explicitly. Following this approach, clinicians 1) attempt to assess the overall level of violence *risk* to determine the corresponding intensity of supervision or intervention necessary and 2) identify specific targets, risk factors, or treatment *needs* for intervention. Depending on the context, clinicians may later reassess individuals to gauge *response* to intervention, as well as changes in risk factors, any of which may lead to changes in the risk management plan. Although clinicians in general practice are less likely to specifically reference the RNR model, they often adopt, at least implicitly, a similar approach. That is, they may administer a structured risk assessment measure at the start of treatment so as to more accurately assess risk, gauge the overall degree of intervention necessary, and delineate specific risk factors for treatment, monitoring, and reduction. Clinicians cannot entirely delegate these tasks to structured violence risk assessment tools, but clinicians can often perform these tasks better using these tools.

Certain instruments are better than others for establishing a baseline risk estimate and guiding treatment. Generally, structured violence risk assessment tools that include dynamic (changeable) risk factors and describe risk state will be more useful than tools that prioritize static (historical) risk factors and describe only risk status. In particular, measures based on the SPJ model, such as the HCR-20, will help clinicians consider carefully both the static and the dynamic empirically supported risk factors potentially relevant to an individual. The COVR, although more structured, also guides clinicians in a manner that ensures broad coverage of relevant risk variables. Indeed, the broad and systematic review required by such structured measures can serve a useful function by directing the clinician's attention beyond the most obvious risk factors to others that may play important (but less obvious) roles. Both the HCR-20 and the COVR guide the clinician toward a final risk estimate (the COVR even provides explicit mathematical estimates based on the large research sample from which the instrument was derived), but both leave room for the clinician to consider factors beyond the instrument before offering a final risk appraisal.

Therefore, several structured measures help clinicians to reach an initial risk estimate and to identify many potential risk factors (or treatment *needs* in the RNR model) that warrant focus. The HCR-20, in particular, also directs the clinician to anticipate the challenges and stressors of the patient's anticipated context and resources (labeled "risk management factors" in the instrument manual) and to develop risk-reduction plans accordingly.

With respect to firearm policies in particular, structured violence risk assessments to gauge baseline risk and design intervention are probably the best response for situations in which courts or other systems request a formal risk assessment to inform decisions about restricting or restoring firearm rights. Decisions about firearm restrictions are probably best informed by considering empirically demonstrated risk factors for violence, rather than broad and heterogeneous categorical restrictions (e.g., history of receiving mental health treatment). Structured risk assessment approaches help clinicians identify, and sometimes even quantify, known violence risk factors, whether or not they relate to mental illness. Doing so provides a more transparent and face-valid approach to decisions about firearm restriction and restoration. That is, decisions about risk are linked to specific, known risk factors rather than broad conceptions of mental illness or dangerousness.

Furthermore, a structured assessment strategy that carefully identifies known risk factors and, when appropriate, identifies them as targets for intervention lays the groundwork for a plan to restore firearm access. All parties involved in removal or restoration proceedings would have a clearer understanding of the factors that necessitated firearm restriction and the progress or improvements necessary for restoration. Such a detailed approached, rooted in a structured violence risk measure, is more transparent and congruent with due process than less individualized or less structured approaches that occur without structured assessment.

Monitoring Risk and Tailoring Treatment Over Time

Proper violence risk management always requires ongoing reassessment of risk (Conroy and Murrie 2007). Clinicians may need to shift the focus of treatment as risk state changes and as some risk factors become more or less salient. Many clinicians monitor risk and modify treatment using less formal and more intuitive methods, but structured risk measures make monitoring risk more comprehensive and consistent. Regularly readministering the same structured risk measure over the course of treatment ensures that clinicians are considering the same risk factors and assessing them on the same "metric," so that their impressions regarding treatment progress or relapse are more reliable. Likewise, regular reassessment ensures that clinicians are considering an individual's response to intervention (the *responsivity* in the RNR model).

For clinicians monitoring risk over the course of treatment, SPJ measures such as the HCR-20 are almost always preferable to actuarial measures. Whereas brief actuarial measures are preferable for single-instance estimates of risk status based primarily on static factors, the SPJ measures require explicit attention to dynamic (changing) risk factors and risk management plans.

There are no fixed rules regarding how often clinicians should reassess risk, although authorities suggest biannual evaluations as a starting point (Douglas et al. 2013). The authors of the HCR-20V3 (Douglas et al. 2013) provide some particularly helpful guidance regarding formal reassessment for purposes of monitoring risk. Specifically, they suggest that the evaluator recommend a date for regular reassessment of risk, and be watchful for any developments that should prompt an earlier reassessment. The rationale for reassessment is that risk fluctuates over time, particularly for people living in the community. Even one development can prompt significant changes in perceived risk. As the developers of the HCR-20V3 advise,

> The timing of risk assessments typically is determined by three considerations. The first is any applicable laws, statutes, or policies, which may mandate reassessment at fixed times. The second is whether the person resides in the community or in an institution. In general, risk should be evaluated more frequently if there are frequent as opposed to infrequent changes in the person's living situation, be it in the community or in the institution. The third and final consideration is case prioritization. In general, the higher the case prioritization, the more frequently risk should be re-assessed. (Douglas et al. 2013, p. 64)

The field often and appropriately emphasizes that reassessment is crucial to identifying situations when risk is increasing and more intense intervention is necessary. Regular reassessment also (and perhaps even more often) reveals ways in which risk has decreased, allowing individuals to receive more autonomy and fewer restrictive interventions. In sum, regular reassessment with a structured risk measure helps ensure that the clinician remains attuned to changes in risk state and responds appropriately.

With respect to firearm policies in particular, structured violence risk assessments appear to be the most fair and thorough approaches to considering the removal or restoration of firearm rights. Specifically, evaluators can consider the presence of and change in known risk factors, as well as gauge overall changes in risk, using the same metric at each assessment. The transparency of this process makes it particularly suitable to high-stakes, potentially disputed decisions that may involve extending or restricting freedoms (e.g., civil commitment, conditional release, restoration or restriction of firearm rights).

Conclusion

Structured violence risk assessment instruments offer clinicians an empirically supported method of identifying individuals at relatively higher risk for violence and planning effective risk management. Although far from perfect, well-designed instruments with empirical support offer clear advantages over other methods, particularly unstructured assessment approaches or behavioral "profiling." Also, despite the fact that there is no violence risk assessment tool specific to *gun* violence, the best available instruments can nevertheless contribute to efforts to reduce gun violence.

When used properly, structured violence risk assessment methods shift the focus of assessments from prediction of violence to prevention of violence. Both the public and many professionals have a vested interest in *prediction*—that is, picking out those relatively few individuals who will commit acts of gun violence. Although clinicians do engage in prediction for circumscribed purposes, most clinical roles emphasize *prevention.* This latter task is less circumscribed and therefore more complex, but likely has a far greater impact on reducing gun violence, among individuals either with or without mental illness. Using structured violence risk assessment methods, many of which are well suited to guiding risk management strategies, can help shift the conversation away from simply identifying at-risk individuals and toward effectively intervening to create an overall reduction in gun violence.

Selecting the most appropriate risk assessment tool will depend on the nature and goals of the assessment. Although no single structured violence risk assessment tool consistently outperforms all others, this does not mean that all tools are equally suited to all purposes. Different tasks call for different risk assessment tools. Clinicians should consider the context of the assessment, particularly the distinction between delineating groups based on risk status and conducting a thorough risk assessment to plan and monitor ongoing risk management efforts.

Policies intended to identify individuals at relatively higher risk for gun violence should use some form of structured violence risk assessment. Structured violence risk assessments, particularly actuarial approaches, are an effective way to classify groups of people based on their risk status, primarily distinguishing between groups of much-higher-risk and much-lower-risk individuals. In this way, members of the former group can be targeted for ongoing assessment and intervention, and members of the latter group can effectively be screened out. Structured violence risk assessments based on the SPJ model can help clinicians evaluate both static and dynamic risk factors and develop risk-reduction interventions. These tools facilitate clinicians' use of the RNR model, which is a framework for tailoring intervention efforts to individuals' unique needs and for monitoring their progress.

All mental health clinicians considering risk of gun violence should have a basic literacy in structured violence risk assessment approaches. Empirical studies, as well as best-practice guides (e.g., Buchanan et al. 2012; Conroy and Murrie 2007; Heilbrun 2009), clearly support the role of structured violence risk assessment in evaluating risk of violence, including gun violence. Mental health clinicians considering a patient's risk for committing violence should have a basic familiarity with the risk assessment literature and some working knowledge of structured approaches. Although advanced expertise in structured violence risk assessment is not necessary for many clinicians, all clinicians should have adequate resources (including consultation) to guide their selection of instruments and overall appraisal of risk during routine practice. Particularly difficult, sensitive, or high-stakes assessments may be best handled by more specialized clinicians (typically described as forensic psychologists or psychiatrists) rather than treating clinicians.

In summary, violence risk assessment will always be a challenging and imperfect process. Although there are no special procedures for assessing risk of *gun* violence, among individuals with or without mental illness, there are well-established, evidence-based best practices for general violence risk assessment. One key theme in these best practices involves the use of structured violence risk assessment measures, not because these perfectly predict those individuals who will become violent, but because they help clinicians to make more accurate appraisals of risk and to conduct better risk management. To the extent that the justice and mental health systems are concerned with preventing gun violence, it may help to consider implementing these structured approaches when making systemic decisions or plans regarding individuals who may be at risk for gun violence.

Suggested Interventions

- Clinicians conducting violence risk assessments, including assessments for risk of gun violence, should use structured violence risk assessment tools as part of the assessment process.
- Structured violence risk assessment approaches should be a routine—but not the only—component when assessing risk of violence, including gun violence, in clinical practice.
- Regular structured violence risk assessment should inform treatment and risk management of individuals at risk for gun violence.
- Clinicians should use structured violence risk assessment tools to assist in informing interventions to reduce violence risk (by identifying key risk factors), as well as in monitoring risk level over

time (this helps clinicians review the most risk-relevant data) to gauge the impact of risk-reduction interventions.

- Legal or judicial interventions—such as restricting gun rights for certain individuals and restoring those rights—should incorporate structured violence risk assessment tools to assess an individual's level of risk, rather than broadly categorizing members of certain groups as prohibited categories of gun owners.

References

Ægisdóttir S, White MJ, Spengler PM, et al: The meta-analysis of clinical judgment project: fifty-six years of accumulated research on clinical versus statistical prediction. Couns Psychol 34(3):341–382, 2006

American Psychological Association: Gun Violence: Prediction, Prevention, and Policy. Panel of Experts Report. Washington, DC, American Psychological Association, 2013

Andrews DA, Bonta J: The Psychology of Criminal Conduct, 4th Edition. Newark, NJ, Routledge, 2006

Andrews DA, Dowden C: Risk principle of case classification in correctional treatment: a meta-analytic investigation. Int J Offender Ther Comp Criminol 50(1):88–100, 2006 16397124

Andrews DA, Bonta J, Hoge R: Classification for effective rehabilitation: rediscovering psychology. Crim Justice Behav 17(1):19–52, 1990

Blanchard AJE, Shaffer CS, Douglas KS: Decision support tools in the evaluation of risk of violence, in The Oxford Handbook of Behavioral Emergencies and Crises. Edited by Kleespies PM. New York, Oxford University Press (in press)

Buchanan A: Risk of violence by psychiatric patients: beyond the "actuarial versus clinical" assessment debate. Psychiatr Serv 59(2):184–190, 2008 18245161

Buchanan A, Binder R, Norko M, et al: Psychiatric violence risk assessment. Am J Psychiatry 169(3):340, 2012 22407122

Campbell MA, French S, Gendreau P: The prediction of violence in adult offenders: a meta-analytic comparison of instruments and methods of assessment. Crim Justice Behav 36(6):567–590, 2009

Coid J, Yang M, Ullrich S, et al: Most items in structured risk assessment instruments do not predict violence. J Forens Psychiatry Psychol 22(1):3–21, 2011

Conroy MA, Murrie DC: Forensic Evaluation of Violence Risk: A Guide to Risk Assessment and Risk Management. Hoboken, NJ, Wiley, 2007

Cooke DJ, Michie C: Limitations of diagnostic precision and predictive utility in the individual case: a challenge for forensic practice. Law Hum Behav 34(4):259–274, 2010 19277854

Dawes RM, Faust D, Meehl PE: Clinical versus actuarial judgment. Science 243(4899): 1668–1674, 1989 2648573

Douglas KS, Reeves K: Historical-Clinical-Risk Management–20 (HCR-20) violence risk assessment scheme: rationale, application, and empirical overview, in Handbook of Violence Risk Assessment (International Perspectives on Forensic Mental Health). Edited by Otto R, Douglas KS. New York, Routledge/Taylor & Francis, 2010, pp 147–186

Douglas KS, Skeem JL: Violence risk assessment: getting specific about being dynamic. Psychol Public Policy Law 11(3):347–383, 2005

Douglas KS, Webster CD: Predicting violence in mentally and personality disordered individuals, in Psychology and Law: The State of the Discipline. Edited by Roesch R, Hart SD, Ogloff JRP. New York, Kluwer Academic/Plenum Publishers, 1999, pp 175–239

Douglas KS, Hart SD, Webster CD, et al: HCR-20V3: Assessing Risk for Violence: User Guide. Burnaby, BC, Canada, Mental Health, Law, and Policy Institute, Simon Fraser University, 2013

Elbogen EB, Calkins C, Scalora MJ, et al: Perceived relevance of factors for violence risk assessment: a survey of clinicians. Int J Forensic Ment Health 1(1):37–47, 2002

Fazel S, Grann M: The population impact of severe mental illness on violent crime. Am J Psychiatry 163(8):1397–1403, 2006 16877653

Fazel S, Singh JP, Doll H, et al: Use of risk assessment instruments to predict violence and antisocial behaviour in 73 samples involving 24,827 people: systematic review and meta-analysis. BMJ 345:e4692, 2012 22833604

Grove WM, Meehl PE: Comparative efficiency of informal (subjective impressionistic) and formal (mechanical, algorithmic) prediction procedures: the clinical-statistical controversy. Psychol Public Policy Law 2(2):293–323, 1996

Grove WM, Zald DH, Lebow BS, et al: Clinical versus mechanical prediction: a meta-analysis. Psychol Assess 12(1):19–30, 2000 10752360

Guy LS: Performance indicators of the structured professional judgment approach for assessing risk for violence to others: a meta-analytic survey. Unpublished doctoral dissertation, Simon Fraser University, Burnaby, BC, Canada, 2008

Hanson RK, Howard PD: Individual confidence intervals do not inform decision-makers about the accuracy of risk assessment evaluations. Law Hum Behav 34(4):275–281, 2010 20556495

Hanson RK, Morton-Bourgon KE: The accuracy of recidivism risk assessments for sexual offenders: a meta-analysis of 118 prediction studies. Psychol Assess 21(1):1–21, 2009 19290762

Harris AJ: Risk assessment and sex offender community supervision: a context-specific framework. Fed Probat 70(2):36–43, 2006

Harris GT, Rice ME: Characterizing the value of actuarial violence risk assessments. Crim Justice Behav 34(12):1638–1658, 2007

Harris GT, Rice ME, Cormier CA: Prospective replication of the Violence Risk Appraisal Guide in predicting violent recidivism among forensic patients. Law Hum Behav 26(4):377–394, 2002 12182529

Harris GT, Rice ME, Quinsey VL, et al: A multisite comparison of actuarial risk instruments for sex offenders. Psychol Assess 15(3):413–425, 2003 14593842

Hart S, Michie C, Cooke D: Precision of actuarial risk assessment instruments: evaluating the “margins of error” of group v. individual predictions of violence. Br J Psychiatry 49:s60–s65, 2007 17470944

Heilbrun K: Prediction versus management models relevant to risk assessment: the importance of legal decision-making context. Law Hum Behav 21(4):347–359, 1997 9335193

Heilbrun K: Evaluation for Risk of Violence in Adults. New York, Oxford University Press, 2009

Heilbrun K, Douglas K, Yasuhara K: Violence risk assessment: core controversies, in Psychological Science in the Courtroom: Controversies and Consensus. Edited by Skeem J, Douglas K, Lilienfeld S. New York, Guilford, 2009, pp 333–357

Heilbrun K, Yasuhara K, Shah S: Approaches to violence risk assessment: overview and critical analysis, in Handbook of Violence Risk Assessment (International Perspectives on Forensic Mental Health). Edited by Otto R, Douglas KS. New York, Routledge/Taylor & Francis, 2010, pp 1–17

Hilton NZ, Harris HT, Rice ME: Sixty-six years of research on the clinical versus actuarial prediction of violence. Couns Psychol 34(3):400–409, 2006

Hurducas C, Singh JP, de Ruiter C, et al: Violence risk assessment tools: a systematic review of clinical surveys. Int J Forensic Ment Health 13(3):181–192, 2014

Kraemer HC, Kazdin AE, Offord DR, et al: Coming to terms with the terms of risk. Arch Gen Psychiatry 54(4):337–343, 1997 9107150

Kroner DG, Mills JF, Reddon JR: A coffee can, factor analysis, and prediction of antisocial behavior: the structure of criminal risk. Int J Law Psychiatry 28(4):360–374, 2005 15936077

Lidz CW, Mulvey EP, Gardner W: The accuracy of predictions of violence to others. JAMA 269(8):1007–1011, 1993 8429581

Meehl P: Clinical Versus Statistical Prediction: A Theoretical Analysis and a Review of the Evidence. Minneapolis, University of Minnesota Press, 1954

Menzies RJ, Webster CD, Sepejak DS: Hitting the forensic sound barrier: predictions of dangerousness in a pre-trial psychiatric clinic, in Dangerousness: Probability and Prediction, Psychiatry and Public Policy. Edited by Webster CD, Ben-Aron MH, Hucker SJ. New York, Cambridge University Press, 1985, pp 115–143

Mercy JA, O'Carroll PW: New directions in violence prediction: the public health arena. Violence Vict 3(4):285–301, 1988 3154184

Monahan J: The Clinical Prediction of Violent Behavior. Washington, DC, U.S. Government Printing Office, 1981

Monahan J: Structured risk assessment of violence, in Textbook of Violence Assessment and Management. Edited by Simon R, Tardiff K. Washington, DC, American Psychiatric Publishing, 2008, pp 17–33

Monahan J: The classification of violence risk, in Handbook of Violence Risk Assessment (International Perspectives on Forensic Mental Health). Edited by Otto R, Douglas KS. New York, Routledge/Taylor & Francis, 2010, pp 187–198

Monahan J, Skeem JL: The evolution of violence risk assessment. CNS Spectr 19(5):419–424, 2014 24679593

Monahan J, Steadman HJ: Extending violence reduction principles to justice-involved persons with mental illness, in Using Social Science to Reduce Violent Offending. Edited by Dvoskin JA, Skeem JL, Novaco RW, Douglas KS. New York, Oxford University Press, 2012, pp 245–261

Monahan J, Steadman HJ, Silver E, et al: Rethinking Risk Assessment: The MacArthur Study of Mental Disorder and Violence. Oxford, UK, Oxford University Press, 2001

Monahan J, Steadman HJ, Robbins PC, et al: An actuarial model of violence risk assessment for persons with mental disorders. Psychiatr Serv 56(7):810–815, 2005 16020812

Monahan J, Steadman HJ, Appelbaum PS, et al: The classification of violence risk. Behav Sci Law 24(6):721–730, 2006 17171769

Mossman D, Sellke T: Avoiding errors about "margins of error" (letter). Br J Psychiatry 191:561, author reply 561–562, 2007 18055965

Norris DM, Price M, Gutheil T, et al: Firearm laws, patients, and the roles of psychiatrists. Am J Psychiatry 163(8):1392–1396, 2006 16877652

O'Toole ME: The School Shooter: A Threat Assessment Perspective. Washington, DC, Federal Bureau of Investigation, 1999. Available at http://www.fbi.gov/stats-services/publications/school-shooter. Accessed August 11, 2015.

Otto RK, Douglas KS (eds): Handbook of Violence Risk Assessment (International Perspectives on Forensic Mental Health). New York, Routledge/Taylor & Francis, 2010

Quinsey VL, Harris GT, Rice ME, et al: Violent Offenders: Appraising and Managing Risk. Washington, DC, American Psychological Association, 1998

Quinsey VL, Harris GT, Rice ME, et al: Violent Offenders: Appraising and Managing Risk, 2nd Edition. Washington, DC, American Psychological Association, 2006

Rice ME, Harris GT: Comparing effect sizes in follow-up studies: ROC area, Cohen's d, and r. Law Hum Behav 29(5):615–620, 2005

Shah SA: Dangerousness and civil commitment of the mentally ill: some public policy considerations. Am J Psychiatry 132(5):501–505, 1975 1119609

Shah S: Dangerousness: conceptual, prediction, and public policy issues, in Violence and the Violent Individual. Edited by Hays JR, Robert TK, Solway KS. New York, SP Medical & Scientific, 1981, pp 151–178

Simpson JR: Bad risk? An overview of laws prohibiting possession of firearms by individuals with a history of treatment for mental illness. J Am Acad Psychiatry Law 35(3):330–338, 2007 17872555

Singh JP, Grann M, Fazel S: A comparative study of violence risk assessment tools: a systematic review and metaregression analysis of 68 studies involving 25,980 participants. Clin Psychol Rev 31(3):499–513, 2011 21255891

Singh JP, Desmarais SL, Hurducas C, et al: Use and perceived utility of structured violence risk assessment tools in 44 countries: findings from the IRiS Project. Int J Forensic Ment Health 13:193–206, 2014

Skeem J, Monahan J: Current directions in violence risk assessment. Curr Dir Psychol Sci 20(1):38–42, 2011

Skeem J, Mulvey E: Monitoring the violence potential of mentally disordered offenders being treated in the community, in Care of the Mentally Disordered Offender in the Community. Edited by Buchanan A. New York, Oxford University Press, 2002, pp 111–142

Steadman HJ, Mulvey EP, Monahan J, et al: Violence by people discharged from acute psychiatric inpatient facilities and by others in the same neighborhoods. Arch Gen Psychiatry 55(5):393–401, 1998 9596041

Swanson JW: Mental disorder, substance abuse, and community violence: an epidemiological approach, in Violence and Mental Disorder. Edited by Monahan J, Steadman H. Chicago, IL, University of Chicago Press, 1994, pp 101–136

Swanson JW, Robertson AG, Frisman LK, et al: Preventing gun violence involving people with serious mental illness, in Reducing Gun Violence in America: Informing Policy With Evidence and Analysis. Edited by Webster DW, Vernick JS. Baltimore, MD, Johns Hopkins University Press, 2013, pp 33–51

Tolman AO, Mullendore KB: Risk evaluations for the courts: is service quality a function of specialization? Prof Psychol Res Pr 34(3):225–232, 2003

Van Dorn R, Volavka J, Johnson N: Mental disorder and violence: is there a relationship beyond substance use? Soc Psychiatry Psychiatr Epidemiol 47:487–503, 2012 21359532

Webster CD, Douglas KS, Eaves D, et al: HCR-20: Assessing Risk for Violence (Version 2). Burnaby, BC, Canada, Mental Health, Law, and Policy Institute, Simon Fraser University, 1997

Yang M, Wong SC, Coid J: The efficacy of violence prediction: a meta-analytic comparison of nine risk assessment tools. Psychol Bull 136(5):740–767, 2010 20804235

10

Decreasing Suicide Mortality

Clinical Risk Assessment and Firearm Management

Robert I. Simon, M.D.
Liza H. Gold, M.D.

Common Misperceptions

- ☒ The most significant association between firearms and violence is mass shootings committed by young men with severe mental illness.
- ☒ Clinicians can predict whether someone will commit suicide.
- ☒ People who want to commit suicide do not seek treatment.
- ☒ People who want to kill themselves will find a way to do it, so restricting access to firearms is futile.

Evidence-Based Facts

- ☑ The most statistically significant connection between firearms and mental illness is suicide by firearm.
- ☑ Clinicians cannot predict if or when a given individual will commit suicide. However, identification of evidence-based risk factors and mental health treatment can reduce the risk of suicide.

☑ Many people have seen their primary care providers or mental health treatment providers in the weeks and months prior to committing suicide, but are not adequately screened for risk of suicide.

☑ When access to firearms is limited, suicide rates decrease. No evidence suggests that a substantial number of people will substitute another method. Even when substitution does occur, other methods are less lethal. Consequently, suicide rates decrease.

Although many people believe that the most likely acts of gun violence perpetrated by individuals with serious mental illness are mass shootings, in actuality individuals with serious mental illness who commit gun violence are most likely to use a firearm to commit suicide, not homicide. Although rare in absolute terms, suicide is significantly more common than mass shootings, which are the least common of all types of gun violence. In 2013, for example, of the nearly 33,000 people who died from gun violence, over 21,000 died from suicide (American Association of Suicidology 2014; Centers for Disease Control and Prevention 2015). In contrast, in the same year, mass shootings perpetrated by individuals with or without mental illness accounted for less than 1% of firearm deaths (see Table 2 in "Introduction" at the beginning of this book).

Almost all people who commit suicide have a diagnosable mental illness. The presence of a psychiatric disorder is among the most consistently reported risk factors for suicidal behavior (Nock et al. 2008). Firearms are the most common method used to commit suicide in the United States (American Association of Suicidology 2014). For the past decade, firearms have consistently been associated with more suicide deaths than have all other means of suicide combined (Centers for Disease Control and Prevention 2015).

Suicide is the result of a variety of different psychiatric, environmental, and cultural factors. Chance and stressful life events can also contribute to suicidal behavior. Nevertheless, suicide is preventable, and as with any behavior for which multiple factors contribute, a variety of interventions can potentially decrease the number of suicide deaths. However, only two interventions have been empirically demonstrated to be effective in decreasing suicide mortality: physician education in suicide risk assessment and treatment, and restriction of lethal means (Mann et al. 2005; Miller and Hemenway 2008).

Strategies for suicide prevention fall into two categories. *Population-based strategies* typically require systemwide design and implementation by professionals in a variety of disciplines and institutional organizations as well as general community support. *Individual-level strategies* related to reduce suicide involve improving the ability to recognize suicide risk and intervene appropriately. The individual-level interventions to prevent suicide are not limited to professionals and institutions; they are also available to the high-risk person's acquaintances, family, and friends (Deisenhammer et al. 2009), who often are the first to suspect or have knowledge of an impending crisis.

The profound connection among suicide, mental illness, and firearms underscores the need for mental health and primary care clinicians to acquire and use clinical risk assessment skills. This connection also emphasizes the need for clinicians to include inquiries regarding access to firearms and to discuss firearm risk management in interactions with patients and their families on a routine basis, but particularly when patients are in crisis.

Suicide in the United States

In the United States, suicide is now the tenth leading overall cause of death. In 2013, suicide was the cause of death for 41,149 people (Table 10–1). On average, about 113 people kill themselves every day, an average of one person every 13 minutes (American Foundation for Suicide Prevention 2014; Centers for Disease Control and Prevention 2015).

Certain demographic groups are at particularly high risk for suicide. The suicide rate in 2013, for example, was highest among Caucasians (14.9 per 100,000) and lowest among African Americans (5.4 per 100,000) and Hispanics (5.3 per 100,000) (American Association of Suicidology 2014). Gender also influences vulnerability to suicide, although women make more suicide attempts than men. The suicide rate is about four times higher among men than among women; in 2013, males accounted for 77.9% of the suicide deaths (American Foundation for Suicide Prevention 2014).

Age is also a significant demographic factor in suicide deaths. White males ages 65–84 had a suicide rate of 31.9 per 100,000, and white males age 85 and older had a rate of 52.6 per 100,000. In contrast, white females age 85 and older had a rate of 3.5 per 100,000. The young are also particularly vulnerable to suicide. Suicide is the second leading cause of death among young people, accounting for 17% of all deaths for those ages 15–24 (American Association of Suicidology 2014).

Suicide, Mental Illness, and Alcohol Use

Beyond demographics, the strongest individual risk factors for suicide are psychiatric disorders and substance use disorders (Ilgen et al. 2008; Miller and Hemenway 1999; Nock et al. 2008). Approximately 90%–95% of suicide victims have a diagnosable psychiatric disorder at the time of death (Cavanagh et al. 2003; Nock et al. 2008). Kessler et al. (2005a), using data collected from the National Comorbidity Study, found that 82% of individuals who reported suicidal ideation, 95% of individuals who reported making suicide plans, and 88% of individuals who reported making suicide attempts had symptoms that met the criteria for one or more DSM disorders. In a meta-analysis, Arsenault-Lapierre

TABLE 10–1. Means of suicide, by percentage of total suicide deaths, 2003–2013

Year	Total suicide deaths	Firearm	Suffocation[a]	Poisoning[b]	Falls	Cutting/ piercing	Drowning
2013	41,149	51.5	24.5	16.1	2.37	1.9	0.1
2012	40,600	50.9	24.9	16.6	2.34	1.8	1.1
2011	39,518	50.6	25.1	16.6	2.04	1.7	0.9
2010	38,364	50.6	24.7	17.2	2.04	1.8	1.1
2009	36,909	50.8	24.4	17.3	1.86	1.8	1.1
2008	36,035	50.6	23.8	17.9	1.97	1.9	1.1
2007	34,598	50.2	23.6	18.4	2.11	1.8	1.0
2006	33,300	50.7	22.5	18.4	2.18	1.8	1.2
2005	32,637	52.1	22.2	17.6	2.09	1.8	1.2
2004	32,439	51.6	22.6	17.9	2.08	1.8	1.1
2003	31,484	53.7	21.1	17.4	2.30	1.8	1.1

[a]Including hanging.
[b]Including medication overdose.
Source. Centers for Disease Control and Prevention 2015.

et al. (2004) found that on average, 87.3% of individuals who committed suicide had a mental disorder, and persons who completed suicide were more likely to have symptoms that met criteria for more than one psychiatric diagnosis.

Affective, substance-related, personality, and psychotic disorders accounted for most of the diagnoses among suicide completers (Arsenault-Lapierre et al. 2004). Of these, mood disorders, particularly depression, are most common among suicide decedents, followed closely by alcohol use disorders, with the highest risk among individuals with comorbid affective disorders and alcohol use disorders (Arsenault-Lapierre et al. 2004; Cavanagh et al. 2003). Suicide is, in fact, one of the leading types of injury mortality linked with alcohol consumption (Conner et al. 2014). Individuals with alcohol dependence who come to clinical attention are at approximately nine times higher risk of completed suicide compared with the general population (Kaplan et al. 2013).

Acute use of alcohol in the hours preceding suicidal behavior, regardless of the presence of an alcohol use disorder, is also highly prevalent, and is a powerful independent risk factor beyond the risk conferred by chronic alcohol use (Dahlberg et al. 2004; Kaplan et al. 2013; Powell et al. 2001). One meta-analytic study found that 37% of suicides were preceded by acute use of alcohol (Cherpitel et al. 2004). An analysis of the National Violent Death Reporting System data (Conner et al. 2014) found that alcohol was present at the time of death in one-third of suicides by firearms, hanging, and poisoning, the three methods that constitute over 90% of suicide deaths in the United States. Moreover, blood alcohol concentrations (BACs) in suicide decedents were high, with the mean exceeding 80 mg/dL, the legal limit for drinking and driving (Conner et al. 2014).

Notably, suicide decedents who died by firearms had the highest mean BACs compared with those who died by hanging or poisoning (Conner et al. 2014). Blumenthal (2007) found a positive BAC in 40% of firearm suicide cases reviewed. Smith et al. (1999) found that 31.5% of firearm suicide decedents were acutely intoxicated, with BACs of 100 mg/dL or higher. Branas et al. (2011) found that individuals who had any level of acute alcohol consumption were 5.9 times more likely to commit firearm suicide than were those who had no acute alcohol consumption, and in cases with excessive acute alcohol consumption, 77.1 times more likely to commit firearm suicide.

Suicide and Firearms

Firearms are obviously not the only means by which people commit suicide; however, they are the most common suicide method in the United States (see Table 10–1; see also Chapter 2, "Firearms and Suicide in the United States"). Between 2003 and 2013, firearm suicide consistently accounted for over 50% of suicide deaths in the United States, more than double the number of the next most common method, suffocation, which includes hanging (Centers for Disease Control and Prevention 2015). In contrast, in other high-income countries, firearms account for only 4.5% of suicides (World Health Organization 2014).

Guns are the most lethal method of suicide (see Chapter 2). As levels of means lethality increase, the chances of rescue with medical treatment dramatically decrease and mortality is substantially more likely (Kolla et al. 2011). Ninety percent of all suicidal acts with firearms are fatal. In contrast, less than 3% of all suicidal acts by intentional overdose or cutting are fatal (Chapdelaine et al. 1991; Elnour and Harrison 2008; Miller et al. 2013b; Shenassa et al. 2003) (also see Chapter 2). In teens ages 15–19, for example, only 1 of every 760 cases of nonfirearm injuries resulted in death in 2013, whereas almost 1 in 4 youth firearm injuries, including suicides, were fatal (Child Trends Data Bank 2015).

The likelihood that a specific method of suicide will lead to death is also related to accessibility (Yip et al. 2012). Firearm ownership is more prevalent in the United States than in any other high-income country. There are more than 310 million privately owned firearms in the United States, representing about one gun per person (Krouse 2012; L.H.G. personal communication with W.J. Krouse, February 13, 2015). In data from a nationally representative survey, Swanson et al. (2015) found that 36.5% of people reported having at least one gun in their home. Approximately 34% of U.S. households have guns (Pew Research Center 2013), and a member of a household often owns more than one firearm (Krouse 2012; Swanson et al. 2015).

An increased risk of suicide is conferred almost immediately by access to a firearm. Wintemute et al. (1999) found that purchase of a handgun was associated with a significant increase in the risk of suicide by firearm as well as by any other method, with risk increasing within 1 week after purchase of a handgun and remaining increased for at least 6 years. Similarly, Grassel et al. (2003) found that among adults who died in California in 1998, handgun purchasers constituted only 0.5% of the study population but were involved in 14.2% of gun suicides.

Approximately 75% or more of suicides occur in the victims' homes (Anglemyer et al. 2014; Dahlberg et al. 2004; Kellermann et al. 1992). Substantial evidence indicates that the presence of firearms in the home is associated with significantly increased risk of suicide in the home (Anglemyer et al. 2014; Brent et al. 2013; Grassel et al. 2003; Shenassa et al. 2003). Studies have found anywhere from a 2 to 10 times greater risk of suicide in homes with guns than in those without guns, depending on the sample population and on methods of firearm storage (Miller et al. 2012, 2013a). This higher risk applies to the gun owners, their spouses, and their children (Dahlberg et al. 2004; Miller and Hemenway 2008; Miller et al. 2013a; Sorenson and Vittes 2008) and persists for years after purchase (Miller and Hemenway 2008; Wintemute 2013).

Individuals with access to firearms in the home, particularly adolescents, are more likely to die by firearm-related suicide than by any other method. Studies have consistently found that most adolescent suicides occur in the home with a firearm owned by a parent (Dahlberg et al. 2004; Johnson et al. 2010; Shah et al. 2000; Wright et al. 2008). Among adolescents with a suicide plan, those with a firearm in the home were more than seven times more likely to have a plan involving firearms than those without a firearm in the home (Betz et al. 2011).

Elderly people are also more likely to suffer self-inflicted gunshot wounds, either intentional or accidental, especially to the head (Kapp 2013). Rates of firearm suicides as a percentage of total suicide deaths are highest for the 65-and-older age group (Richardson and Hemenway 2011). The use of firearms has become the most common suicide method for both elderly men and elderly women, with the rates highest among those age 75 and older (Kapp 2013; Mertens and Sorenson 2012).

The association between higher rates of overall suicide and firearm suicide and higher rates of gun ownership is independent of psychopathology. Compared with people who live in homes without firearms, people who live in homes with firearms are not more likely to have psychosocial distress or any of the major psychopathological disorders known to increase suicide risk. They are not more likely to have suicidal thoughts or to have made suicide attempts (Betz et al. 2011; Hemenway and Miller 2002; Ilgen et al. 2008; Miller et al. 2009, 2012, 2013b; Sorenson and Vittes 2008).

Individuals with mental illness are as likely to have access to guns as individuals without mental illness (Ilgen et al. 2008; Kolla et al. 2011; McNiel et al. 2007). The link between guns and suicide is therefore unlikely to be explained solely by higher levels of gun access among higher-risk individuals. Instead, higher-risk individuals may simply be more likely to use guns that they possess to harm themselves (Ilgen et al. 2008). For example, many early adolescent suicide victims do not show clear evidence of a mental disorder. One of the only risk factors found for these young suicide decedents is the presence of a loaded gun in the home (Brent et al. 2013).

Reducing Suicide Mortality

A significant amount of empirical evidence supports two complementary approaches to decreasing suicide mortality. The first is reducing the number of suicide attempts by recognizing suicide risk factors and associated mental illness and providing treatment. The second is reducing the probability that suicide attempts will prove fatal by reducing access to lethal means.

Recognizing Suicide Risk Factors and Providing Treatment

Prevention, Not Prediction

The detection of suicide risk, the determination of risk level, and the treatment decisions that are dependent on that determination are important judgments clinicians make (Berman and Silverman 2014). Unfortunately, no method of suicide risk assessment can reliably predict which individuals will attempt or complete suicide (sensitivity) and which will not (specificity) (Simon 2012b).

Although suicide is the tenth leading cause of death in the United States, it is a statistically rare event; the overall national rate of suicide in 2013 was 0.013% of the population (American Association of Suicidology 2014). The *absolute risk* that any individual will commit suicide is low, because the vast majority of people, even those who have general risk factors and those who express suicidal thoughts or behaviors, do not go on to commit suicide. Therefore, efforts to predict who will die by suicide lead to a large number of false positives and false negatives (Simon 2006b, 2012b; Swanson 2011).

As a result, professionals evaluating people who might commit suicide now focus on prevention by assessing risk, rather than prediction. The assessment of *relative risk* is based on the fact that people with mental illness are significantly more likely to commit suicide than people who do not have mental illness (Swanson 2011). Only the *risk* of suicide is determinable (Simon 2012b). Additionally, the concept of *imminent risk* implies temporal prediction; although the term is still frequently used to describe potential suicide behavior—for example, in civil commitment statutes—no evidence-based risk factors help in identifying a suicide as imminent (Simon 2006a).

Suicide risk assessment is a complex, difficult, and challenging clinical task. Suicide is not a diagnosis but rather a behavior that may be associated with many different psychiatric diagnoses. Although the presence of a psychiatric diagnosis can be a risk factor, even patients with similar diagnoses are at varying degrees of risk for suicide. In addition, the level of risk can change rapidly and often without notice (Simon 2012b).

Conceptually, suicide risk assessment is a process that identifies and prioritizes evidence-based acute or short-term risk factors, chronic or long-term risk factors, and protective factors. Short-term risk factors are those found prospectively and statistically significant within 1 year of assessment (Fawcett et al. 1990). These include panic attacks, anxiety, loss of pleasure or interest, agitated depression, decreased concentration, and insomnia. Long-term risk factors, derived from association with completed suicides 2–10 years following assessment, include suicidal ideation, suicide intent, severe hopelessness, and prior attempts (Fawcett et al. 1990, 1993). Protective factors are those that decrease risk of suicide, such as close, supportive family relationships and treatment compliance, among others.

The information from a suicide risk assessment is synthesized into a clinical formulation of foreseeable risk of suicidal behavior (Jacobs et al. 2003; Silverman 2014; Simon 2006b). The level of risk dictates the need for and types of treatment intervention. Systematic suicide risk assessment is therefore critical to clinical decision making, including safety planning and management, triage decisions, treatment planning (especially regarding voluntary or involuntary hospitalization), and overall risk management (Silverman and Berman 2014; Simon 2012b).

Competency in suicide risk assessment and management is expected of all mental health professionals (Hung et al. 2012; Wortzel et al. 2013). It is a core competency (Jacobs et al. 2003; Rudd 2014; Silverman 2014; Simon 2012b) for both psychiatrists (Accreditation Council for Graduate Medical Education 2014) and psychologists (Cramer et al. 2013). To date, no current methods for conducting a standardized suicide risk assessment have been widely agreed on or adopted by a professional organization or training curriculum as a standard professional guideline or teaching tool.

Nevertheless, a wide range of clinical approaches and a number of suicide risk assessment models are available and may be effectively used in systematic suicide risk assessment (Simon 2012b). Suicide risk assessments should include inquiries about and review of demographic risk factors, short- and long-term risk factors, and the individual patient's unique risk factors and protective factors (Simon 2012b). No single risk factor is pathognomonic for suicide. A single suicide risk factor, or even a combination of risk factors, does not have the statistical significance on which to base an overall risk assessment, due to the infrequency (i.e., low absolute risk) of suicide (Jacobs et al. 2003; Simon 2012b).

Suicide risk assessment has been approached through a variety of methodologies. Many mental health professionals rely on the clinical interview alone to assess risk. Others rely on structured or semistructured checklists, which generally list suicide risk factors and sometimes list protective factors. Patient self-surveys, asking about suicidal ideation and history, are also used. The use of any of these methods alone, however, does not constitute an adequate suicide risk assessment. For example, many clinicians continue to rely on unaided clinical judgment in assessing suicide risk. Although clinical experience and judgment are an essential part of suicide risk assessment, greater experience does not necessarily result in better judgment or improved competence (Berman and Silverman 2014; Silverman 2014). Unaided and unstructured clinical judgment and intuition are especially vulnerable to the influence of personal and social biases and are highly subject to error (Simon 2006b).

Many semistructured suicide assessment scales and checklists are available, but these alone are also not effective suicide risk assessment methodologies (Jacobs et al. 2003; Simon 2012b). Checklists are overly sensitive and lack specificity. None have been tested for reliability and validity (Silverman 2014; Silverman and Berman 2014; Simon 2009). In addition, checklists cannot encompass all the relevant risk factors present for a given patient (Simon 2012b). Patient self-report instruments cannot be considered adequate by themselves because patients may conceal suicidal thoughts or intent.

Ideally, routine, systematic suicide risk assessments combine semistructured tools, self-report surveys, and the clinical interview, which together increase opportunities for capturing significant information. For example, because suicidal ideation, suicide intent, and suicide planning may be difficult for some patients to disclose directly, the inclusion of self-report measures provides another potential opportunity for detecting thoughts of suicide (Silverman and Berman 2014). Semistructured screening instruments complement and improve routine clinical assessments and can provide support and corroboration for a well-conducted clinical suicide risk assessment (Homaifar et al. 2013; Silverman 2014; Silverman and Berman 2014; Simon 2009, 2012b; Wortzel et al. 2013). Important risk and protective factors are easily overlooked in the absence of systematic assessment (Simon 2006b). A "checklist" of risk and protective factors can prompt clinicians to systematically review all relevant factors.

The assessment of overall suicide risk involves an understanding of how risk factors interact, exacerbate, and otherwise contribute to a heightened or lowered risk of suicide (Berman and Silverman 2014), and incorporates information from a number of sources (Simon 2006b). Many factors are not simply present or absent but may vary in degrees of severity. In addition, some factors may contribute to risk in some individuals but not in others or may be relevant only when they occur in combination with particular psychosocial stressors (Jacobs et al. 2003). The clinician's judgment is central in identifying and assigning clinical weight to the risk and protective factors identified through systematic assessment (Berman and Silverman 2014; Simon 2012b).

Once risk factors are identified, clinicians can consider treatment interventions based on whether or not factors are modifiable. Although immutable factors such as demographic characteristics and family history are important to identify, they cannot be the focus of intervention. Modifiable and treatable suicide risk factors should be identified as early as possible and treated aggressively. For example, anxiety, depression, insomnia, and psychosis may respond rapidly to medications as well as psychosocial interventions. Clinicians should also identify, support, and when possible enhance protective factors. Psychosocial interventions, for example, can help a patient mobilize existing social supports (Jacobs et al. 2003; Rudd 2014; Simon 2012b).

Importantly, suicide risk assessment is a process, not a singular event. Most individuals with suicidal ideation have varying levels of ambivalence about committing suicide. Suicide intent can increase with accumulation of stressors or decrease as effective interventions are implemented. The accuracy of any suicide risk assessment therefore decreases over time as circumstances and clinical risk factors change. Consequently, suicide risk assessment needs to be repeated according to the clinical needs of the patient, particularly when a treatment decision, such as discharge from inpatient treatment, is considered (Jacobs et al. 2003; Silverman and Berman 2014; Simon 2012b).

TABLE 10–2. Suicide risk assessment: approach to data gathering

1. Identify distinctive individual suicide risk factors.
2. Identify acute suicide risk factors.
3. Identify protective factors.
4. Evaluate medical history, including laboratory data if available.
5. Obtain information from other clinical care providers such as primary care providers.
6. Interview patient's significant others.
7. Speak with current or prior mental health treatment providers, including, if inpatient, treatment team.
8. Review patient's current and prior hospital records.

Source. Simon 2012a.

Data Collection

Systematic risk assessment also serves as a prompt for gathering essential information about patients, because it reminds clinicians to consider multiple data sources. Some of the most significant risk factors for completed suicide are suicidal ideation, suicide plans, and a history of previous attempts. However, any number of patients at risk for suicide, particularly individuals who are intent on dying, may deny having suicidal thoughts or suicide plans or may conceal or minimize a history of suicidal behavior (Nock et al. 2008; Rudd 2014; Silverman 2014; Simon 2012a). Several studies have found that the majority of patients who die by suicide denied having suicidal thoughts when last asked, although they may have communicated their risk through behaviors preceding suicide (see Silverman and Berman 2014). Simon (2012b) has suggested one approach to collecting the necessary data in a suicide risk assessment (Table 10–2).

Collateral information may be a key element in suicide risk assessment, particularly when a patient denies ideation, intent, or plans. Family members should be consulted if possible, because they may be aware of changes in behavior or warning signs that the patient does not report (Simon 2012b). Additional collateral information can be obtained from the medical record, the patient's medical and mental health providers, friends, and possibly others sources, such as police records (Silverman and Berman 2014; Simon 2012b).

Models for Suicide Risk Assessment

A variety of models and frameworks for systematic suicide risk assessment have been suggested, each of which should be considered a tool designed to encourage and facilitate systematic assessment. Rudd (2014) has suggested that seven clinical domains or "core competencies" provide the essential foundations and basic levels of skills for clinicians working with suicidal patients. Rudd asserts that effective assessment and clinical management require this broad skill set and expansive knowledge base with competency in skills associated with all these related core competencies, which he identifies as:

1. Attitudes and approach
2. Understanding suicide
3. Collecting accurate assessment information
4. Formulating risk
5. Developing a treatment plan
6. The clinical management of care, and
7. Understanding the legal and regulatory issues related to suicide.

Rudd proposes a general framework for conducting suicide risk assessments, based on empirical evidence and clinical experience identifying risk and protective factors. This framework, a critical element of Rudd's suggested core competencies of collecting accurate information and formulating risk, identifies eight categories of risk factors that require review, as well as a ninth essential but often overlooked category in suicide risk assessments, that of protective factors (see Table 10–3). The model suggested by this outline provides a basis for a systematic risk assessment. However, as noted above, any model or method of gathering information should be considered an aid or guide to a thorough and systematic clinical assessment. Use of any list alone does not constitute an adequate suicide risk assessment (Simon 2009).

Rudd's (2014) model specifically distinguishes between suicide risk factors and warning signs. A *suicide risk factor* is defined as a factor empirically demonstrated to correlate with suicide, regardless of when it first becomes present. The presence of chronic or long-term risk factors, for example, establishes lifetime vulnerability to suicide risk. In contrast, *suicide warning signs* are the earliest detectable signs that indicate acute heightened risk for suicide. Suicide intent is fluid in nature; however, warning signs, some of which are also short-term risk factors, provide observable markers consistent with potentially increased intent. The presence of one or more warning signs is indicative of increased suicide risk in the context of lifetime vulnerability (Berman and Silverman 2014; Rudd 2014).

Rudd (2014) and others (Berman and Silverman 2014; Simon 2012b) suggest weighting risk and protective factors and overall suicide risk on a dimensional scale of low, moderate, or high risk. As a general rule, as symptom severity and complexity increase, so does suicide intent, with the emergence of distinct warning signs and the presence of associated suicidal behaviors such as preparation, rehearsals, or attempts (Rudd 2014). Higher versus lower levels of judged

TABLE 10–3. Suicide risk assessment: proposed model outline (based on Rudd 2014)

Category	Examples of category-specific risk factors*
I. Predisposition to suicidal behavior	Psychiatric history, demographic considerations, (age, gender, gender orientation, ethnicity); history of sexual, physical, or emotional abuse
II. Identifiable precipitants or stressors (most can be conceptualized as losses)	Financial, stability of interpersonal relationships; loss of social support; acute or chronic health problems
III. Symptomatic presentation	Symptoms of depression, anxiety, psychosis; borderline and antisocial personality disorder features
IV. Hopelessness	Severity, duration
V. Nature of suicidal thinking and behaviors	Ideation, plan, availability and lethality of means, intent
VI. Previous suicide attempts and history of self-injury	Frequency, perceived lethality, preparatory behaviors including rehearsal, reactions to previous attempts
VII. Impulsivity and self-control	Subjective perception of self- control; objective control as demonstrated by behaviors such as substance abuse and aggression
VIII. Presence of warning signs	Active suicidal thinking; preparation and rehearsal behavior; recklessness, dramatic mood changes, acute anxiety and agitation, increase in alcohol or drug use
IX. Protective factors	Availability and accessibility of social support; problem solving and coping skills; participation in treatment; children in the home; intact reality testing

*This list of examples is not exhaustive. For Rudd's complete list and suggested format for suicide risk assessment forms to facilitate gathering information and formulating level of risk, see Rudd 2014, pp. 325–329.

risk carry greater imperatives for aggressive treatment planning, triage, and intervention (Berman and Silverman 2014).

A dimensional rating scale is obviously not a precise method for conveying suicide risk. As observed by Berman and Silverman (2014), standardized, operational definitions of these levels of risk are difficult to find. Nevertheless, most clinicians caution practitioners against relying on models based on quantifiable scores (Simon 2009; Wortzel et al. 2013). Numerical scoring systems are arbitrary and idiosyncratic, and they create an illusion of scientific accuracy that can be misleading (Simon 2009).

Low risk is characterized by mild psychiatric symptoms with no associated suicidal intent or features. *Moderate risk* emerges as symptoms escalate, warning signs start to emerge, and evidence of subjective intent is identified. *High risk* is characterized by four essential elements: serious psychiatric symptoms, the presence of active intent (subjective or objective), the presence of warning signs, and limited protective factors. Once objective evidence of suicide intent is identified, such as preparation and rehearsal behaviors, a high-risk designation is more likely to be assigned (Rudd 2014).

Suicide Risk Factors and Protective Factors

Empirically identified risk and protective factors associated with suicide are listed in Table 10–3. A detailed discussion of all risk and protective factors and the strength of the empirical evidence behind them is beyond the scope of this discussion. As mentioned in the introduction to this chapter, however, mental illness is one of the strongest risk factors for suicide. The following discussion focuses on some other factors with strong evidence bases.

Suicidal ideation and related behaviors, including warning signs and intent, are among the most significant suicide risk factors. In the National Comorbidity Survey, Kessler et al. (1999) found that approximately 90% of unplanned suicide attempts and 60% of planned first attempts occurred within 1 year of the onset of suicidal ideation. The probability of transitioning from suicidal ideation to suicide plan was 34%; the probability of transitioning from a plan to an attempt was 72%.

When assessing suicidal ideation, clinicians should consider specific content, intensity, duration, and prior episodes (Berman and Silverman 2014; Rudd 2014; Simon 2012a). Fleeting, nonspecific suicidal thoughts with no associated subjective or objective intent are not evidence of risk escalation beyond an individual's chronic baseline level. Reduced duration frequently translates to reduced specificity, less severity, and lower intent, along with lower risk (Rudd 2014). However, the presence or absence of suicidal thinking is not a particularly good indicator of escalating suicide risk, particularly in multiple attempters and individuals experiencing chronic suicidal ideation (Rudd 2014; Simon 2012b).

Major interpersonal stressful life events may increase suicide risk, particularly among adults with alcohol use disorders or other compromised coping skills and psychiatric or psychological vulnerabilities (Hawton 2007; Nock et al. 2008; Owens et al. 2003). For such individuals, an adverse event may lead to a suicide attempt within a relatively short period of time. Examples of such events include loss of a significant relationship, financial or employment setbacks, involvement in legal or disciplinary problems, and perceived public shame or humiliation. One study (Owens et al. 2003) found that half of all suicide decedents had suffered at least one adverse life event in their final month of life, most commonly involving relationships, money, and work.

Although less research regarding factors that protect against suicide is available, such factors are critically important because they can decrease the probability of a fatal outcome. Protective factors, like risk factors, vary with the distinctive clinical presentation of the individual patient at risk (Simon 2012b). Arguably, the most important protective factor is accessible and available family and/or other social supports. The ability to engage in treatment is also an essential protective factor. Additional examples of protective factors include feelings of responsibility to family, child-related concerns, strong religious beliefs, and cultural sanctions against suicide (Nock et al. 2008; Simon 2012b). Nevertheless, for any individual, a delicate balance may exist between suicide risk and protective factors, and acute high suicide risk may nullify protective factors (Berman and Silverman 2014; Simon 2012b).

Suicide and Impulsivity

Although suicidal ideation and suicide planning are major risk factors for suicide, many suicide attempts also demonstrate a strong component of impulsivity. For example, according to Rimkeviciene et al. (2015), the majority of studies of impulsivity and suicide have found an absence of proximal planning or an abruptness of attempt in over 50% of cases. Seventy-five percent of attempts occur within 3 hours of the time of initial suicidal ideation, suicide planning, or decision to carry out the suicide act. The length of time from first thought to the suicide act has been found to be as little as a few minutes to a few hours (Ilgen et al. 2008; Shenassa et al. 2004; Simon et al. 2001; Yip et al. 2012).

Studies assessing preparation behaviors or indicators of extensive planning mostly reported that these are absent in more than two-thirds of attempts. The absence of proximal planning and the suddenness of suicide attempt were related to the absence of mental disorder, the presence of fewer comorbid conditions, and the presence of alcohol use disorders (Rimkeviciene et al. 2015). However, adverse life events are common precursors to suicide and suicide attempts, particularly after recent alcohol consumption (Powell et al. 2001). Intense negative emotions, specifically anger, rage, shame, and guilt, that may arise quickly in a crisis situation can lead to an unplanned suicide attempt (Rimkeviciene et al. 2015).

Transient personal crises can create considerable emotional distress. Suicidal ideation among impulsive attempters may be more transient and temporary than that experienced by persons with chronic depression (Simon et al. 2001). Often, as the acute phase of a crisis passes, the urge to commit suicide decreases (Deisenhammer et al. 2009; Miller and Hemenway 1999; Miller et al. 2012; Yip et al. 2012). One seminal study, for example, examined what had become of 515 people who were prevented from attempting suicide at the Golden Gate Bridge between 1937 and 1971. After more than 26 years on average, 94% were still alive or had died of natural causes (Seiden 1978).

The impulsive and unplanned nature of many suicides strongly suggests that individuals are inclined to use the method most readily accessible to them. Firearms, especially if stored unlocked and loaded, are easily accessed and highly lethal, and require little preparation to be effective. They therefore may be chosen over less lethal methods of suicide, particularly when the suicide is impulsive (Dahlberg et al. 2004; Miller et al. 2012; Rimkeviciene et al. 2015).

Suicide Risk Assessment and Physician Training

Each patient contact with a medical or mental health treatment provider is potentially an opportunity to decrease suicide risk through appropriate assessment and intervention. Assessing suicide risk is a clinical skill necessary in all mental health and primary care settings. Contact with primary care providers and mental health providers prior to suicide is common (Ahmedani et al. 2014; Silverman and Berman 2014). For example, Luoma et al. (2002) found that in the year prior to death by suicide, approximately 32% of their study cohort made contact with a mental health care provider and 77% made contact with a primary care provider. For example, Luoma et al. (2002) found that in the year prior to death by suicide, approximately 32% of their study cohort made contact with a mental health care provider and 77% made contact with a primary care provider.

Nevertheless, regardless of specialty, physicians often lack basic skills and adequate training in suicide risk assessment and do not appear to regularly and systematically assess suicide risk. For example, training of most mental health professionals, including psychiatrists, in the assessment and management of suicidal patients is limited (Schmitz et al. 2012), and many mental health professionals appear to lack the requisite training and skills to assess appropriately for suicide risk (Hung et al. 2012; Schmitz et al. 2012; Silverman 2014).

The absence of formal, systematic, and evidence-based skills training is one important factor that contributes to the suboptimal competency in this critical clinical skill (Jacobson et al. 2012). Suicide risk assessment is a core competency in psychiatric residency training (Jacobs et al. 2003). Despite the fact that as many as 90 psychiatry residency programs offer some teaching on the care of suicidal patients, reviews of the nature of this training have found it lacking.

One survey study found that on average, only 3.6 seminar sessions or lectures were provided during psychiatric residency, and the specific content covered was characterized as often vague and nondescript. Many of the responding residents in this study were of the opinion that attention in clinical training to suicide intervention was insufficient (Schmitz et al. 2012). Only about half of psychological graduate-level trainees receive didactic training on suicide (Cramer et al. 2013; Schmitz et al. 2012). Where training is available, many psychology internship trainees indicate that training quality is low or poor (Cramer et al. 2013).

Primary care physicians play an even more significant role in providing care for potentially suicidal patients than do mental health care providers (Hooper et al. 2012; Luoma et al. 2002; Schulberg et al. 2004). One large-scale study found that 83% of those who died by suicide had received primary care health services in the year prior to death and half had made a medical visit within 4 weeks of death (Ahmedani et al. 2014). Nevertheless, depression and other psychiatric disorders are underrecognized and undertreated in the primary care setting (Mann et al. 2005).

Even when seeing patients with depressive symptoms, primary care providers do not consistently inquire about suicidal ideation or suicide plans (Feldman et al. 2007; Graham et al. 2011; Kaplan et al. 1998). Hooper et al. (2012) found that only 36% of primary care physicians evaluated reported they would conduct a suicide risk assessment when treating a patient presenting with major depression with moderate levels of severity. Such research has led to recommendations for increased training, particularly of primary care providers, in the recognition and management of suicide risk (Cavanagh et al. 2003; Hung et al. 2012; Mann et al. 2005).

Improving Physician Education: Population-Based and Individual-Level Strategies

To date, all comprehensive approaches to suicide prevention that have reduced suicide rates include the training of health professionals as a critical component of their strategies (Alexopoulos et al. 2009; Coffey 2007; Mann et al. 2005; Schmitz et al. 2012). Available studies suggest that suicide risk assessment training can enhance clinicians' knowledge, practical skills, and attitudes (Jacobson et al. 2012; Mann et al. 2005; McNiel et al. 2008; Pisani et al. 2011; Schmitz et al. 2012; Silverman 2014).

On an individual level, clinical care providers can access training opportunities to improve their abilities to detect and assess suicide risk and to implement appropriate suicide risk management interventions. Training is offered by professional organizations such as the American Psychiatric Association and American Psychological Association, as well as other clinical professional organizations. The Suicide Prevention Resource Center (www.sprc.org) and the American Association of Suicidology (www.suicidology.org) also offer training opportunities.

Population-based strategies for improving training in suicide risk assessment and management need to be aggressively pursued. Health care professionals and their professional organizations should take a leading role in promoting increased training. For example, methods for teaching and evaluating suicide risk assessment competency are being developed and researched (e.g., Berman and Silverman 2014; Hung et al. 2012; Schmitz et al. 2012). These models should include recommendations for a standardized curriculum integrated into primary care and mental health professional training programs. For example, an updated version of the American Psychiatric Association's *Practice Guideline for the Assessment and Treatment of Patients With Suicidal Behaviors* (Jacobs et al. 2003) reflecting current and evidence-based best practices could become the basis for a standardized training curriculum for psychiatric residencies and could be modified as needed for other mental health and primary care specialties.

Novel population-based strategies are emerging. For instance, the suicide death of a prominent Seattle attorney in February 2011 prompted scrutiny of mental health professionals' suicide prevention skills. Evidence that the majority of clinicians were unprepared to assess and treat suicidal individuals led to Washington State's 2012 passage of House Bill 2366, the first legislation requiring certain health professionals to obtain continuing medical education in suicide risk assessment and treatment (Stuber and Quinnett 2013). Psychologists and other mental health professionals must have a minimum of 6 hours of continuing education every 6 years to obtain and maintain professional licensure. (Despite recognition that psychiatrists and primary care providers also required additional training, these groups were excluded from the mandated requirement [Stuber and Quinnett 2013].)

Reducing Access to Lethal Means: Suicide, Firearms, and Firearm Safety Management

Population-Based Strategies

General restriction of access to common means of suicide is a population-based suicide prevention strategy with multiple advantages. Removal of access to a lethal method precludes potentially fatal actions or forces the use of a less lethal method (Yip et al. 2012). In addition, population-level means restriction is not dependent on individual assessment or professional skills. Applied to the population as a whole, means restriction affects people whose suicide risk might go undetected or who do not seek assistance.

Population-wide restriction of lethal means has been demonstrated to be an effective strategy to reduce suicide when the method is both highly lethal and common and when the restriction is supported by the community (Mann et al. 2005; Reisch et al. 2013; Yip et al. 2012). For example, suicides in the United States and other countries due to poisoning decreased dramatically after restrictions were placed on the availability of pesticides; domestic gas was detoxified; packaging of over-the-counter medication was modified; and new lower-toxicity antidepressants replaced older, more toxic antidepressants (Mozaffarian et al. 2013).

Similarly, when restrictions are placed on access to firearms, rates of suicide by firearm decrease, particularly in youth, as do overall suicide rates. Studies have demonstrated reduced rates of both firearm-related and overall suicide following legislation and policy changes reducing access to firearms in Australia (Brent et al. 2013; Large and Nielssen 2010), Switzerland (Reisch et al. 2013), New Zealand (Beautrais et al. 2006), and Israel (Lubin et al. 2010; Miller et al. 2012).

Restricting access to firearms has also been found effective in decreasing rates of suicide in the United States. Among men and women, and in every age group including children, states with more firearm restrictions and lower rates of gun ownership have lower rates of both overall suicide and firearm suicide (Barber 2005; Conner and Zhong 2003; Fleegler et al. 2013; Price et al. 2004). States with fewer restrictions on firearm ownership and higher rates of gun ownership have higher rates of firearm-related suicides (Miller and Hemenway 2008; Miller et al. 2013b). Notably, suicide attempt rates were similar in both high- and low-gun-ownership states, but mortality rates were twice as high in high-gun-ownership states. The differences in mortality were entirely attributable to differences in firearm suicide rates (Miller et al. 2013b).

Even small relative declines in the use of firearms in suicide acts could result in large reductions in the number of suicides. Miller et al. (2006) found that each 10% decline in household firearm ownership was associated with a 4.2% decline in the rate of all firearm suicides and, more notably, an 8.3% decline in the firearm suicide rate among children and adolescents ages 0–19. The 10% decline in firearm ownership was also associated with a 2.5% decline in the rate of overall suicides. In contrast, changes in nonfirearm suicide were not associated with changes in firearm ownership (Miller et al. 2006). Over the same time period, no national changes in suicidal tendencies were found (Kessler et al. 2005b).

Substitution. Many people, including many physicians, believe that restricting access to firearms does not prevent suicide. Despite data showing powerful population effects, the beliefs that a person intent on committing suicide will inevitably find a way to do so and that if people lack access to one method they will simply substitute another are common (Miller and Hemenway 2008; Yip et al. 2012). However, most studies have shown that restriction of one method of suicide does not inevitably lead to a compensating rise in the use of other methods (Yip et al. 2012). The reduced overall suicides rates and reduced rates of firearm suicides, particularly among children, that result from reduction in household firearm ownership do not support arguments that people will simply resort to means substitution if firearms are less available.

Moreover, where method substitution occurs, chances for surviving a suicide attempt increase. Almost all other methods of suicide are less lethal than firearms, and therefore individuals who substitute another means of suicide for use of a firearm typically use a less lethal method (Conner and Zhong 2003). From the perspective of public health and injury prevention, the choice of a less lethal method of suicide can be advantageous if the attempt proves to be nonfatal, as it increases chances of intervention to prevent mortality (Yip et al. 2012). For example, even if we were to make the conservative assumption that every individual intent on committing suicide using a firearm would, if denied access to a firearm, substitute suffocation, the second most lethal method of committing suicide, suicide mortality among minors alone could be reduced by as much as 32% (Shenassa et al. 2003).

Population-based strategies to restrict firearms in the United States. To date, almost no studies have examined how gun violence prevention policies focused on persons with mental illness affect suicide (McGinty et al. 2014). However, evidence-based population-level strategies for reducing access to firearms among a population at high risk for suicide have been suggested.

Several studies have found that the first year after discharge from psychiatric hospitalization is associated with a significantly elevated risk of suicide (Bickley et al. 2013; Deisenhammer et al. 2009; Dougall et al. 2014; Owen-Smith et al. 2014; Qin and Nordentoft 2005). Kessler et al. (2015) found that access to firearms was one of the strongest predictors of suicide after psychiatric hospitalization. Although individuals who are involuntarily committed to psychiatric treatment are prohibited from purchasing or possessing firearms, they may petition to have those rights restored (see Chapter 13, "'Relief From Disabilities': Firearm Rights Restoration for Persons Under Mental Health Prohibitions"). The evidence of high risk during the first year following discharge led the Consortium for Risk-Based Firearm Policy (2013a, 2013b) to recommend that federal and state laws require a minimum waiting period of 1 year before these individuals are allowed to petition for restoration of firearm rights.

Similarly, some states have adopted a population-level restriction strategy through mandated waiting periods between the time of purchase and the physical transfer of the firearm. In addition to allowing time to complete background checks, these laws are intended to decrease or prevent impulsive acts of violence, including suicide (Law Center to Prevent Gun Violence 2013). Ten states and the District of Columbia have waiting periods, varying from 24 hours (Illinois) to 14 days (Hawaii), that apply to the purchase of some or all firearms. Additional states require firearm purchasers to obtain a license or permit prior to purchase. Licensing laws such as these play a similar role to waiting period laws (Law Center to Prevent Gun Violence 2013).

Broad means restriction of access to firearms through this kind of regulation requires federal or state legislation as well as community support. Such support is difficult to mobilize when the benefits of the legislation will be small or nonexistent for most people (Yip et al. 2012). Moreover, even proposed minor changes in firearm laws are politically and socially controversial. Thus, use of population-level prevention measures is likely to meet with substantial resistance, despite data supporting large population effects (Yip et al. 2012). Therefore, although broad evidence-based reforms of firearm regulations are a potential strategy for reducing suicide that have yet to be exhausted, means-restriction strategies focused on individuals at risk of suicide must be considered.

Individual Strategies for Lethal Means Restriction

Approaches to reducing access to lethal means of suicide on an individual basis are not means specific. Identifying individuals at high risk for suicide can be challenging for mental health and primary care clinicians, even for those with adequate training and clinical experience. However, utilizing individual strategies offers the advantage of opportunities to include supportive family and friends in a patient's care. A suicidal individual's social support network can be just as important as or even more important than clinicians in preventing suicide (Deisenhammer et al. 2009). Mental health professionals and primary care providers can work with high-risk patients and their families to remove potentially lethal methods from the immediate environment, even if only temporarily. Such interventions can make a difference literally between life and death, because family, friends, and concerned others may recognize signs of an impending crisis.

The potential for success of this individual-level strategy lies in the empirical evidence, discussed above (see subsection "Suicide and Impulsivity"), that many acts of suicide have a significant impulsive component and that decreasing access to lethal means results in decreased suicide mortality. Reducing the availability of lethal means during a suicidal crisis can prolong the period between the initial decision to commit suicide and the suicidal act. During this time, suicidal impulses and intent may decrease and opportunities to access assistance can increase, thereby averting fatal outcomes (Miller and Hemenway 1999; Shenassa et al. 2004; Simon et al. 2001; Yip et al. 2012).

Empirical data support the efficacy of individual-level means restriction. Shenassa et al. (2004) found that firearm owners who had kept their firearms locked or unloaded were at least 60% less likely to die from firearm-related suicide than those who stored their firearms unlocked or loaded. In fact, a dose-response relationship is consistently found in suicides that occur in the home, with ease of firearm access creating a hierarchy of suicide risk (Miller and Hemenway 2008). People in homes with loaded firearms were at higher risk of suicide than people in homes with unloaded firearms, and people in households in which a gun was stored unlocked were at higher risk than people in homes in which all guns were stored locked (Brent 2001; Grossman et al. 2005; Kellermann et al. 1993; Miller et al. 2012).

Firearm Safety Planning as Part of Suicide Risk Assessment and Management

The relative unavailability of population-level means restriction in regard to firearms makes physicians' involvement in and management of high-risk patients' safety in regard to suicide and access to firearms all the more imperative. Suicide risk assessment is the first step in implementing a firearms safety plan, which is an individual-level intervention that restricts access to the most lethal means of suicide, for people at higher risk of suicide. Proactive intervention on a case-by-case basis to limit a suicidal patient's access to firearms may decrease the risk of a fatal outcome in the event of a suicide attempt. Table 10–4 summarizes the key elements of a firearm safety plan.

Questions regarding access to lethal means when assessing risk of suicide should not be limited to firearms; however, given the widespread availability of firearms, their common use as means of suicide, and their high lethality, suicide risk assessments should specifically include queries regarding access to firearms. Important inquiries include whether the patient owns guns, has access to guns in the home owned by someone else, and has plans to purchase any firearms (Simon 2012a; Wintemute et al. 1999).

Discussions regarding firearm safety management should be based on an explicit acknowledgment of concern regarding the patient's safety. A collaborative team approach that includes supportive family members or friends is highly recommended (Homaifar et al. 2013; Simon 2012a). Designing and implementing a firearm safety plan may require one or more meetings with the patient and concerned family or friends. The patient and involved others need to understand that an individual in crisis may be impulsive and reactive, and that the presence of a firearm in the home increases the likelihood that a suicide attempt will be fatal. The role of drugs or alcohol in increasing risk of impulsive suicide and fatal outcomes should also be reviewed with both patients and families.

Patients at risk for suicide may refuse authorization for clinicians to speak with others regarding the need to secure firearms. Patients may not want family members or concerned others to know that they have been having suicidal thoughts or that they have access to firearms. Clinicians will then have to determine whether the situation is an emergency necessitating a breach of confidentiality (Simon 2012a).

If a patient or concerned other reports access to firearms, regardless of the presence or absence of other risk factors, steps should be taken to separate the individual at risk from the firearms. Clinicians should discuss with the patient and concerned others methods for delaying or preventing access to guns during

TABLE 10–4. Restricting access to lethal means: example of a firearm safety plan

1. Ask patients at risk for suicide (and ask significant others) about guns at home or elsewhere, such as car or workplace. Patients who have a gun at home often have more than one gun.
2. Consider invoking emergency exception to consent if a patient at high risk for suicide withholds consent to contact significant others.
3. Involve significant others and the patient, if possible, in designing a firearm safety plan. Include discussions of clinical criteria to be considered for return of firearms.
4. Use this opportunity to educate all involved of the increased risks of a fatal suicide with access to firearms or use of drugs or alcohol, and inform them that the safest option is removal of guns from home, even if only temporarily. Discuss clinical criteria that will be evaluated in regard to restoring access to firearms.
5. Designate a willing, responsible individual, usually a family member or partner, to follow through with the gun safety plan as instructed by the clinician.
6. Confirm via callback from the responsible, designated person that the gun safety plan has been implemented. For example, confirm that all guns and ammunition were separated, removed from the home, and safely secured in a location unknown to the patient.
7. Document that the designated individual implemented the gun removal plan and that a callback was received from that individual confirming the removal of the guns according to the plan.
8. Repeat suicide risk assessments as often as clinical circumstances indicate, particularly before a treatment decision that may restore access to firearms.

Source. Adapted from Simon 2012a.

high-risk periods (Ilgen et al. 2008; Miller and Hemenway 2008; Simon 2012a). Suicide prevention contracts are not to be relied on, especially in regard to firearm safety. No evidence exists that such contracts reduce or eliminate suicide risk (Simon 2012a).

As a clinical axiom, clinicians should understand that there is no such thing as safe gun storage at a suicidal patient's home. Firearm removal, even temporarily, is the safest option. However, suicidal patients should not be handling firearms, even to remove them from the home. A supportive family member or friend should be tasked, if at all possible, with arranging for removal and storage of firearms until the patient's suicide risk decreases. Some local law enforcement agencies will also store weapons, but before suggesting this option, clinicians should know if this possibility is in the patient's community.

Some patients who may not agree to removal of firearms may accept limiting access through safe storage. Access can be delayed through four specific practices:

keeping guns 1) locked and 2) unloaded, and storing ammunition 3) locked and 4) in a separate location. Each of these delaying tactics is associated with a protective effect for suicide, and decreasing levels of risk and mortality are associated with each additional step (Grossman et al. 2005). Hiding firearms and ammunition in an unlocked area is the least effective intervention. Experience has repeatedly demonstrated that an individual intent on finding the firearms is likely to be able to do so (Grossman et al. 2005; Simon 2012a).

Verification that the plan has been implemented is an essential element of a firearm safety plan. Clinicians should not assume that patients or family members have followed through with firearm removal (Simon 2008). Whichever method of firearm safety management is adopted, it should include a prearranged callback verification from a responsible, designated person (Simon 2012a). If no callback is received as prearranged, or the patient has refused to comply with the plan, the patient's firearm safety plan is no longer reliable and the clinician may need to reassess both the level of risk and the feasibility of the safety plan. A fallback plan should be implemented, if possible (Simon 2012a).

Limiting a patient's access to firearms does not have to be permanent. If the decision is made to remove access to firearms through secured storage, the firearm safety plan should include a discussion, again collaboratively with involved others if possible, of the clinical criteria that will be considered in the decision to restore access to firearms to the patient (Simon 2012a). Suicide risk assessment should continue on an ongoing basis (Homaifar et al. 2013) and be repeated as often as necessary or clinically indicated. Clinicians should be certain to repeat suicide risk assessments prior to any clinical or treatment decisions that may alter a patient's level of risk or result in restoring access to firearms.

The Effect of Firearm Restriction on Suicide Rates

Studies of clinical practice in regard to asking about access to firearms and making efforts to eliminate access have been discouraging (Yip et al. 2012). For example, in one study (Carney et al. 2002), only 6% of psychiatric patients in an outpatient setting reported screening for access to firearms. In a survey of psychiatrists regarding the provision of anticipatory guidance about firearm safety (Price et al. 2007), only 27% of psychiatrists reported having a routine system for identifying patients who owned firearms, even among suicidal patients. One of the most common reasons cited by psychiatrists in this study for not providing firearm safety guidance was "lack of expertise."

Similarly, in a survey of psychiatric residency training directors (Price et al. 2010), only 13% reported providing firearm injury prevention training to residents; 79% reported that they had not seriously thought about providing such training. The following were the most significant barriers reported by residency training directors to providing firearm injury prevention training to residents:

- Lack of standardized teaching material for resident training (50%)
- Lack of faculty expertise on firearm issues (49%)
- Lack of guidelines for training residents on firearm issues (47%)
- Absence of curriculum competencies or guidelines approved by the American Psychiatric Association or the Accreditation Council for Graduate Medical Education (42%)

Price et al. (2010) and others (see, e.g., Coverdale et al. 2010; Kolla et al. 2011; Miller and Hemenway 2008; Traylor et al. 2010) have called for the development of curricular guidelines or models for postgraduate psychiatric and psychological training that include access to firearms as part of routine suicide risk assessment and management training. As Schmitz et al. (2012) noted, the "scientific literature is beginning to demonstrate that empirically based skills taught in a brief continuing education format can change clinic policy, confidence in risk assessment, and confidence in management of suicidal patients, with changes sustained at a 6-month follow-up" (p. 296).

In addition, some studies have indicated that physician involvement and education can result in changes in firearm storage practice. One study of family practice patients found that gun owners who were counseled by a doctor about safe firearm storage were 2.2 times more likely to improve their practices than those who were not counseled (Albright and Burge 2003). Brent et al. (2013) reviewed several intervention studies that support the potential to decrease suicide rates among youth by limiting access to lethal means. These studies have demonstrated that a 1-minute intervention as part of well-child care, with an offer of free trigger locks, substantially improves the safety of firearm storage. One nationwide randomized controlled trial found that patients who were counseled by their pediatrician about gun safety and who were offered free cable locks were 22% more likely (compared with a control group of patients who did not receive training and locks) to report 6 months later that they were still following the recommended gun storage protocol (Barkin et al. 2008).

Regardless of levels of training, physicians have only limited ability to ensure that patients comply with recommendations for firearm safety (Simon 2012a). Physicians are all too aware that many health and injury prevention suggestions go unheeded. For example, one study (Brent et al. 2013) found that more than three-fourths of parents responded positively toward physicians providing gun safety counseling; however, only 17% were willing to actually remove the guns from their homes. Studies providing data regarding individual-level suicide education and lethal means restriction, particularly for those at higher risk of suicide, are needed. Nevertheless, although many patients and their families may not benefit from more routine and proactive physician firearm injury prevention counseling, the benefits of averting even a small number of tragic suicide and accidental injury deaths, especially among children and teens, are incalculable.

Therefore, mental health professionals, professional organizations, and organizations that oversee training programs should prioritize the development of standardized curricula or guidelines for suicide risk assessment. These curricula should include education regarding lethal means, the benefit of lethal means restriction especially at times of crisis, and firearm safety management for patients at risk of suicide. These curricula should be required as core competencies for mental health professionals and primary care physicians, and offered both during postgraduate training and in continuing education settings. Given the data regarding the profound risks associated with firearms, psychiatric illness, and substance use, the continued failure to adequately train clinicians underserves patients, families, and communities and leaves families and caring clinicians vulnerable to the consequences of patient suicides.

"Physician Gag Laws"

Perhaps individual-level restriction of access to firearms could be more successful in preventing suicide deaths if routine screening for firearms in the home and counseling regarding associated risks were standard practice and not considered only at times of crisis. Other common physician inquiries, such as whether patients use tobacco or seat belts, have been part of the successful public health campaigns to reduce the morbidity and mortality associated with cigarette smoking and motor vehicles. Patients and families with firearms present in their homes can be counseled on a one-to-one basis regarding suicide risk associated with access to firearms, especially in homes where someone has a psychiatric disorder and/or a substance use problem.

A number of clinicians and physician professional organizations have called for increased routine screening of psychiatric and primary care patients for access to firearms as a form of preventive care (e.g., Dolan et al. 2011; Fleegler et al. 2012; Ilgen et al. 2008; Price et al. 2010; Silverman and Berman 2014). The American College of Physicians (ACP) has stated that physicians have a responsibility to discuss with their patients the risks of having a firearm in the home and recommend ways to mitigate such risks, including best practices to reduce injuries and deaths (Butkus et al. 2014). The ACP emphasizes that this responsibility is imperative when children, adolescents, people with dementia, people with mental illnesses, people with substance use disorders, or others who are at increased risk of harming themselves or others are present in the home.

However, as with almost any aspect of the debate regarding firearm safety, recommendations for routine patient screening and counseling for risk of injury due to firearms has resulted in social and political controversy. In 2011, Florida adopted the Firearm Owner's Privacy Act, creating the Florida statute entitled "Medical Privacy Concerning Firearms" (Fla. Stat. §§790.338, 381.026), thus becoming the first state to enact a "physician gag law" regarding firearms (National Physicians Alliance and the Law Center to Prevent Gun Violence

2013). Among other provisions, the Florida law states that health care practitioners "shall respect a patient's right to privacy" by refraining from

1. making a written inquiry or asking questions concerning the ownership of a firearm or ammunition by the patient or by a family member of the patient;
2. making a written inquiry or asking questions concerning the presence of a firearm in a private home or other domicile of the patient or a family member of the patient;
3. unnecessarily harassing a patient about firearm ownership during an examination; and
4. entering any disclosed information concerning firearm ownership into the patient's medical record.

unless the health care practitioner "in good faith" believes the information is "relevant to the patient's medical care or safety or the safety of others" (Fla. Stat. §790.338). Health care practitioners who violate this law are subject to disciplinary action by the Florida Board of Medicine, including suspension or revocation of their medical licenses as well as a fine of up to $10,000 for each offense (Fla. Stat. §456.072).

One month after the Firearm Owners' Privacy Act was signed into law, a group of Florida physicians and medical professional organizations challenged its constitutionality in federal court (*Wollschlaeger v. Governor of Florida,* Vol. 760 F.3d 1195, 2014). When the case reached the Eleventh Circuit Court of Appeals, the American Psychiatric Association, the American Medical Association, and several other physician organizations submitted amicus curiae briefs opposing the law. Although the federal district judge ruled the law unconstitutional, the Eleventh Circuit Court in 2014 overturned the lower court's decision and ruled the law constitutional (*Wollschlaeger et al. v. Governor of Florida,* 760 F.3d 1195 [11th Cir. 2014]). An en banc appeal was filed, and in July 2015, the Eleventh Circuit Court, although substantially revising their 2014 opinion, in a 2–1 decision again upheld the Act (Case No. 12–14009, decided July 28, 2015).

Since Florida passed its "physician gag law" in 2011, approximately a dozen other states have introduced similar legislation. The majority of such proposed legislation has not been enacted. Nevertheless, Montana in 2013 passed a weaker version of the Florida law, prohibiting physicians from refusing to treat a patient if the patient refuses to answer questions about firearm ownership (2013 H.B. 459). In 2014, Missouri passed a law (S.B. 656), stating, among other provisions, that health care professionals cannot be required to ask about a patient's ownership of firearms, but may do so if medically indicated. Additionally, health care professionals may not use an electronic medical record program that requires entry of data regarding whether or not a patient owns, has access to, or lives in a home containing a firearm, in order to complete and save a medical record.

In addition, at the time of this discussion, Texas is considering a bill introduced in March 2015 that provides that "A physician, other than a psychiatrist, may not:

1. inquire into, or ask a patient to disclose, whether a firearm is located or stored on property owned by or under the patient's control, including the patient's home; and
2. require that [this information] be disclosed before providing treatment to the patient.

As in Florida, the proposed Texas law allows the Texas Medical Board to take disciplinary action against a physician who violates these provisions (Texas HB No. 2823).

Attempts to prevent physicians from routine discussions with patient regarding safe firearm storage practices have not been limited to state legislation (National Physicians Alliance and the Law Center to Prevent Gun Violence 2013). The Affordable Care Act (ACA), signed into law by President Obama in 2010, also contained restrictions on medical care providers' ability to discuss firearm safety and injury prevention with patients. The section of the ACA entitled "Ensuring the quality of care" [42 USC §300-17] mandates, among other provisions, the implementation of wellness and health promotion activities (42 USC §300-17[a][1][d]). Certain public and personal health problems are specifically names as appropriate subjects for health and wellness programs, including smoking cessation, weight management, physical fitness, and even "healthy lifestyle support" (see 42 USC §300-17[b][1–8]). However, the section immediately following this list is entitled "Protection of Second Amendment gun rights" [42 USC §300-17(c)], which states that such programs "may not require the disclosure or collection of any information relating to the presence or storage of a lawfully-possessed firearm or ammunition in the residence or on the property of an individual or the lawful use, possession or storage of a firearm or ammunition by an individual" (42 USC §300-17[c][1]).

The federal government abandoned this position relatively quickly. *The Washington Post* on December 30, 2012 reported that "the deal [with the National Rifle Association] to add gun language to the health-care bill was struck so quietly that several top officials in the Obama administration and in Congress had no idea the passages had been added until approached by the Washington Post" (Wallsten and Hamburger 2012). President Obama signed 23 executive actions to reduce gun violence on January 16, 2013. One of these included an order to "clarify that the Affordable Care Act does not prohibit doctors asking their patients about guns in their homes" (The White House 2013). On January 24, 2013, the Centers for Medicare & Medicaid Services issued this clarification, indicating that the provisions of the ACA do not prohibit or otherwise limit communications between health care professionals and their patients concerning firearms or ammunition. This clarification continues, “Health care providers can play an important role in promoting gun safety” (Centers for Medicare & Medicaid Services 2013).

State legislators have adopted a different and more troubling attitude towards their “physician gag laws,” focusing on exceptions to “medically nonrelevant” inquiries regarding firearms. The proposed Texas law makes an explicit exception for such inquiries for psychiatrists. The relevance exception in the Florida and Missouri laws will likely to apply to mental health professionals performing standard psychiatric evaluations, which routinely include screening for suicide risk.

However, many people obtain mental health care from primary care providers, who must be prepared to assess the mental stability and safety of their patients. Preventive care, even in absence of obvious risk, is central to physician practice. This includes screening patients for common psychiatric problems such as depression and substance use, as well as suicide risk, even if these are not a patient’s chief complaints. The “relevance” exception that might be considered to apply primarily to psychiatrists actually should extend to all physicians providing patient care (Cooke et al. 2012), given the numbers of firearm injuries and deaths due to firearm suicide (as well as homicide related to interpersonal violence and accidental injuries).

Concerns regarding “physician gag laws” center around two primary issues. The first is the role of government regulation of physicians and intrusions into the physician-patient relationship (see e.g., Harvard Law Review 2015). One psychiatric expert stated in regard to the 11th Circuit Court’s 2014 decision in *Wollschlaeger,* “[T]he judges have decided that asking routinely about the presence of guns is contrary to good medical practice and hence can be prohibited by the state. When courts set the standards for clinical interactions rather than leaving that task in medical hands, the inevitable result is harmful to the public’s health” (Psychiatric News Alert 2014).

The second central issue raised by “physician gag laws” was articulated by the dissenting judges in both the first and second 11th Circuit Court opinions in *Wollschlaeger.* In the first opinion, the dissenting judge opined, “As a result of the Act, there is no doubt that many doctors in Florida will significantly curtail, if not altogether cease, discussions with patients about firearms and firearm safety.” In the second opinion, the dissenting judge emphasized this concern and called out the political motivation behind the legislation. He stated, “The Act does significantly limit doctors’ ability to speak to their patients in ways that they believe will protect the public and save lives. The poor fit between what the Act actually does and the interests it purportedly serves belies Florida’s true purpose in passing this Act: silencing doctors’ disfavored message about firearm safety.... The district court properly invalidated the Act as a ... restriction that ‘chills practitioners’ speech in a way that impairs the provision of medical care and may ultimately harm the patient.’”

Many have voiced concerns that these laws will inhibit physicians from asking questions and offering guidance regarding safe firearm storage practices out of fear that such questions might result in a complaint to the Board of Medicine (Lowes 2011). If physicians "routinely" ask about firearm ownership, they risk disciplinary action. As Cooke et al. (2012) observed, the fear of disciplinary action is a "compelling reason not to inquire about firearms ownership" (p. 405). However, ethical obligations such as acting in the best interest of patients' health and promoting patient autonomy compel "routine" inquiries and education regarding firearms risks and injury prevention that maximizes patients' informed decision-making" (Murtagh and Miller 2011).

Physicians and their professional organizations have opposed any laws restricting health care providers from routine inquiries regarding firearm ownership and safety. A multidisciplinary group of the leaders of eight health professional organizations (including the American Psychiatric Association) and the American Bar Association, representing the official policy positions of their organizations, has called for the elimination of physician gag laws, among other measures, to reduce the consequences of firearm morbidity and mortality (Weinberger et al. 2015). The American Psychiatric Association has also independently stated that actions to minimize firearm injuries and violence should include "assuring that physicians and other health care professionals are free to make clinically appropriate inquiries of patients and others about possession of and access to firearms and take necessary steps to reduce the loss of life by suicide, homicide, and accidental injury" (American Psychiatric Association 2014).

New Approaches to Individual Lethal Means Restriction

Limiting access to firearms on a case-by-case basis requires novel approaches toward public education and community participation. As Brent et al. (2013) cautioned, "Although we support the need for rapid access to mental health care for those at risk, it is unrealistic to place complete emphasis on mental health access, triage and care, because of the difficulty in assessing imminent risk for suicide" (p. 335). Innovative approaches that mobilize groups other than mental health professionals to be aware of signs of increasing risk in those people with access to firearms on individual levels need to be designed and explored.

One such promising program, focusing on increasing education for both buyers and sellers of firearms, has been implemented in New Hampshire. Gun advocates, firearm retailers, and public health professionals have collaborated in the design of suicide prevention tip sheets, posters, brochures, and other materials, voluntarily made available at stores that sell firearms. These education materials are based on a social marketing model, similar to the "designated driver" and "friends don't let friends drive drunk" public education campaigns. This campaign encourages a social norm in which friends and family hold on to one another's guns during a mental health crisis, just as they would hold onto the car keys of someone who was drunk and attempting to drive (Vriniotis et al. 2015).

This collaboration builds on the culture of gun safety promoted by many firearm retailers and owners. It encourages people to be alert to signs of suicide in loved ones and to keep firearms from them while they may be most vulnerable. The New Hampshire program is already being replicated in other states (see Chapter 2, "Firearms and Suicide in the United States"). One major advantage of this approach is that it avoids the need for any legislation or public policy initiative. Another is that it demonstrates that areas of agreement, collaboration, and community support can be found between people who own and sell firearms and those who advocate firearm safety when it comes to reducing mortality due to firearm suicide (Vriniotis et al. 2015).

Another innovative approach uses a combination of population-level and individual-level interventions for individual firearm restriction. Mental health and primary care clinicians may not be aware of sudden changes in their patients' level of risk, especially when level of risk changes in relation to an unexpected personal crisis or change in behavior. Many individuals do not consult clinicians regularly. Families and concerned others are often acutely aware of an individual's deteriorating clinical condition and increasing risk of committing firearm suicide (and at times homicide).

Recognizing the potential of individual-level lethal means restriction interventions initiated by families and friends, the Consortium for Risk-Based Firearm Policy has proposed a new type of legislation, the gun violence restraining order (GVRO), discussed in detail in Chapter 12, "Preventing Gun Violence." Briefly, the GVRO is a civil restraining order, a legal process modeled on the domestic violence restraining order. The GVRO would allow family members to petition a court to request that firearms be temporarily removed from another family member or intimate partner who poses a credible risk of harm to self or others (Consortium for Risk-Based Firearm Policy 2013a, 2013b). To date, California is the only state that has adopted this legislation (Calif. AB-1014), which will become effective on January 1, 2016.

The GVRO empowers families by providing a mechanism through which law enforcement will be able to separate individuals, with or without mental illness, from their firearms during times of crisis. The GVRO is a population-level intervention, in that it requires a change in state or federal law that will apply to everyone equally. However, the effect of such legislation is to allow individual, case-by-case intervention, initiated by those who may have more information about an individual's behavioral and psychological state than do clinicians or law enforcement. In addition, the GVRO does not focus on or stigmatize individuals with mental illness; unlike involuntary commitment laws, for example, the presence of a psychiatric disorder is not required for this intervention to be utilized.

These new approaches hold promise for decreasing firearm suicide rates. The individual-level interventions described in this section are so new that no empirical evidence regarding their efficacy is available. Hopefully, research will be designed that allows evaluation of the implementation and outcomes of these new types of intervention in lethal means restriction. Such research can inform modifications of these and other interventions as well as suggest avenues for additional interventions, on both a population-level and an individual-level basis.

Conclusion

Calls from politicians, firearm legislation reform advocates, pro-gun advocates, and the media to restrict firearm access to those with "dangerous mental illness" are not intended to decrease rates of firearm suicide. Compared with mass shootings, firearm suicide is statistically more frequent; unlike mass shootings, suicide is almost always associated with psychiatric illness. Nevertheless, political and social rhetoric regarding firearm restriction and mental illness is intended to decrease the perceived high risk that those with serious mental illness will commit mass shootings.

The only two interventions that have been empirically demonstrated to reduce the incidence of suicide are 1) physician education and training in suicide risk assessment and risk management and 2) restriction of access to lethal means. Postgraduate medical training, regardless of specialty, needs to significantly improve clinical training in suicide risk assessment and management skills. Professional organizations need to develop and adopt standardized suicide risk assessment guidelines. These practice guidelines need to emphasize the importance of evaluating access to lethal means, particularly firearms.

The presence of a gun in the home, no matter how it is stored, is a risk factor for completed suicide for everyone who lives in the home. The rates of firearm morbidity and mortality are such that all mental health patients and primary care patients should be queried regarding their access to firearms and counseled regarding firearm safety. Laws intended to curb physician inquiries serve neither public health concerns presented by rates of firearm suicide morbidity or mortality nor the welfare of patients.

Patients at risk for suicide also require active implementation of a clinical gun safety management plan. The mental health prohibitions on legal access to firearms do not capture the population at high risk of firearm suicide and do little more than reinforce the stigma associated with mental illness. Nevertheless, population-wide restrictions of access to firearms that would apply equally to all individuals are difficult to implement in the current political and social climate, despite the data that indicate the efficacy of such restrictions in decreasing rates of firearm suicide as well as overall suicide.

Individual-level interventions require the design and implementation of novel strategies based on common areas of agreement. The need for intervention on a case-by-case basis further emphasizes the need for clinical suicide risk assessment and firearm safety management skills and counseling in all mental health and primary care specialties. In addition, individually based interventions to prevent suicide can include family and concerned others, a powerful source of social support. As yet, little or no empirical data regarding outcomes of individual-level efforts in communities are available.

Decreasing levels of firearm suicide morbidity and mortality will require multiple interventions on multiple levels. Without question, more research on population and individual levels and improved training and skills on the part of mental health and primary care providers are needed. Increasing public education through campaigns on recognizing increased risks of suicide in loved ones and the high risk of a fatal outcome should a person have access to firearms at a time of crisis holds promise of changing social norms. Educating family members and gun owners about the importance of storing firearms properly is essential. Identifying those at risk of suicide, developing effective treatment plans, and implementing safety strategies can save many lives.

Suggested Interventions

- *Increase postgraduate and public education in suicide risk assessment and management, including firearm risk assessment and safety:* Professional organizations, including those overseeing postgraduate education, should design, adopt, and use a standardized suicide risk assessment and management curriculum and practice guidelines. This curriculum should include firearm risk assessment and safety management and should be implemented as soon as possible into all training for mental health and primary care providers. State licensing boards should require continuing education in suicide risk assessment and firearm safety management for accreditation for license renewal by every mental health professional and primary care physician.

- *Conduct routine suicide risk and firearm risk assessment screening of all patients:* Mental health professionals and primary care clinicians should conduct routine suicide assessment screening and screening for access to firearms, even for patients for whom risk of suicide seems low. Patients and possibly family members should be advised of the increased risk of fatal injury, intentional and unintentional, associated with firearms in the home, and should be advised regarding safe storage practices.

- *Advise removal of firearms from the home of people at high risk of suicide:* All physicians should understand and emphasize to their patients that if patients or others in their home have a psychiatric illness and use substances, particularly alcohol, safe storage of firearms in the home is *not* possible. Under these circumstances, concerned others should do everything possible to remove firearms from the home, even if only on a temporary basis.
- *Advocate against "physician gag laws":* Medical professionals and their professional organizations should continue to advocate against so-called physician gag laws. These laws intrude into the physician-patient relationship and will have a chilling effect on physicians in regard to screening patients as well as increase risk of death and injury due to firearms, despite the exception for "relevant inquiries."
- *Partner with community organizations, including groups that promote firearm ownership, to find common ground regarding suicide prevention interventions:* Mental health professionals and their professional organizations should seek opportunities to partner with members of the firearm community to increase public education regarding suicide, firearm access, and firearm safety at points of access to firearms.

References

Accreditation Council for Graduate Medical Education: ACGME Program Requirements for Graduate Medical Education in Psychiatry. Chicago, IL, Accreditation Council for Graduate Medical Education, 2014. Available at: http://www.acgme.org/acgmeweb/Portals/0/PFAssets/ProgramRequirements/400_psychiatry_07012014.pdf. Accessed August 18, 2015.

Ahmedani BK, Simon GE, Stewart C, et al: Health care contacts in the year before suicide death. J Gen Intern Med 29(6):870–877, 2014 24567199

Albright TL, Burge SK: Improving firearm storage habits: impact of brief office counseling by family physicians. J Am Board Fam Pract 16(1):40–46, 2003 12583649

Alexopoulos GS, Reynolds CF III, Bruce ML, et al: Reducing suicidal ideation and depression in older primary care patients: 24-month outcomes of the PROSPECT study. Am J Psychiatry 166(8):882–890, 2009 19528195

American Association of Suicidology: Facts & Statistics. Washington, DC, American Association of Suicidology, 2014. Available at: http://www.suicidology.org/resources/facts-statistics. Accessed January 13, 2015.

American Foundation for Suicide Prevention: Understanding Suicide: Facts and Figures. Washington, DC, American Foundation for Suicide Prevention, 2014. Available at: https://www.afsp.org/understanding-suicide/facts-and-figures. Accessed March 7, 2015.

American Psychiatric Association: Position Statement on Firearm Access, Acts of Violence, and the Relationship to Mental Illness and Mental Health Services. Arlington, VA, American Psychiatric Association, 2014. Available at: http://www.psychiatry.org/File%20Library/Learn/Archives/Position-2014-Firearm-Access.pdf. Accessed January 9, 2015.

Anglemyer A, Horvath T, Rutherford G: The accessibility of firearms and risk for suicide and homicide victimization among household members: a systematic review and meta-analysis. Ann Intern Med 160(2):101–110, 2014 24592495

Arsenault-Lapierre G, Kim C, Turecki G: Psychiatric diagnoses in 3275 suicides: a meta-analysis. BMC Psychiatry 4:37, 2004 15527502

Barber CW: Fatal connection: the link between guns and suicide. Advancing Suicide Prevention 1(2):25–26, 2005

Barkin SL, Finch SA, Ip EH, et al: Is office-based counseling about media use, timeouts, and firearm storage effective? Results from a cluster-randomized, controlled trial. Pediatrics 122(1):e15–e25, 2008 18595960

Beautrais AL, Fergusson DM, Horwood LJ: Firearms legislation and reductions in firearm-related suicide deaths in New Zealand. Aust NZ J Psychiatry 40(3):253–259, 2006 16476153

Berman AL, Silverman MM: Suicide risk assessment and risk formulation, part II: suicide risk formulation and the determination of levels of risk. Suicide Life Threat Behav 44(4):432–443, 2014 24286521

Betz ME, Barber C, Miller M: Suicidal behavior and firearm access: results from the Second Injury Control and Risk Survey. Suicide Life Threat Behav 41(4):384–391, 2011 21535097

Bickley H, Hunt IM, Windfuhr K, et al: Suicide within two weeks of discharge from psychiatric inpatient care: a case-control study. Psychiatr Serv 64(7):653–659, 2013 23545716

Blumenthal R: Suicidal gunshot wounds to the head: a retrospective review of 406 cases. Am J Forensic Med Pathol 28(4):288–291, 2007 18043013

Branas CC, Richmond TS, Ten Have TR, et al: Acute alcohol consumption, alcohol outlets, and gun suicide. Subst Use Misuse 46(13):1592–1603, 2011 21929327

Brent DA: Firearms and suicide. Ann NY Acad Sci 932:225–239, discussion 239–240, 2001 11411188

Brent DA, Miller MJ, Loeber R, et al: Ending the silence on gun violence. J Am Acad Child Adolesc Psychiatry 52(4):333–338, 2013 23571100

Butkus R, Doherty R, Daniel H, et al: Reducing firearm-related injuries and deaths in the United States: executive summary of a policy position paper from the American College of Physicians. Ann Intern Med 160(12):858–860, 2014 24722815

Carney CP, Allen J, Doebbeling BN: Receipt of clinical preventive medical services among psychiatric patients. Psychiatr Serv 53(8):1028–1030, 2002 12161681

Cavanagh JT, Carson AJ, Sharpe M, et al: Psychological autopsy studies of suicide: a systematic review. Psychol Med 33(3):395–405, 2003 12701661

Centers for Disease Control and Prevention: Injury Prevention & Control: Data & Statistics (WISQARS). Atlanta, GA, Centers for Disease Control and Prevention, 2015. Available at: http://www.cdc.gov/injury/wisqars/index.html. Accessed February 11, 2015.

Centers for Medicare & Medicaid Services, The Center for Consumer Information & Insurance Oversight: Affordable Care Act Implementation FAQs–Set 11. Available at: https://www.cms.gov/CCIIO/Resources/Fact-Sheets-and-FAQs/aca_implementation_faqs11.html. Accessed August 22, 2015.

Chapdelaine A, Samson E, Kimberley MD, et al: Firearm-related injuries in Canada: issues for prevention. CMAJ 145(10):1217–1223, 1991 1933704

Cherpitel CJ, Borges GLG, Wilcox HC: Acute alcohol use and suicidal behavior: a review of the literature. Alcohol Clin Exp Res 28(5):18S–28S, 2004 15166633

Child Trends Data Bank: Teen Homicide, Suicide, and Firearm Deaths: Indicators on Children and Youth. Bethesda, MD, Child Trends, March 2015. Available at: http://www.childtrends.org/wp-content/uploads/2014/10/70_Homicide_Suicide_Firearms.pdf. Accessed April 3, 2015.

Coffey CE: Building a system of perfect depression care in behavioral health. Jt Comm J Qual Patient Saf 33(4):193–199, 2007 17441556

Conner KR, Zhong Y: State firearm laws and rates of suicide in men and women. Am J Prev Med 25(4):320–324, 2003 14580634

Conner KR, Huguet N, Caetano R, et al: Acute use of alcohol and methods of suicide in a U.S. national sample. Am J Public Health 104(1):171–178, 2014 23678938

Consortium for Risk-Based Firearm Policy: Guns, Public Health, and Mental Illness: An Evidence-Based Approach for Federal Policy. Baltimore, MD, Johns Hopkins Center for Gun Policy and Research, 2013a

Consortium for Risk-Based Firearm Policy: Guns, Public Health, and Mental Illness: An Evidence-Based Approach for State Policy. Baltimore, MD, Johns Hopkins Center for Gun Policy and Research, 2013b

Cooke BK, Goddard ER, Ginory A, et al: Firearms inquiries in Florida: "medical privacy" or medical neglect? J Am Acad Psychiatry Law 40(3):399–408, 2012 22960923

Coverdale JH, Roberts LW, Balon R: The public health priority to address the accessibility and safety of firearms: recommendations for training. Acad Psychiatry 34(6):405–408, 2010 21041461

Cramer RJ, Johnson SM, McLaughlin J, et al: Suicide risk assessment training for psychology doctoral programs: core competencies and a framework for training. Train Educ Prof Psychol 7(1):1–11, 2013 24672588

Dahlberg LL, Ikeda RM, Kresnow MJ: Guns in the home and risk of a violent death in the home: findings from a national study. Am J Epidemiol 160(10):929–936, 2004 15522849

Deisenhammer EA, Ing CM, Strauss R, et al: The duration of the suicidal process: how much time is left for intervention between consideration and accomplishment of a suicide attempt? J Clin Psychiatry 70(1):19–24, 2009 19026258

Dolan MA, Fein JA; Committee on Pediatric Emergency Medicine: Pediatric and adolescent mental health emergencies in the emergency medical services system. Pediatrics 127(5):e1356–e1366, 2011 21518712

Dougall N, Lambert P, Maxwell M, et al: Deaths by suicide and their relationship with general and psychiatric hospital discharge: 30-year record linkage study. Br J Psychiatry 204:267–273, 2014 24482439

Elnour AA, Harrison J: Lethality of suicide methods. Inj Prev 14(1):39–45, 2008 18245314

Fawcett J, Scheftner WA, Fogg L, et al: Time-related predictors of suicide in major affective disorder. Am J Psychiatry 147(9):1189–1194, 1990 2104515

Fawcett J, Clark DC, Busch KA: Assessing and treating the patient at risk for suicide. Psychiatr Ann 23(5):244–255, 1993

Feldman MD, Franks P, Duberstein PR, et al: Let's not talk about it: suicide inquiry in primary care. Ann Fam Med 5(5):412–418, 2007 17893382

Fleegler EW, Monuteaux MC, Bauer SR, et al: Attempts to silence firearm injury prevention. Am J Prev Med 42(1):99–102, 2012 22176854

Fleegler EW, Lee LK, Monuteaux MC, et al: Firearm legislation and firearm-related fatalities in the United States. JAMA Intern Med 173(9):732–740, 2013 23467753

Graham RD, Rudd MD, Bryan CJ: Primary care providers' views regarding assessing and treating suicidal patients. Suicide Life Threat Behav 41(6):614–623, 2011 22145822

Grassel KM, Wintemute GJ, Wright MA, et al: Association between handgun purchase and mortality from firearm injury. Inj Prev 9(1):48–52, 2003 12642559

Grossman DC, Mueller BA, Riedy C, et al: Gun storage practices and risk of youth suicide and unintentional firearm injuries. JAMA 293(6):707–714, 2005 15701912

Harvard Law Review: Wollschlaeger v. Governor of Florida. Harv Law Rev 128(3):1045, 2015

Hawton K: Restricting access to methods of suicide: rationale and evaluation of this approach to suicide prevention. Crisis: The Journal of Crisis Intervention and Suicide Prevention 28 (suppl 1):4–9, 2007

Hemenway D, Miller M: Association of rates of household handgun ownership, lifetime major depression, and serious suicidal thoughts with rates of suicide across U.S. census regions. Inj Prev 8(4):313–316, 2002 12460969

Homaifar B, Matarazzo B, Wortzel HS: Therapeutic risk management of the suicidal patient: augmenting clinical suicide risk assessment with structured instruments. J Psychiatr Pract 19(5):406–409, 2013 24042246

Hooper LM, Epstein SA, Weinfurt KP, et al: Predictors of primary care physicians' self-reported intention to conduct suicide risk assessments. J Behav Health Serv Res 39(2):103–115, 2012 22218814

Hung EK, Binder RL, Fordwood SR, et al: A method for evaluating competency in assessment and management of suicide risk. Acad Psychiatry 36(1):23–28, 2012 22362432

Ilgen MA, Zivin K, McCammon RJ, et al: Mental illness, previous suicidality, and access to guns in the United States. Psychiatr Serv 59(2):198–200, 2008 18245165

Jacobs DG, Baldessarini RJ, Conwell Y, et al: Practice Guideline for the Assessment and Treatment of Patients With Suicidal Behaviors. Arlington, VA, American Psychiatric Association, November 2003. Available at: http://psychiatryonline.org/pb/assets/raw/sitewide/practice_guidelines/guidelines/suicide.pdf. Accessed April 3, 2015.

Jacobson JM, Osteen P, Jones A, et al: Evaluation of the Recognizing and Responding to Suicide Risk training. Suicide Life Threat Behav 42(5):471–485, 2012 22924960

Johnson RM, Barber C, Azrael D, et al: Who are the owners of firearms used in adolescent suicides? Suicide Life Threat Behav 40(6):609–611, 2010 21198329

Kaplan MS, Adamek ME, Rhoades JA: Prevention of elderly suicide: physicians' assessment of firearm availability. Am J Prev Med 15(1):60–64, 1998 9651640

Kaplan MS, McFarland BH, Huguet N, et al: Acute alcohol intoxication and suicide: a gender-stratified analysis of the National Violent Death Reporting System. Inj Prev 19(1):38–43, 2013 22627777

Kapp MB: Geriatric patients, firearms, and physicians. Ann Intern Med 159(6):421–422, 2013 23836076

Kellermann AL, Rivara FP, Somes G, et al: Suicide in the home in relation to gun ownership. N Engl J Med 327(7):467–472, 1992 1308093

Kellermann AL, Rivara FP, Rushforth NB, et al: Gun ownership as a risk factor for homicide in the home. N Engl J Med 329(15):1084–1091, 1993 8371731

Kessler RC, Borges G, Walters EE: Prevalence of and risk factors for lifetime suicide attempts in the National Comorbidity Survey. Arch Gen Psychiatry 56(7):617–626, 1999 10401507

Kessler RC, Berglund P, Borges G, et al: Trends in suicide ideation, plans, gestures, and attempts in the United States, 1990–1992 to 2001–2003. JAMA 293(20):2487–2495, 2005a 15914749

Kessler RC, Demler O, Frank RG, et al: Prevalence and treatment of mental disorders, 1990 to 2003. N Engl J Med 352(24):2515–2523, 2005b 15958807

Kessler RC, Warner CH, Ivany C, et al: Predicting suicides after psychiatric hospitalization in U.S. Army soldiers: the Army Study to Assess Risk and Resilience in Servicemembers (Army STARRS). JAMA Psychiatry 72(1):49–57, 2015 25390793

Kolla BP, O'Connor SS, Lineberry TW: The base rates and factors associated with reported access to firearms in psychiatric inpatients. Gen Hosp Psychiatry 33(2):191–196, 2011 21596213

Krouse WJ: Gun Control Legislation. Washington, DC, Congressional Research Service, 2012

Large MM, Nielssen OB: Suicide in Australia: meta-analysis of rates and methods of suicide between 1988 and 2007. Med J Aust 192(8):432–437, 2010 20402605

Law Center to Prevent Gun Violence: Waiting Periods Policy Summary. San Francisco, CA, Law Center to Prevent Gun Violence, 2013. Available at: http://smartgunlaws.org/waiting-periods-policy-summary/. Accessed April 7, 2015.

Lowes R: Physicians fight Florida "gag law" on gun questions. Medscape, June 8, 2011

Lubin G, Werbeloff N, Halperin D, et al: Decrease in suicide rates after a change of policy reducing access to firearms in adolescents: a naturalistic epidemiological study. Suicide Life Threat Behav 40(5):421–424, 2010 21034205

Luoma JB, Martin CE, Pearson JL: Contact with mental health and primary care providers before suicide: a review of the evidence. Am J Psychiatry 159:909–916, 2002 12042175

Mann JJ, Apter A, Bertolote J, et al: Suicide prevention strategies: a systematic review. JAMA 294(16):2064–2074, 2005 16249421

McGinty EE, Webster DW, Barry CL: Gun policy and serious mental illness: priorities for future research and policy. Psychiatr Serv 65(1):50–58, 2014 23852317

McNiel DE, Weaver CM, Hall SE: Base rates of firearm possession by hospitalized psychiatric patients. Psychiatr Serv 58(4):551–553, 2007 17412859

McNiel DE, Fordwood SR, Weaver CM, et al: Effects of training on suicide risk assessment. Psychiatr Serv 59(12):1462–1465, 2008 19033175

Melton BB, Coverdale JH: What do we teach psychiatric residents about suicide? A national survey of chief residents. Acad Psychiatry 33(1):47–50, 2009 19349444

Mertens B, Sorenson SB: Considerations about the elderly and firearms. Am J Public Health 102:396–400, 2012 22390501

Miller M, Hemenway D: The relationship between firearms and suicide: a review of the literature. Aggress Violent Behav 4(1):59–75, 1999

Miller M, Hemenway D: Guns and suicide in the United States. N Engl J Med 359(10):989–991, 2008 18768940

Miller M, Azrael D, Hepburn L, et al: The association between changes in household firearm ownership and rates of suicide in the United States, 1981–2002. Inj Prev 12(3):178–182, 2006 16751449

Miller M, Barber C, Azrael D, et al: Recent psychopathology, suicidal thoughts and suicide attempts in households with and without firearms: findings from the National Comorbidity Study Replication. Inj Prev 15(3):183–187, 2009 19494098

Miller M, Azrael D, Barber C: Suicide mortality in the United States: the importance of attending to method in understanding population-level disparities in the burden of suicide. Annu Rev Public Health 33:393–408, 2012 22224886

Miller M, Azrael D, Hemenway D: Firearms and violent death in the United States, in Reducing Gun Violence in America: Informing Policy With Evidence and Analysis. Edited by Webster DW, Vernick JS. Baltimore, MD, Johns Hopkins University Press, 2013a, pp 3–20

Miller M, Barber C, White RA, et al: Firearms and suicide in the United States: is risk independent of underlying suicidal behavior? Am J Epidemiol 178(6):946–955, 2013b 23975641

Mozaffarian D, Hemenway D, Ludwig DS: Curbing gun violence: lessons from public health successes. JAMA 309(6):551–552, 2013 23295618

Murtagh L, Miller M: Censorship of the patient-physician relationship: a new Florida law. JAMA 306(10):1131–1132, 2011 21835978

National Physicians Alliance and the Law Center to Prevent Gun Violence: Gun Safety & Public Health: Policy Recommendations for a More Secure America. San Francisco, CA, Law Center to Prevent Gun Violence, 2013. Available at: http://smartgunlaws.org/gun-safety-public-health-policy-recommendations-for-a-more-secure-america. Accessed March 11, 2015.

Nock MK, Borges G, Bromet EJ, et al: Suicide and suicidal behavior. Epidemiol Rev 30:133–154, 2008 18653727

Owens C, Booth N, Briscoe M, et al: Suicide outside the care of mental health services: a case-controlled psychological autopsy study. Crisis 24(3):113–121, 2003 14518644

Owen-Smith A, Bennewith O, Donovan J, et al: "When you're in the hospital, you're in a sort of bubble." Understanding the high risk of self-harm and suicide following psychiatric discharge: a qualitative study. Crisis 35(3):154–160, 2014 24698726

Pew Research Center: Why Own a Gun? Protection Is Now Top Reason. Washington, DC, Pew Research Center, 2013

Pisani AR, Cross WF, Gould MS: The assessment and management of suicide risk: state of workshop education. Suicide Life Threat Behav 41(3):255–276, 2011 21477093

Powell KE, Kresnow MJ, Mercy JA, et al: Alcohol consumption and nearly lethal suicide attempts. Suicide Life Threat Behav 32(1 suppl):30–41, 2001 11924693

Price JH, Thompson AJ, Dake JA: Factors associated with state variations in homicide, suicide, and unintentional firearm deaths. J Community Health 29(4):271–283, 2004 15186014

Price JH, Kinnison A, Dake JA, et al: Psychiatrists' practices and perceptions regarding anticipatory guidance on firearms. Am J Prev Med 33(5):370–373, 2007 17950401

Price JH, Thompson AJ, Khubchandani J, et al: Firearm anticipatory guidance training in psychiatric residency programs. Acad Psychiatry 34(6):417–423, 2010 21041464

Psychiatric News Alert: Court says Florida's ban on physicians discussing gun ownership is legal. Psychiatric News, July 29, 2014

Qin P, Nordentoft M: Suicide risk in relation to psychiatric hospitalization: evidence based on longitudinal registers. Arch Gen Psychiatry 62(4):427–432, 2005 15809410

Reisch T, Steffen T, Habenstein A, et al: Change in suicide rates in Switzerland before and after firearm restriction resulting from the 2003 "Army XXI" reform. Am J Psychiatry 170(9):977–984, 2013 23897090

Richardson EG, Hemenway D: Homicide, suicide, and unintentional firearm fatality: comparing the United States with other high-income countries, 2003. J Trauma 70:238–243, 2011 20571454

Rimkeviciene J, O'Gorman J, De Leo D: Impulsive suicide attempts: a systematic literature review of definitions, characteristics and risk factors. J Affect Disord 171:93–104, 2015 25299440

Rudd MD: Core competencies, warning signs, and a framework for suicide risk assessment in clinical practice, in The Oxford Handbook of Suicide and Self-Injury. Edited by Nock MK. New York, Oxford University Press, 2014, pp 323–336

Schmitz WM Jr, Allen MH, Feldman BN, et al: Preventing suicide through improved training in suicide risk assessment and care: an American Association of Suicidology Task Force report addressing serious gaps in U.S. mental health training. Suicide Life Threat Behav 42(3):292–304, 2012 22494118

Schulberg HC, Bruce ML, Lee PW, et al: Preventing suicide in primary care patients: the primary care physician's role. Gen Hosp Psychiatry 26(5):337–345, 2004 15474633

Seiden RH: Where are they now? A follow-up study of suicide attempters from the Golden Gate Bridge. Suicide Life Threat Behav 8(4):203–216, 1978 217131

Shah S, Hoffman RE, Wake L, et al: Adolescent suicide and household access to firearms in Colorado: results of a case-control study. J Adolesc Health 26(3):157–163, 2000 10706163

Shenassa ED, Catlin SN, Buka SL: Lethality of firearms relative to other suicide methods: a population based study. J Epidemiol Community Health 57:120–124, 2003 12540687

Shenassa ED, Rogers ML, Spalding KL, et al: Safer storage of firearms at home and risk of suicide: a study of protective factors in a nationally representative sample. J Epidemiol Community Health 58(10):841–848, 2004 15365110

Silverman MM: Suicide risk assessment and suicide risk formulation: essential components of the therapeutic risk management model. J Psychiatr Pract 20(5):373–378, 2014 25226200

Silverman MM, Berman AL: Suicide risk assessment and risk formulation, Part I: a focus on suicide ideation in assessing suicide risk. Suicide Life Threat Behav 44(4):420–431, 2014 25250407

Simon OR, Swann AC, Powell KE, et al: Characteristics of impulsive suicide attempts and attempters. Suicide Life Threat Behav 32(1 suppl):49–59, 2001 11924695

Simon RI: The myth of "imminent" violence in psychiatry and the law. Univ Cincinnati Law Rev 75(2):631–644, 2006a

Simon RI: Suicide risk: assessing the unpredictable, in The American Psychiatric Publishing Textbook of Suicide Assessment and Management. Edited by Simon RI, Hales RE. Washington DC, American Psychiatric Publishing, 2006b, pp 1–32

Simon RI: Clinically based risk management of potentially violent patients, in Textbook of Violence Assessment and Management. Edited by Simon RI, Tardiff K. Washington, DC, American Psychiatric Publishing, 2008, pp 555–565

Simon RI: Suicide risk assessment forms: form over substance? J Am Acad Psychiatry Law 37(3):290–293, 2009 19767492

Simon RI: Patient safety and freedom of movement: coping with uncertainty, in The American Psychiatric Publishing Textbook of Suicide Assessment and Management, 2nd Edition. Edited by Simon RI, Hales RE. Washington, DC, American Psychiatric Publishing, 2012a, pp 331–346

Simon RI: Suicide risk assessment: gateway to treatment and management, in The American Psychiatric Publishing Textbook of Suicide Assessment and Management, 2nd Edition. Edited by Simon RI, Hales RE. Washington, DC, American Psychiatric Publishing, 2012b, pp 3–28

Smith GS, Branas CC, Miller TR: Fatal nontraffic injuries involving alcohol: a metaanalysis. Ann Emerg Med 33(6):659–668, 1999 10339681

Sorenson SB, Vittes KA: Mental health and firearms in community-based surveys: implications for suicide prevention. Eval Rev 32(3):239–256, 2008 18456876

Stuber J, Quinnett P: Making the case for primary care and mandated suicide prevention education. Suicide Life Threat Behav 43(2):117–124, 2013 23331347

Swanson JW: Explaining rare acts of violence: the limits of evidence from population research. Psychiatr Serv 62(11):1369–1371, 2011 22211218

Swanson JW, Sampson NA, Petukhova MV, et al: Guns, impulsive angry behavior, and mental disorders: results from the National Comorbidity Survey Replication (NCS-R). Behav Sci Law Apr 8, 2015 25850688 (Epub ahead of print)

Traylor A, Price JH, Telljohann SK, et al: Clinical psychologists' firearm risk management perceptions and practices. J Community Health 35(1):60–67, 2010 20094905

Vriniotis M, Barber C, Frank E, et al: A suicide prevention campaign for firearm dealers in New Hampshire. Suicide Life Threat Behav 45(2):157–163, 2015 25348506

Wallsten P, Hamburger T: NRA fingerprints in landmark health-care law. The Washington Post, December 30, 2012. Available at: http://www.washingtonpost.com/politics/nra-fingerprints-in-landmark-health-care-law/2012/12/30/e6018656-5066-11e2-950a-7863a013264b_story.html. Accessed August 22, 2015.

Weinberger SE, Hoyt DB, Lawrence HC, et al: Firearm-related injury and death in the United States: a call to action from 8 health professional organizations and the American Bar Association. Ann Intern Med 162(7):513–516, 2015

The White House: Now is the time: gun violence reduction executive actions, 2013. Available at: https://www.whitehouse.gov/sites/default/files/docs/wh_now_is_the_time_ actions.pdf. Accessed August 22, 2015.

Wintemute GJ: Responding to the crisis of firearm violence in the United States: comment on "Firearm legislation and firearm-related fatalities in the United States." JAMA Intern Med 173(9):740–741, 2013 23467768

Wintemute GJ, Parham CA, Beaumont JJ, et al: Mortality among recent purchasers of handguns. N Engl J Med 341(21):1583–1589, 1999 10564689

World Health Organization: Preventing Suicide: A Global Imperative. Geneva, World Health Organization, 2014.

Wortzel HS, Matarazzo B, Homaifar B: A model for therapeutic risk management of the suicidal patient. J Psychiatr Pract 19(4):323–326, 2013 23852108

Wright MA, Wintemute GJ, Claire BE: Gun suicide by young people in California: descriptive epidemiology and gun ownership. J Adolesc Health 43(6):619–622, 2008 19027653

Yip PS, Caine E, Yousuf S, et al: Means restriction for suicide prevention. Lancet 379(9834):2393–2399, 2012 22726520

11

Treatment Engagement, Access to Services, and Civil Commitment Reform

Would These Strategies Help Reduce Firearm-Related Risks?

Debra A. Pinals, M.D.

Common Misperceptions

- ☒ People with mental illness can be hospitalized easily even if they do not want to be hospitalized.
- ☒ People with serious mental illness are always able to recognize the importance of treatment to minimize their risk of harm to self or others and maximize their functioning.
- ☒ People with mental illness are by far more dangerous to others than people without mental illness, especially with regard to firearm violence.

The opinions expressed in this chapter are the author's and do not reflect the views or opinions of any agency or entity with which the author is affiliated.

☒ People with mental illness who commit gun violence are not in treatment because nobody has recognized that they have serious mental illness and tried to get them into treatment.

Evidence-Based Facts

☑ Laws related to civil commitment are varied, but most rely heavily on a need to prove risk of harm to self or others due to active symptoms of mental illness. These narrow criteria can be difficult to prove, even if individuals are experiencing acute symptoms of mental illness. Therefore, for an individual who does not wish to be hospitalized even if he or she could benefit from it, involuntary commitment can be a limited option.

☑ People with serious mental illness often lack insight into their condition and thus are likely to decline services. They therefore might not adhere to treatment despite experiencing significant social, personal, and economic consequences from their illness.

☑ Persons with mental illness present a small increased risk of violence compared to people without mental illness, but substance use and trauma histories can compound these risks. When people with mental illness become dangerous, they are more often dangerous to themselves than to others, particularly in regard to use of firearms. Suicide deaths by firearms far outnumber homicides related to firearms.

☑ For the small number of individuals with mental illness who commit gun violence against others, attempts to access care may or may not have taken place. Even when illness is recognized, the individual may be unwilling to access services, and forced treatment may not be available or appropriate for the particular issue at hand. When illness is unrecognized, access to care may not have been sought.

Media coverage of mass shootings seems to continually turn societal attention to questions about the perpetrators' mental health. This trend occurs, in part, because heinous acts often belie explanation, yet we as a society tend to try to put some rational label or construct on horrific events in a way that deflects notions of evil, anger, and poor but competent choice. However, the motivation and premorbid functioning or mental health symptoms of many mass shooters may never be fully understood. As mentioned repeatedly in this text, most individuals with serious mental illness are not violent, and the frequency of firearm use related to mental illness is estimated to be very low (Pinals et al.

2014). Additionally, the low base rate of mass shooting incidents makes it difficult to identify patterns and risk factors that would lead to reliable strategies to predict who will someday commit such alarming offenses.

Nevertheless, incidents involving "active shooters"—that is, individuals "actively engaged in killing or attempting to kill people in a confined and populated area" (Blair and Schweit 2014, p. 5)—have been increasing since 2000, leading to media coverage and public discussion that reinforce stereotypes of individuals with mental illness as dangerous. A clarion call for solutions has included efforts to preclude individuals thought to be at high risk from purchasing firearms as well as the investment of federal and state dollars in databases that seek to identify such individuals. Additionally, there has been an effort to focus solutions on mental health care in the broadest sense, including early identification of children with emotional disturbances.

This chapter addresses aspects of proposed solutions that some have suggested might mitigate risks related to firearms among individuals with mental disturbances. In particular, it focuses on examining the potentials and limitations related to involuntary commitment, as well as the fundamental need to take a broad public health approach to gun violence. Strategies to improve access to appropriate services and better engage individuals in treatment should be considered just some of these public health approaches.

Mass Shooters: Challenges to Prediction and Prevention

As one looks at the stories of mass shooters, generally an evolution of difficulties has taken place for these individuals that may be noticed by family and significant others but nevertheless may culminate in the moment when firearm shots sound. Sometimes, the difficulties seem to involve social isolation, anger, and typical teenage frustration; at times, they may emerge out of developmental difficulties, a social rupture, and an impaired ability to develop coping strategies to stressors; and at still other times, they appear as classic serious mental illness that has gone untreated. Every case has a unique story, but there is a common perception, in hindsight, that perhaps an earlier intervention could have thwarted a deadly event. Some of the most widely reported cases of mass shooters serve as examples.

> On April 20, 1999, two young men entered their high school in Columbine, Colorado, armed with several types of firearms and with coordinated explosive devices. They shot and killed 12 students and one teacher, and another 24 were injured, before the perpetrators killed themselves (Wikipedia 2014b). Later, it was learned that one of the shooters had been taking an antidepressant medication, and many speculated whether the other had had depressive symptoms as well.

On April 16, 2007, a young man shot and killed 32 people and wounded 17 others before shooting himself at the Virginia Polytechnic Institute and State University (Virginia Tech) in Blacksburg, Virginia (Friedman 2009). Following this massacre, many raised questions about his mental state at the time of the killing spree. In addition, even though the perpetrator of the Virginia Tech shootings had been involuntarily committed to a course of outpatient treatment approximately 2 years earlier, mechanisms for tracking his adherence to the court-ordered treatment were lacking, as was reporting regarding his prohibited firearm status.

Despite his involuntary commitment and his prohibited firearm purchaser status, the Virginia Tech shooter did not access treatment, there was no outreach or monitoring to ensure his follow-up, and he was able to purchase the firearms he used in the shootings (Swartz and Swanson 2008). Reports indicated discrepancies between state and federal statutory language and interpretation of these statutes, and raised questions about the operationalization of the commitment statutes at the level of actual firearm purchase. These circumstances resulted in a reexamination of the legal landscape pertaining to commitment laws in Virginia (Lo 2007) and ultimately led to significant reform of Virginia's mental health commitment statutes (Bonnie et al. 2009).

On January 8, 2011, a young man began shooting at a crowd, killing six and injuring several other people, including U.S. Representative Gabrielle Giffords (Lacey 2011). In subsequent trial proceedings, the shooter was found to have had active symptoms of mental illness that had gone untreated for several years. He was initially found incompetent to stand trial but ultimately pled guilty. He is now serving a life sentence for his offenses (Santos 2012).

On July 20, 2012, in Aurora, Colorado, in the midst of a theater showing of the movie *The Dark Knight Rises,* a man set off tear gas and fired shots into the audience, killing 12 and injuring 70 individuals (Wikipedia 2014a). The suspect in the case, a graduate student at the University of Colorado Anschutz Medical Campus, was arrested and later pled not guilty by reason of insanity. According to press reports, a university psychiatrist treating him prior to the shootings had become increasingly concerned about his homicidal thoughts and threatening behaviors, and had notified police of these concerns, with limited responses (Connor 2013; Morrissey 2013). The shooter was found guilty in 2015 and was sentenced to life in prison although the prosecution had sought the death penalty (Almasy et al. 2015).

In a tragic event on December 14, 2012, a young man shot and killed his mother at home and then 20 children and six adults at Sandy Hook Elementary School in Newtown, Connecticut, before shooting and killing himself. The exact motivation for the incident will likely never be fully understood. Immediately after the incident, however, the shooter's mental state became a major focus of attention. Over time, data emerged showing that his mother had had increasing worries about her son's mental state, including possible autism-like features, and had difficulty in accessing appropriate school services (Griffin and Kovner 2013).

A subsequent blog related to the events in Newtown went viral, as one mother, identifying with the Newtown shooter's mother, described her own challenges managing her 13-year-old son. This child's differential diagnosis included autism spectrum disorder and oppositional defiant disorder (Long 2012), and his violent behavior required the development of a "safety plan" at home to prevent family members from serious harm. Although not specific to the shooter, the blog raised the public awareness of the challenges in prediction and prevention of tragic events.

In May 2014, a 22-year-old man killed six people (three by stabbing, three by firearms) and injured 13 others using firearms before he shot and killed himself in Santa Barbara, California (Wikipedia 2014c). His parents had become increasingly concerned about his emotional state, especially closer to the time when the acts of violence and suicide took place. News reports and disclosures by family after the events described him as someone who had been in therapy as a youth for social and emotional problems, in part related to bullying experiences. As an adult, however, he reportedly refused recommended mental health care. Following this event, many politicians called for an overhaul of mental health services and laws (Szabo 2014), resulting in the September 2014 passage of California's Gun Violence Restraining Orders bill (California Assembly Bill 1014, as discussed in greater detail in Chapter 12, "Preventing Gun Violence").

These horrific incidents involved individuals who were experiencing or hovering on the edge of depression, personality conflicts, developmental disabilities, some unspecified broad-based emotional disturbances, or even exhibiting frank symptoms of mental illness. The emotions leading to the tragic behaviors did not spontaneously emerge at the moment of the shooting. Although each perpetrator had distinct emotional and mental states, questions remain about prediction and prevention, such as why mental health interventions were not effective or why these individuals were not tightly engaged in mental health services. Because of these frightening and tragic (but statistically infrequent) occurrences, the national debate related to firearm access has been interwoven with mental illness and mental health services, and laws related to each.

Mental Illness, Firearm Risks, and Disqualifiers for Access

In media coverage, individuals with mental illness are often implied to be or explicitly described as being dangerous (Whitley and Berry 2013). In a public opinion survey conducted after the shootings in Newtown, approximately 50% of individuals believed that persons with mental illness are more dangerous than others (Barry et al. 2013). Despite these popular beliefs, mental illness is not the major driver of violence in society. According to research in this area, mental illness accounts for only 3%–5% of violence overall (Swanson 1994). Substance use, trauma histories, personality development, and a variety of factors other than mental illness are variables that are more likely to heighten the risk of violence and criminal behavior, and these variables are more common among individuals with mental illness than those without (Elbogen and Johnson 2009; Fisher et al. 2014; Steadman et al. 1998).

In contrast to risk of homicide, suicide risk is strongly associated with mental illness, a fact that receives much less public recognition and discussion. Factors other than mental illness can also increase the risk of suicide (see Chapter 2, "Firearms and Suicide in the United States," and Chapter 10, "Decreasing Suicide Mortality"), including demographic factors such as being an elderly male, a married woman, or an African American (American Psychiatric Association 2003).

Data also clearly indicate that firearm access increases the risk of morbidity and death, especially by suicide (Anglemyer et al. 2014). Firearm-related suicides are a major public health issue. In 2010, suicide was the tenth leading cause of all deaths, with more than 19,000 suicides total (Bendery 2013). Of the deaths due to firearms in 2010, most (about 61%) were attributable to suicide, and half the suicides that year involved firearm usage (Murphy et al. 2013). Therefore, concerns about suicide should be kept at the forefront of examination of risk-reduction interventions related to firearm use.

Death and injury due to crimes and accidents involving firearms is also a public health concern. In 2011, of the 478,400 fatal and nonfatal violent crimes committed with a firearm, just over 11,000 resulted in homicides. Although this reflects a significant decline from the number of crime-related firearm homicides in 1993, these statistics are similar to those for the years 2004–2014 (Planty and Truman 2013). In addition, according to the Centers for Disease Control and Prevention, firearm deaths are the third leading cause of injury-related deaths, with poisoning and motor vehicle accidents being the only two that are higher (Centers for Disease Control and Prevention 2014).

In the United States, Second Amendment protections of the right of private citizens to bear arms, separate from access by those in the military (U.S. Constitution), underlie debates regarding interventions to reduce firearm-related deaths and injuries. In light of the provisions of the Second Amendment, in the case of *District of Columbia v. Heller* (554 U.S. 570, 583, 2008), the U.S. Supreme Court ruled unconstitutional the District of Columbia's Firearms Control Regulation Act of 1975, a statute that banned household ownership of certain firearms. As a result of this decision, activists and lobbyists who support unlimited public access to firearms gained firm ground for their position. Nevertheless, even these activists support certain restrictions on public access to firearms based on group identifications (see Chapter 6, "Mental Illness and the National Instant Criminal Background Check System").

As described throughout this volume, individuals with a history of mental illness are one group that has been a focus for firearm restrictions. The laws related to disqualifying criteria are discussed principally in Chapter 6. Suffice it to say that limiting firearm access for individuals with mental disorders who actually are dangerous may be politically expedient and can even be appropriate if the dangerousness is clear-cut. Statistically speaking, if purchasing prohibitions work at all, limiting firearm access by persons with mental illness may be more effective in preventing a suicide than in preventing a rare act of violence toward others, and thus may reflect sound policy for more than one reason. That said, the problems with limiting access to firearms on the basis of an individual's categorization in a database as a way to decrease the incidence of gun violence, particularly mass shootings, are far more complicated than these legal prohibitions suggest.

Some of the complexities of trying to limit firearm access to those with mental illness as a way to prevent mass shootings are demonstrated in the highly publicized cases reviewed in the previous section. For one thing, several of the shooters did not use firearms registered in their names, so a database list would have had no impact on their ability to access guns. Also, approaches to limiting firearm access that single out a large group of people for general characteristics that may not actually mean they are at greater risk of using firearms for mass killings are likely to have limited impact on reducing risks overall. Moreover, as discussed in previous chapters, such an approach raises concerns that the creation of large databases of persons with mental illness for purposes of firearm restrictions can increase stigma and further reluctance to seek mental health care.

Recently, alternative ideas have been suggested to improve mechanisms of firearm restrictions that would have a more meaningful impact on risk reduction. For example, approaches that permit the contemporaneous removal of a firearm from an individual who is at known heightened risk have been described (Consortium for Risk-Based Firearm Policy 2013). Other mechanisms for firearm removal in dangerous situations have also been proffered. One of these, as noted in the description of the Santa Barbara shooting above, was adopted in California in 2014: A gun violence restraining order (GVRO) is a type of familial or other civil temporary restraining order specific to limiting firearm access. This intervention could be initiated by family members or friends when they become frightened or concerned that the individual might harm self or others (Consortium for Risk-Based Firearm Policy 2013; see also Chapter 13, "'Relief From Disabilities': Firearm Rights Restoration for Persons Under Mental Health Prohibitions"). In specific situations, the GVRO would prohibit an individual respondent from purchasing or possessing firearms for the duration of the order (Martinez 2014).

Regarding the complex interplay between firearm access and safety as it relates to the mental health of the individuals at risk of perpetrating harm to themselves or others, solutions under consideration include a wide-ranging array of initiatives that attempt to make a meaningful difference in firearm-associated risks. The legal interventions discussed in this section seek to mitigate risk in an emergency and focus on firearms themselves. Alternative additional approaches that could enhance access to care at the front end, where an individual is seen as needing help and before an emergency and/or dangerous act occurs, are also important to consider. Several such strategies are described in the following sections.

Mental Health Services and Access to Care as Components of a Comprehensive Firearm Risk–Reduction Strategy

An entire array of public health interventions is needed to help prevent gun violence and to reduce, to the extent possible, the risk of harm to others and the more significant risk of firearm-related suicide by individuals with mental illness. Treatment services for those individuals with mental illness who present elevated risks of harm to themselves or others are an important component of public health policy and should be a public health priority. Other strategies include community-based planning, education, research, appropriate funding of an array of educational and social services, and interventions discussed in other chapters.

Although strides are being made with regard to access to mental health services, there is room for improvement. In 2002, President George W. Bush issued a report from the New Freedom Commission on Mental Health, in which the mental health system was described as "fragmented and in disarray…lead[ing] to unnecessary and costly disability, homelessness, school failure and incarceration" (President's New Freedom Commission on Mental Health 2003, p. 3). As discussed in Chapter 8, "Accessing Mental Health Care," during the 1960s and 1970s a number of factors, in addition to efforts to close state hospitals, contributed to the changing trends in how mental health services were delivered and where they were delivered. Contrary to popular belief, the closing of state hospitals was not the sole issue responsible for the situation identified in this commission report. Other political forces at play included the criminalization of drug use and harsh related sentences, as well as evolving laws pertaining to involuntary civil commitment.

Additionally, over recent decades, a major shift has taken place in how public funding for mental health services has been provided, moving from a state-funded state hospital system toward blended federal- and state-funded community-based systems of care. In part related to complex funding and treatment structures, individuals with mental disorders and substance use disorders who move among behavioral health, correctional, and forensic systems have disruptions in treatment. Some of this population may be at heightened risk of violence, including firearm violence, especially given other high-risk variables such as criminal behavior and substance use often found in this group. Recognition of these problems has resulted in recent efforts at developing collaborative approaches across behavioral health, forensic, and justice systems (Pinals 2014). Although these innovations are promising, when mental illness is present among individuals at heightened risk for violence, treatment can only work if a means to get the person into care exists. For example, in the cases of mass shooters described above, some apparently had access to mental health care but seemingly did not follow up with treatment. Others may not have been able to access sufficient or appropriate care.

Every state has mechanisms to initiate involuntary psychiatric commitment. Is this a reasonable approach among the array of public health options to help thwart those mass shootings that are in fact committed by individuals with mental illness? Views vary regarding the best role of involuntary commitment in the provision of mental health care, and each perspective has some valid supporting arguments. The Bazelon Center for Mental Health Law, for example, strongly advocates against involuntary treatment of any kind, viewing it as a massive curtailment of liberty that flies in the face of the rights of individuals with mental illness. The Bazelon Center (2014) instead believes that the vast majority of individuals with mental illnesses would be best served by full access to appropriate voluntary services. These strongly held opinions help highlight the important tension between public health concerns and individual liberties in regard to individuals with severe mental illness. They serve as a reminder that involuntary commitment is necessarily intended to address the mental health problems of only the very small percentage of individuals for whom a justification exists to use an involuntary treatment approach.

With that caveat in mind, involuntary commitment laws, as a means of protecting individuals with mental illness, protecting the public, and assisting some individuals to get treatment, and the legal and social rationales that support these laws have existed for centuries. Despite this long history, however, the commitment provisions represent very narrowly tailored options. Given the higher prevalence of firearm-related suicide and its relationship to mental illness, involuntary commitment may be most commonly used as an intervention for an individual who is at acute firearm-related suicide risk. Nevertheless, its use, limited to circumscribed situations, serves as one tool when an individual presents with risk to others due to mental illness.

Civil Commitment Laws: History and Current Landscape

Services for mental health care, like services for medical care, are for the most part voluntarily sought and received by patients. Exceptions to voluntary treatment include circumstances in which an individual has been adjudicated as incompetent to make treatment decisions. Although this situation is a relatively rare outcome of mental illness, legal procedures and processes generally are in place for alternative decision makers, such as health care proxies or guardians, to step in and make specific treatment decisions for the incompetent person who is in need of care.

Another exception to voluntary care is involuntary commitment. Involuntary civil commitment represents an order by a court to a form of care, usually but not always in an inpatient setting, as the vehicle to mandate into treatment specific individuals with mental illness. These individuals typically do not want mental health care but meet some (usually risk-related) criteria that justify society's authority to mandate such an involuntary approach. Although individuals can refuse medical hospitalization, involuntary psychiatric commitment laws allow and provide due process for requiring that an individual with mental illness be hospitalized or comply with outpatient services. Whether care provided under involuntary commitment statutes includes mandated medications varies across jurisdictions, although involuntary medication administration generally follows separate legal provisions and pathways.

Involuntary civil commitment is complex, and its role and limitations are often not well understood. Some of the high-profile mass killings, such as the Virginia Tech shootings in 2007, have catalyzed reexamination and revision of mental health commitment laws (Bonnie et al. 2009; Szabo 2014). The reforms in Virginia included efforts to enhance the management of persons with mental illness at risk of harm; some of these reforms specifically addressed the gaps in the civil commitment system identified as a result of the shootings (Bonnie et al. 2009).

Although individual liberty and autonomy are core principles that drive the American legal system and social culture, two fundamental doctrines, *parens patriae* and police powers, provide the rationale that justifies the intrusive intervention of involuntary commitment of individuals with mental illness (see Chapter 7, "Mental Illness, Dangerousness, and Involuntary Commitment"; see also Appelbaum and Gutheil 2007; Pinals and Mossman 2012). The doctrine of *parens patriae* holds that the government (or king, in days of monarchies), acting as parent of last resort, is responsible for caring for citizens who are incapable of caring for themselves. The doctrine of police powers justifies involuntary civil commitment and detention when, as a result of mental illness, individuals are posing a risk of harm to themselves or others. Deference to state powers in this regard entitles each state to define the circumstances under which civil commitment may occur. These statutory criteria can be overridden only if they do not pass some constitutional muster.

For the purpose of civil commitment, *mental illness* is usually defined in statutes or regulations and involves, for example, some substantial disorder of mood, thought, perception, orientation, or memory (Pinals and Mossman 2012) as a threshold criterion. Dangerousness that would warrant commitment must flow from a mental illness. Dangerousness unrelated to mental illness (e.g., when an individual seeks revenge for a debt and breaks a neighbor's leg) does not meet this threshold for civil commitment. A dangerous act in the absence of mental illness results in a criminal charge and incapacitation through incarceration. Some states incorporate or have distinct statutes allowing for civil commitment of individuals related to other issues, such as substance use or sex offenses (Pinals and Mossman 2012; Williams et al. 2014).

Dangerousness in regard to commitment criteria for mental illness is also principally defined in state laws, which vary from state to state. Generally, statutory definitions that would meet criteria for dangerousness due to mental illness include risk of harm to self (by suicide), grave disability (when an individual is at risk due to an inability to care for self), and/or risk of harm to others related to violence. Less commonly, some state statutes include in the definition of *dangerousness* a risk of deterioration, a risk to property, and/or need for treatment (Pinals and Mossman 2012).

Over time, the basis for commitment and the decision-making authority surrounding the commitment determination have shifted between deference to medical judgment and deference to legal processes. In 1948, the Group for the Advancement of Psychiatry raised concerns about how previously treatment-focused civil commitment processes had become too legalistic (Group for the Advancement of Psychiatry, Committee on Forensic Psychiatry 1948). The group raised issues about various problematic aspects of commitment proceedings, including the lack of privacy for patients exposed to a public commitment hearing, the conflation of incompetence and need for hospitalization, and the use of a lay jury in some jurisdictions to determine who needed to be committed.

The 1952 U.S. Draft Act Governing Hospitalization of the Mentally Ill (U.S. Public Health Service 1952) came about in response to such concerns (Appelbaum 2000). This legislation considered both *parens patriae* and police powers rationales in commitment determinations. This act required that individuals under consideration for involuntary commitment either have demonstrable risk of harm to self or others or simply need care and treatment related to mental illness that the individuals lacked the capacity to seek independently (U.S. Public Health Service 1952).

Despite these efforts at reform, involuntary civil commitment laws have increasingly focused on due process and have narrowed the circumstances under which commitment can occur. For example, in 1966, the case of *Lake v. Cameron* (364 F. 2d 657, D.C. Cir., 1966) spelled out the need to consider the "least restrictive alternative" available to meet an individual's needs before allowing an involuntary commitment to a hospital. *Lessard v. Schmidt* (349 F. Supp. 1078, 1972), a transformative landmark case on this issue, hallmarked the need for strict procedural protections for individuals who might be subject to civil commitment. In this case, a federal district court ruled the existing Wisconsin commitment law to be unconstitutional, establishing that involuntary commitment should be limited to situations in which an "extreme" likelihood existed that the person would be an immediate danger to self or others if not committed.

The *Lessard* ruling, in addition to highlighting dangerousness as opposed to a need for treatment as the rationale for commitment, held that the same protections offered to a criminal defendant should be required in a civil commitment proceeding, including a right to an attorney, and set the standard of proof of the need for commitment to beyond a reasonable doubt. *Lessard* led many other states to reform their civil commitment laws using similar provisions, although the U.S. Supreme Court later held that the standard of proof for civil commitment should at a minimum be "clear and convincing evidence" (*Addington v. Texas,* 441 U.S. 418, 1979). Over time, much was written about the pendulum swinging too far in the direction of basing civil commitment statutes almost entirely on dangerousness and a police powers rationale, rather than considering those individuals who needed treatment but were unwilling or unable to seek care (Treffert 1985).

Approximately a decade before *Lessard* resulted in widespread changes in state laws, President Kennedy signed into law the Mental Retardation and Community Mental Health Centers Construction Act of 1963 (P.L. 88-164, 77 Stat 282). This legislation sought to shift the delivery of mental health services toward community-based programs, although the reality of community mental health services did not ultimately live up to the idealized approaches envisioned for persons with serious mental illness. As such, at the same time that commitment laws were being reshaped, more individuals with mental illness were living in the community with insufficient or dyscoordinated services, making access to needed care more difficult.

The case of *Olmstead v. L.C.* (527 U.S. 581, 1999) resulted in a push to further develop community-based services to help individuals with disabilities to live full and meaningful lives in their communities, even if doing so necessitates offering and funding additional appropriate supports. These trends have resulted in the values of autonomy, individual rights, and self-determination becoming even more deeply embedded in legal and social principles related to the treatment of mental illness. With the tidal shift that has occurred over the past 40 years, approaches that might expand involuntary inpatient commitment require even more deliberative consideration.

Involuntary Outpatient Commitment

While mechanisms for involuntary commitment to inpatient treatment seem to have become more limited, some states have been expanding the potential for involuntary commitment to outpatient treatment. These new laws have generally been based on the views that some individuals with serious mental illness have not fared well in community settings and, as a result, revolve in and out of hospitals and other institutions. In an effort to address this problem and maximize adherence to care, outpatient mental health commitment (also called assisted outpatient treatment in some places) has emerged over the last several decades as an alternative for individuals who meet some threshold criteria that require a court mandate for community-based oversight. Some of the laws related to outpatient commitment came to public attention after an individual with mental illness engaged in a dangerous act (although interestingly for this discussion, these acts in the majority of cases did not involve firearms). Other statutes were already part of a legal landscape that may or may not have been in use.

Outpatient commitment reduces institutional costs associated with more expensive inpatient care and complies with requirements that treatment, even if involuntary, take place in the least restrictive alternative setting possible. Under outpatient commitment statutes, nonadherence to court orders in the community results in some action, up to and including involuntary hospitalization. As of 1999, forty states plus the District of Columbia had legislation authorizing outpatient commitment, but only about half had a means of utilizing it (American Psychiatric Association 1999). More recent estimates indicate that 45 states have such laws (Treatment Advocacy Center 2011).

Involuntary outpatient commitment presents some unique complexities that some states are still sorting out. For example, criteria for outpatient and inpatient commitment do not always differ significantly, in that both often require some level of danger to self, danger to others, or inability to care for self (Swartz and Swanson 2008). Thus, distinguishing who meets criteria for inpatient as opposed to outpatient commitment can be clinically and legally challenging. In addition, enforcement and monitoring strategies may not exist, as was noted earlier with regard to the Virginia Tech shooter (Swartz and Swanson 2008). Questions therefore remain regarding how specific outpatient commitment criteria might evolve and be refined with regard to their legal construction and systematic implementation and enforcement.

Some reports have raised questions about whether outpatient commitment yields positive effects beyond what might come from enhancing voluntary community-based services (Kisely et al. 2011). In England, the Oxford Community Treatment Order Evaluation Trial compared individuals conditionally released from a psychiatric hospital (i.e., using means based on hospital procedure after an involuntary inpatient commitment order but with no separate outpatient commitment order) and individuals directly committed to outpatient treatment (i.e., using a mandated civil legal mechanism specific to outpatient commitment). This study found no significant difference in rates of subsequent hospitalization between the two groups (Burns et al. 2013).

In contrast, research from jurisdictions within the United States has demonstrated positive outcomes for outpatient commitment when used for a properly and narrowly tailored population, and in conjunction with appropriate community-based intervention strategies for specified periods of time. For example, the most rigorous studies, examining outpatient commitment outcomes in North Carolina and New York, have demonstrated that outpatient commitment as an intervention, delivered with a range of community services, can be effective in reducing admissions to hospitals and in keeping individuals in treatment in the community (Swartz et al. 1999, 2010). This may be especially true for a subgroup of individuals with mental illness who have shown cyclical patterns of treatment nonadherence and reinstitutionalization (Swanson and Swartz 2014). Further research on the effectiveness of outpatient commitment statutes and implementation is needed to help shed light on benefits, limitations, and best practices if the use of this intervention is to expand.

Beyond Civil Commitment: Alternative Legal Mechanisms That Lead to Treatment

As alternatives to civil commitment, conditional release from an inpatient commitment and the use of guardianship have been proposed as legal approaches to maximize treatment (Morrissey et al. 2014). These interventions could serve to help support and enhance the probability of ongoing care and treatment for individuals in their communities who might not otherwise readily avail themselves of such care and who may justifiably better fall under other legal provisions. Morrissey et al. (2014) describe conditional release as a type of outpatient commitment, but one that does not involve a "separate court order mandating the outpatient phase of treatment" (p. 813).

Guardianship is used for individuals who have been determined by a court to lack decision-making capacity. After deeming an individual to be incapacitated, the court appoints a guardian to make best-interest determinations for that individual. In this way, danger to self and others is not a formal part of the process (although courts may look to that type of data to assess issues in question such as poor decision making and judgment). A judge must make a determination of incapacity for a guardian to be assigned, and states have their own statutory language that governs these determinations.

Morrissey et al. (2014) report that overall study results on the impact of guardianship in reducing rates of inpatient hospitalization are somewhat mixed, but some evidence may indicate that guardianship preserves higher levels of functioning. They note, however, that the process of adjudicating an individual incapacitated and in need of a guardian is slow and that finding a guardian can be difficult. Due process issues and appointment of an appropriate guardian differ significantly from due process of outpatient commitment or even conditional release.

The potential alternatives of outpatient commitment, conditional release, and guardianship warrant continued review and consideration. This is especially important because a range of options may be best, given that any option for involuntary care will have necessary and appropriate limitations and constraints, making it more or less applicable in certain scenarios. Overall, further exploration will continue to be relevant as systems search for interventions to improve care for those individuals with serious mental illness who are unable or unwilling to avail themselves of community treatment and are cycling through hospitals and the criminal justice system (Swanson and Swartz 2014).

Limitations of Current Civil Commitment Laws for Reducing Violence to Others: Pros and Cons

Even with a range of options for involuntary treatment, in an ideal world, all individuals in need of care would seek it voluntarily and mental health treatment resources would be readily available. For any number of reasons, not all individuals seek care or recognize their need for it. As stated above (see "Involuntary Outpatient Commitment"), the current narrow legal requirements for involuntary psychiatric commitment demand evidence of dangerousness due to mental illness. This may result in the "day late and a dollar short" phenomenon in which individuals can be mandated into treatment only after they have demonstrated dangerousness and not early enough to help prevent harm.

Examining involuntary commitment as a prevention strategy in the context of mass shootings raises numerous questions. Despite the inevitable speculation regarding the perpetrators' mental health following these incidents, whether the individual perpetrators would have met the narrow legal criteria for some type of involuntary commitment is unclear. Therefore, it would seem that no single legal intervention such as involuntary civil commitment is likely to be sufficient to prevent all such incidents in the future. Given the liberty interests at stake, commitment orders, whether for inpatient or outpatient services, will continue to be narrowly defined and applied. Where available and more applicable, other legal options, such as guardianship, also can be pursued, but each has limitations. Thus, commitment law reform is not a straightforward strategy for firearm violence prevention, and the pros and cons can be complicated.

The American Psychiatric Association (APA) made efforts to raise concerns about the narrowing commitment criteria over three decades ago when it drafted its own model civil commitment legislation (Stone 1975; Stromberg and Stone 1983). This model highlighted a "need for treatment" as a legitimate additional criterion for involuntary commitment (Stromberg and Stone 1983). The model law contained the standard current criteria: that individuals had a mental illness and that they were likely to cause harm to themselves or others. In addition, it offered another potential category of individuals who could be committed involuntarily—namely, those who were likely to suffer deterioration due to mental illness and who lacked the capacity to make a competent decision regarding treatment. According to this model law, under circumstances in which a psychiatrist, through examination, determined that any of these criteria were met and determined that hospitalization would be the needed step to prevent harm or deterioration, the person could be detained for further evaluation (Appelbaum 1985).

The proposed model law received a great deal of commentary. Some thought that criteria for commitment focusing solely on dangerousness are more readily operationalized than the model law criteria and that the APA's proposal for a need-for-treatment criterion ran the risk of being overly vague, broad, and poorly defined (Rubenstein 1985). The reliance on medical judgment of need for involuntary commitment with fewer legal checks and balances was also questioned (Rubenstein 1985). Pierce et al. (1985) commented that expanded criteria such as those proposed by the APA unintentionally could create an increased burden on state hospitals due to a significant increase in admissions. Some others argued that fiscal, administrative, and geographic factors, separate from the legal and medical criteria, would influence commitment determinations (Faulkner et al. 1989).

Despite these concerns, the public health crisis of mental illness and suicide and the public health crisis of gun violence, particularly in regard to suicide, might lead some individuals to feel that the time is ripe to revisit some of these earlier ideas of reforming commitment criteria. For example, it could be suggested that such reform include a more consistently applied need-for-treatment component under limited circumstances, as well as more realistic systems of checks and balances, including monitoring systems if outpatient commitment is used.

If civil commitment criteria were to be reformed based on some degree of recognition of need for treatment, the circumstances that would permit such a deprivation of liberty would need further refining. In the APA's model law criteria, involuntary commitment would require that respondents have demonstrable symptoms of mental illness that put them at risk of mental or physical deterioration and that they lack the capacity to make an informed decision concerning treatment. Whether all individuals at risk of committing mass gun violence, if identified early, would meet those criteria is doubtful; this may be especially true for those individuals with disorders that may not impact decisional capacity. Thus, expansion of commitment criteria would again have limitations in preventing firearm-related violence.

Any expanded criteria for commitment would require careful review in terms of understanding how they would offer something more than guardianship and similar provisions that focus on the core issue of decisional capacity. Furthermore, any change or reform, if pursued, should be undertaken in the context of a nonreactive and well-reasoned process of analysis that is fair and ethical and that incorporates rationales that are clinically and legally sound.

With all these caveats in mind, those who advocate attempts to reform civil commitment laws should remember that the purpose of trying to assist individuals (and their families) who are managing mental illnesses is to provide access to treatment to prevent decompensation and progression of mental illness and potentially heightened risk of harm to themselves or others. Rather than allowing individuals to flounder with active symptoms of mental illness or potentially dangerous emotional dysregulation and, in the worst cases, to engage downstream in serious violence, modified criteria for commitment that incorporate a reconsidered limited need-for-treatment component as well as improved linkages to services might have the impact of securing earlier access to care. However, they can also have the unintended consequence of dissuading people from care because of the very involuntary nature of commitment. Therefore, before this idea is adopted wholesale, the additional caveats described below should be considered.

When expansion of involuntary commitment criteria is being considered, for example, it is also important to examine where the laws leave gaps and to ponder whether the act of commitment, likely to a hospital in the acute situation, would be helpful. Success in providing timely and effective intervention when inpatient or outpatient commitment does occur requires clear delineation and integration of procedures for processing, tracking, monitoring, and following up treatment (Rubenstein 1985). Details must be specified regarding how community-based services would be organized and which agencies would be responsible for arranging which services. In New York, for example, court-ordered assisted outpatient treatment provides mental health practitioners, police, and involved others with specific instructions for serving notice and the procedures to be followed if the individual fails to comply with the assisted outpatient treatment order (Office of Mental Health 2006). Thus, challenges in contemplating civil commitment reform include ascertaining whether appropriate interventions could be operationalized successfully.

Furthermore, any involuntary intervention, with current or expanded criteria, should come with appropriate and sufficiently funded inpatient or community-based services. As discussed in Chapter 8, "Accessing Mental Health Care," in many places, individuals who have been found to meet current criteria for involuntary hospitalization must wait sometimes for days, usually in a hospital emergency department, for a bed to become available. Since their inception, community-based services have struggled with a lack of sufficient funding to provide services for individuals with serious mental illness. The problems involving coordination of resources for people with serious mental illness have at times resulted in overwhelmed hospital emergency departments, as well as increased rates of homelessness, incarceration, and victimization of individuals. Expanding criteria for involuntary inpatient or outpatient commitment might be futile if such changes are not accompanied by funding for the necessary resources, particularly for those individuals in need of acute inpatient or emergency outpatient care.

In addition, treatment issues within the context of the involuntary commitment should not be overlooked. Whether an individual needs medications, psychotherapy to diminish preoccupations with suicide or violent thoughts, and/or ongoing periodic risk assessment would need to be addressed to determine if these are necessary parts of the involuntary commitment intervention. Therefore, if commitment criteria were broadened to provide increased access to treatment for individuals with various mental illnesses, the type of treatment would need to be appropriate, reasonably paced, and designed to meet each individual's unique needs.

Whether coercion into care would inadvertently increase an individual's risks of becoming dangerous to self or others by further alienating the person and leading him or her to resent unrequested care also requires more study. A current and growing body of literature addresses the impact of such coercion on treatment outcome. Steinert and Schmid (2004), for example, demonstrated that functioning and changes in symptoms did not differ across patients who received voluntary or involuntary care. Coercion overall did not appear to result in nonadherence to treatment. Also, perceptions of coercion may have more to do with how one is treated than with the voluntary versus involuntary status of one's treatment (Pinals and Mossman 2012). In a study examining psychiatric patients' experiences of voluntary versus involuntary treatment, patients' views of the care they received were more positive when patients felt treated well by staff (Wallsten et al. 2006). Perceptions of coercion seem connected to a sense of whether patients felt treated respectfully and felt themselves to have a voice in the process (Lidz et al. 1995).

Over time, there should be further study on the impact of coercion for the individual and for the systems that provide care. Research across populations should also be pursued to understand and ensure fair applications of involuntary treatment regardless of race, ethnicity, or socioeconomic status. Overall, however, the findings related to coercion in psychiatric care do give some guidance in regard to approaching involuntary treatment. These findings indicate that involuntary interventions such as inpatient or outpatient commitment should be undertaken with built-in strategies to foster respect, information sharing, and fairness in proceedings to minimize unintended negative consequences such as increasing resistance to needed treatment. Additionally, approaches to both voluntary services and involuntary commitment must be sensitive to helping individuals remain engaged in treatment.

Upstream and Downstream Interventions: Early Screening, Enhanced Treatment Engagement, and Broader Public Health Approaches

As discussed in this and previous chapters, mass shooters constitute too small a group of individuals to permit conclusions regarding patterns or prevalence of mental illness to be reasonably drawn. Some mass shootings could perhaps have been avoided if the perpetrators had been able to benefit from early screening for new-onset or worsening emotional distress and subsequent assessment and strategies to access effective treatment.

Consider, for example, the young man in Santa Barbara, whose father, following media reports of the incident, described his sense of helplessness as his son had grown increasingly isolated and angry over previous months (Wikipedia 2014c). This young man's parents had reportedly used every option available to help their son access treatment and avoid acting on violent thoughts, including maintaining contact with his therapist and reporting their concerns to the police prior to the murders. Given the reported mental health history of the young man and the support of family members, in addition to involuntary treatment for which he may or may not have met the criteria, options to assist the concerned parents in accessing help for their adult child needed to be even broader than what seemed available. Safety-net services may exist that buttress the work of a therapist. However, strict limits (e.g., state entitlements or insurance coverage) often also exist that determine which services, if any, are available in a particular case.

The ability of treatment providers to engage patients and to help them adhere to treatment recommendations is also one of the most important factors in assisting individuals. All too often, discussions of reform of civil commitment laws neglect to consider the issues related to engagement, motivational enhancements for treatment adherence, and the importance of enlisting the assistance of family members and supportive others to help individuals pursue positive goals as part of treatment and services. In all too many circumstances, treatment providers, families, and others may "give up" or feel at a loss when treatment does not seem to be effective or when patients seem uninterested in the particular treatment they are receiving.

Strategies designed to work across an entire support network may further expand the ability to engage individuals in ongoing treatment. Increased use of "peer staff"—that is, employment of individuals with personal experience of substance use or mental illness who can help patients relate to hopeful outcomes—as positive prosocial role models and formal supports is one such approach. Receiving treatment that is sensitive to an individual's vulnerabilities due to trauma exposure might serve to make treatment more palatable for some patients. Additional community engagement strategies may be helpful as well.

In all settings, before moving toward an involuntary commitment intervention for an individual, community efforts should ensure that a broad array of support services can be obtained through the least restrictive means. Involuntary civil commitment cannot protect society from all situations involving an individual with some type of general emotional distress or even from all situations involving an individual with serious mental illness who has access to a firearm. Experience demonstrates that regardless of civil commitment laws, firearm access for persons with and without mental illness will continue in this country; however, because not all firearm access is nefarious, maintaining focus on situations in which dangerousness to others is present is important.

Thus, broader public health approaches for prevention and targeted firearm access restrictions, especially in acute dangerous situations, are extremely important. Additional efforts should include enhanced research and education related to firearm violence and suicide. Clinicians should receive enhanced education regarding firearm-related risk assessment and risk management strategies. Community solutions to improve firearm-related safety will be needed as well, and this should reach far beyond interventions targeting a small population of individuals with mental illness (who likely also have criminogenic features) who may be at elevated risk. Solutions include improved and better-funded educational services, early identification of troubled youth, interventions to help enhance successful prosocial development, and strengthened community safety networks to help point individuals in the direction of care and treatment engagement as soon as signs of distress or signs of other remediable risks are recognized.

Conclusion

In contrast to what the media may have us believe, acts of firearm violence toward others committed by individuals with mental illness are infrequent events compared with firearm violence in general. However, when incidents involving individuals with mental illness and firearm violence occur, we are reminded that mental health care might have been one of a variety of potentially preventive interventions for a small subset of individuals. Mental health interventions should be designed for both upstream and downstream impact and should emphasize dignity, sensitivity, and treatment engagement. Sufficient levels of funding for mental health and substance use services are necessary to mitigate the morbidity and mortality associated with mental illness and substance use disorders. Attempts to decrease stigma surrounding mental illness and substance use and to improve access to treatment services can further the efforts to help individuals with these challenges.

Reform of involuntary civil commitment statutes to include a need-for-treatment component may be helpful in mitigating risk for some individuals who are at risk of firearm-related suicide and the much smaller number of persons with mental illness who are at risk of committing firearm violence against others. However, this type of reform would not be a total solution for gun violence. Broadening criteria for involuntary civil commitment comes with its own legal and treatment nuances that will be different in each jurisdiction. These would require careful study individualized for each state, given the current landscape of existing civil commitment laws, evolving civil rights and attention to self-determination, and the need for coordinated treatment services—services that would necessarily need to be balanced in any reform effort. Taken together, if we are to make a difference and truly reduce the public health crisis of firearm-related suicide and violence, taking a collective, broad public health approach will require consideration of simultaneous and wide-ranging evolving strategies and ongoing national attention.

Suggested Interventions

- Mental health providers should develop enhanced engagement strategies to maximize adherence to voluntary mental health care through the use of interventions such as family inclusion, peer support, trauma-informed services, community outreach, and other avenues to help support individuals in treatment in the least restrictive way possible.
- Discussions regarding inpatient and outpatient commitment should take into account potential gains and unintended negative consequences of any reform efforts that expand commitment criteria.
- Mental health and legal professionals should consider, as alternatives to civil commitment, the use of interventions such as guardianship and conditional release mechanisms where they exist and when necessary, and further examine such mechanisms where they do not exist, because these may be among the options that can be useful in directing individuals into treatment in certain cases.
- State and local agencies and organizations should utilize community- and public health–based education and outreach to improve the ability of families to initiate processes for accessing mental health care for individuals who need it as early as possible.
- The federal government, federal government agencies, and other research sponsors should support and fund medical and public health research and education on firearm-related violence and suicide.

References

Almasy S, O'Neill A, Weisfeldt S, Cabrera A: James Holmes sentenced to life in prison for Colorado movie theater murders. CNN.com, August 8, 2015. Available at: http://www.cnn.com/2015/08/07/us/james-holmes-movie-theater-shooting-jury/. Accessed August 9, 2015.

American Psychiatric Association: Mandatory Outpatient Treatment Resource Document (Ref No 990007). Washington, DC, American Psychiatric Association, 1999

American Psychiatric Association: Practice guidelines for the assessment and treatment of patients with suicidal behaviors. Am J Psychiatry 160(11 suppl):1–60, 2003

Anglemyer A, Horvath T, Rutherford G: The accessibility of firearms and risk for suicide and homicide victimization among household members. Ann Intern Med 160:101–110, 2014 24592495

Appelbaum PS: Special section on APA's model commitment law: an introduction. Hosp Community Psychiatry 36(9):966–968, 1985 11643844

Appelbaum PS: Commentary & analysis: the Draft Act Governing Hospitalization of the Mentally Ill: its genesis and its legacy. Psychiatr Serv 51(2):190–194, 2000 10655001

Appelbaum PS, Gutheil TG: Clinical Handbook of Psychiatry and the Law. Philadelphia, PA, Lippincott Williams & Wilkins, 2007

Barry CL, McGinty EE, Vernick JS, et al: After Newtown—public opinion on gun policy and mental illness. N Engl J Med 368(12):1077–1081, 2013 23356490

Bazelon Center: Where We Stand: Forced Treatment Policy Documents. Washington, DC, Bazelon Center, 2014. Available at: http://www.bazelon.org/Where-We-Stand/Self-Determination/Forced-Treatment/Forced-Treatment-Policy-Documents.aspx#Position_Statement_on_Involuntary_Commitment. Accessed September 14, 2014.

Bendery J: Suicide is leading cause of gun deaths, but largely absent in debate on gun violence. Huffington Post, May 14, 2013. Available at: http://www.huffingtonpost.com/2013/05/14/guns-suicide_n_3240065.html. Accessed July 22, 2014.

Blair JP, Schweit KW: A Study of Active Shooter Incidents in the United States Between 2000 and 2013. Washington, DC, U.S. Department of Justice, Federal Bureau of Investigation, and Texas State University, 2014. Available at: http://www.fbi.gov/news/stories/2014/september/fbi-releases-study-on-active-shooter-incidents/pdfs/a-study-of-active-shooter-incidents-in-the-u.s.-between-2000-and-2013. Accessed November 16, 2014.

Bonnie RJ, Reinhard JS, Hamilton P, et al: Mental health system transformation after the Virginia Tech tragedy. Health Aff (Millwood) 28(3):793–804, 2009 19414889

Burns T, Rugkåsa J, Molodynski A, et al: Community treatment orders for patients with psychosis (OCTET): a randomised controlled trial. Lancet 381(9878):1627–1633, 2013 23537605

Centers for Disease Control and Prevention: QuickStats: death rates for three selected causes of injury, National Vital Statistics System, United States, 1979–2012. MMWR Morb Mortal Wkly Rep, November 21, 63(46);1095, 2014. Available at: http://www.cdc.gov/mmwr/preview/mmwrhtml/mm6346a19.htm. Accessed August 7, 2015.

Connor T: First suit filed against University of Colorado in Aurora shooting. January 16, 2013. Available at: http://usnews.nbcnews.com/_news/2013/01/16/16545060-first-suit-filed-against-university-of-colorado-in-aurora-shooting?lite. Accessed June 3, 2014.

Consortium for Risk-Based Firearm Policy: Firearms, Public Health and Mental Illness: An Evidence-Based Approach for State Policy. Baltimore, MD, Johns Hopkins Center for Gun Policy and Research, 2013. Available at: http://www.jhsph.edu/research/centers-and-institutes/johns-hopkins-center-for-gun-policy-and-research/publications/GPHMI-State.pdf. Accessed July 26, 2014.

Elbogen EB, Johnson SC: The intricate link between violence and mental disorder: results from the National Epidemiologic Survey on Alcohol and Related Conditions. Arch Gen Psychiatry 66(2):152–161, 2009 19188537

Faulkner LR, McFarland BH, Bloom JD: An empirical study of emergency commitment. Am J Psychiatry 146(2):182–186, 1989 2912260

Fisher WH, Hartwell SW, Deng X, et al: Recidivism among released state prison inmates who received mental health treatment while incarcerated. Crime Delinq 60(6):811–832, 2014

Friedman E: Va. Tech shooter Seung-Hui Cho's mental health records released. ABC News, August 19, 2009. Available at: http://www.abcnews.go.com/us/seug-hui-chos-mental-health-records-released/story?id=8278195. Accessed June 2, 2014.

Griffin A, Kovner J: Adam Lanza's medical records reveal growing anxiety. Hartford Courant, June 20, 2013. Available at: http://www.courant.com/news/connecticut/newtown-sandy-hook-school-shooting/hc-adam-lanza-pediatric-records-20130629,0,7137229.story. Accessed June 14, 2013.

Group for the Advancement of Psychiatry, Committee on Forensic Psychiatry: Commitment Procedures, Report 4. New York, Group for the Advancement of Psychiatry, 1948

Kisely S, Campbell LA, Preston NJ: Compulsory community and involuntary outpatient treatment for people with severe mental disorders. Cochrane Database Syst Rev (2):CD004408, 2011 21328267

Lacey M: Suspect in shooting of Giffords ruled unfit for trial (U.S. section). New York Times, May 25, 2011. Available at: http://www.nytimes.com/2011/05/26/us/26loughner.html?pagewanted=alland_r=0. Accessed June 17, 2014.

Lidz CW, Hoge SK, Gardner W, et al: Perceived coercion in mental hospital admission: pressures and process. Arch Gen Psychiatry 52(12):1034–1039, 1995 7492255

Lo M: Cho's mental illness should have blocked gun sale (U.S. section). New York Times, April 20, 2007. Available at: http://www.nytimes.com/2007/04/20/us/20cnd-guns.html?_r=0. Accessed June 20, 2014.

Long L: I am Adam Lanza's mother: it's time to talk about mental illness. Blue Review, December 16, 2012. Available at: https://thebluereview.org/i-am-adam-lanzas-mother. Accessed July 22, 2014.

Martinez M: California lawmakers push "gun violence restraining order" after mass killing. CNN.com, May 29, 2014. Available at: http://www.cnn.com/2014/05/28/us/california-killing-spree-legislation. Accessed July 26, 2014.

Morrissey E: Psychiatrist warned campus police about Aurora shooter a month before mass murder. Hot Air, April 5, 2013. Available at: http://hotair.com/archives/2013/04/05/psychiatrist-warned-campus-police-about-aurora-shooter-a-month-before-mass-murder/. Accessed June 2, 2014.

Morrissey JF, Desmaris SL, Domino ME: Outpatient commitment and its alternatives: questions yet to be answered. Psychiatr Serv 65(6):812–815, 2014

Murphy SL, Xu J, Kochanek KD: Deaths: final data for 2010. Natl Vital Stat Rep 61(4):1–117, 2013 24979972

Office of Mental Health: An Explanation of Kendra's Law. Albany, New York Office of Mental Health, May 2006. Available at: http://www.omh.ny.gov/omhweb/Kendra_web/Ksummary.htm. Accessed July 26, 2014.

Pierce GL, Durham ML, Fisher WH: The impact of broadened civil commitment standards on admissions to state mental hospitals. Am J Psychiatry 142(1):104–107, 1985 3966567

Pinals DA: Forensic services, public mental health policy, and financing: charting the course ahead. J Am Acad Psychiatry Law 42(1):7–19, 2014 24618515

Pinals DA, Mossman D: Evaluation for Civil Commitment. New York, Oxford University Press, 2012

Pinals DA, Appelbaum PS, Bonnie R, et al: Resource Document on Access to Firearms by People With Mental Disorders. Arlington, VA, American Psychiatric Association, 2014

Planty M, Truman JL: Firearm Violence, 1993–2011. Washington, DC, Bureau of Justice Statistics, 2013. Available at: www.bjs.gov/content/pub/pdf/fv9311.pdf. Accessed July 22, 2014.

President's New Freedom Commission on Mental Health: Achieving the Promise: Transforming Mental Health Care in America. Rockville, MD, Substance Abuse and Mental Health Services Administration, 2003. Available at: http://govinfo.library.unt.edu/mentalhealthcommission/reports/FinalReport/FullReport-1.htm. Accessed May 27, 2013.

Rubenstein LS: APA's model law: hurting the people it seeks to help. Hosp Community Psychiatry 36(9):968–972, 1985 4065856

Santos F: Life term for gunman after guilty plea in Tucson killings (U.S. section). New York Times, August 7, 2012. Available at: http://www.nytimes.com/2012/08/08/us/loughner-pleads-guilty-in-2011-tucson-shootings.html. Accessed July 22, 2014.

Steadman HJ, Mulvey EP, Monahan J, et al: Violence by people discharged from acute psychiatric inpatient facilities and by others in the same neighborhoods. Arch Gen Psychiatry 55(5):393–401, 1998 9596041

Steinert T, Schmid P: Effect of voluntariness of participation in treatment on short-term outcome of inpatients with schizophrenia. Psychiatr Serv 55(7):786–791, 2004 15232018

Stone AA: Mental Health and Law: A System in Transition (DHEW Publ No ADM-76-176). Rockville, MD, National Institute of Mental Health, Center for Studies of Crime and Delinquency, 1975

Stromberg CD, Stone AA: A model state law on civil commitment of the mentally ill. Harvard J Legis 20(2):275–396, 1983 11658832

Swanson JW: Mental disorder, substance abuse, and community violence: an epidemiological approach, in Violence and Mental Disorder: Developments in Risk Assessment. Edited by Monahan J, Steadman HJ. Chicago, IL, University of Chicago Press, 1994, pp 101–136

Swanson JW, Swartz MS: Why the evidence for outpatient commitment is good enough. Psychiatr Serv 65(6):808–811, 2014 24881685

Swartz M, Swanson J: Outpatient commitment: when it improves patient outcomes. Current Psychiatry 7(4):25–35, 2008

Swartz MS, Swanson JW, Wagner HR, et al: Can involuntary outpatient commitment reduce hospital recidivism? Findings from a randomized trial with severely mentally ill individuals. Am J Psychiatry 156(12):1968–1975, 1999 10588412

Swartz MS, Wilder CM, Swanson JW, et al: Assessing outcomes for consumers in New York's assisted outpatient treatment program. Psychiatr Serv 61(10):976–981, 2010 20889634

Szabo L: Shooting spree inspires call for mental health overhaul. USA Today, May 27, 2014. Available at: http://www.usatoday.com/story/news/nation/2014/05/27/changing-mental-health-laws/9638529/. Accessed July 26, 2014.

Treatment Advocacy Center: Assisted Outpatient Commitment Laws. Arlington, VA, Treatment Advocacy Center, 2011. Available at: http://www.treatmentadvocacy-center.org/solution/assisted-outpatient-treatment-laws. Accessed June 26, 2014.

Treffert DA: The obviously ill patient in need of treatment: a fourth standard for civil commitment. Hosp Community Psychiatry 36(3):259–264, 1985 3979975

U.S. Public Health Service: A Draft Act Governing Hospitalization of the Mentally Ill (Revised). Washington, DC, U.S. Government Printing Office, 1952

Wallsten T, Kjellin L, Lindström L: Short-term outcome of inpatient psychiatric care—impact of coercion and treatment characteristics. Soc Psychiatry Psychiatr Epidemiol 41(12):975–980, 2006 17080321

Whitley R, Berry S: Trends in newspaper coverage of mental illness in Canada: 2005–2010. Can J Psychiatry 58(2):107–112, 2013 23442898

Wikipedia: 2012 Aurora Shooting. Wikipedia.com, 2014a. Available at: http://en.wikipedia.org/wiki/2012_Aurora_shooting. Accessed July 26, 2014.

Wikipedia: Columbine High School Massacre. Wikipedia.com, 2014b. Available at: http://en.wikipedia.org/wiki/Columbine_High_School_massacre. Accessed June 1, 2014.

Wikipedia: 2014 Isla Vista Killings. Wikipedia.com, 2014c. Available at: http://en.wikipedia.org/wiki/2014_Isla_Vista_killings. Accessed July 26, 2014.

Williams AR, Cohen S, Ford EB: Statutory definitions of mental illness for involuntary hospitalization as related to substance use disorders. Psychiatr Serv 65(5):634–640, 2014 24430580

12

Preventing Gun Violence

Decreasing Access to Firearms During Times of Crisis

Josh Horwitz, J.D.
Anna Grilley, M.S.P.H.
Kelly Ward, J.D.

Common Misperceptions

☒ Gun violence prevention policies cannot stop dangerous people from purchasing or possessing firearms.

☒ The Second Amendment prohibits any new policy interventions to regulate firearms.

☒ Limiting access to firearms during times of crisis will not affect suicidal behavior because people who want to kill themselves will always find another means to do so.

Evidence-Based Facts

☑ Current gun violence prevention policies that are directed at groups with an elevated risk of violent behavior have been demonstrated to be effective. However, there are still individuals at an elevated risk of violence who are not prohibited from purchasing or possessing firearms. Gun violence prevention policies based on evidence of increased risk for these individuals are likely to be effective in reducing gun violence morbidity and mortality.

- ☑ Policy efforts to clarify and improve the categories of individuals who are prohibited from purchasing or possessing firearms are likely to be found constitutional.
- ☑ Overall, more than 50% of the individuals who die from suicide kill themselves with a firearm, and research has clearly indicated that decreasing access to lethal suicide means such as firearms decreases suicide rates.

The frequency of mass shootings in the United States has increased in recent years. The time between mass shootings has decreased from 200 days (the average for the years 1982–2010) to 64 days (the average for the years 2011–2014) (Cohen et al. 2014). These tragic events devastate families and communities. Inevitably, following these massacres policy makers and the media ask what can be done to prevent the next tragedy. This question resonates beyond the all-too-frequent mass shootings. On average, 86 individuals die each day as the result of a gunshot; the majority of these deaths are suicides (Hoyert and Xu 2012).

To address the personal, family, and community tolls caused by mass shootings, as well as the more typical homicides and suicides that occur daily in the United States, policy makers need to ask a more precise question: Are there policy steps that can decrease the morbidity and mortality of gun violence by reducing access to firearms for individuals, with or without mental illness, who are in crisis and therefore at high risk for committing firearm violence, including firearm suicide? In this chapter we answer this question by outlining policies that prohibit individuals at an elevated risk of gun violence from purchasing and possessing firearms. In particular, we focus on a proposed policy development referred to as the *gun violence restraining order* (GVRO), which is intended to provide a tool for families and law enforcement to intervene before violence occurs by petitioning a court to remove guns from a loved one, friend, or other individual in crisis (McGinty et al. 2014a).

Examination of the rates of firearm morbidity and mortality demonstrates that the current law does not adequately focus on those at risk of committing firearm violence. For instance, the federal mental illness prohibition disqualifies from purchasing or possessing firearms those individuals who have been civilly committed to inpatient psychiatric care, have been found incompetent to manage their affairs, or have been found to be incompetent to stand trial or not guilty by reason of insanity (18 U.S.C. § 922[g]; 27 C.F.R. § 478.11; McGinty et al. 2014b). This broad, sweeping disqualification prohibits many individuals with mental illness who may not be violent and misses a large population who are at an elevated risk of committing firearm violence due to other factors (Appelbaum and Swanson 2010).

A different approach is necessary to ensure that those persons at an elevated risk of committing firearm violence may not legally purchase or possess firearms. The Consortium for Risk-Based Firearm Policy (2013) has developed one approach, the GVRO. The GVRO differs from current policy in that it allows temporary removal of firearms from an individual at times of high risk or crisis, whether or not that individual has a psychiatric illness. The GVRO is a proposed intervention that would empower family members, who are often in the best position to recognize a loved one's increasing risk of becoming violent, to take steps to intervene before gun violence occurs.

In outlining this proposed policy in this chapter, we highlight how the GVRO provides an opportunity to change the social assumptions surrounding mental illness and gun violence by reconfiguring the focus from mental illness to times of crisis, when the risk of suicide or violence toward others is highest. We trace the history of gun violence prevention legislation and explore in greater detail how the GVRO addresses the gaps in current policy. We then address potential Second Amendment legal challenges to the GVRO and discuss the relevant case history and evaluation that the policy will likely face. We conclude by outlining why this evidence-based policy should withstand a constitutional challenge and demonstrate how the implementation of the GVRO can help change commonly held but erroneous assumptions about mental illness and violence.

Overview of the Legal History of Firearm Policy

In 1968, Congress passed the Gun Control Act (Pub. L. No. 90-618, 82 Stat. 1213), which was the true genesis for prohibiting the purchase and possession of firearms by select groups of individuals. This landmark legislation significantly expanded on the idea, first asserted in the Firearms Act of 1934, that the federal government can and should regulate the individuals who purchase and possess common types of firearms. Following the Gun Control Act of 1968, members of Congress refined which groups of people they believed should be prohibited from purchasing or possessing firearms. Today, these broad categories of individuals include, but are not limited to, felons, fugitives, unlawful users or addicts of controlled substances, individuals dishonorably discharged from the military, and those who give up U.S. citizenship (18 U.S.C. § 922[g]).

In addition, as noted in the introduction to this chapter, federal law disqualifies certain groups of individuals with mental disorders from owning or possessing firearms. The current archaic and offensive statutory terms defining this group state that firearm ownership or possession is prohibited to an individual "adjudicated as a mental defective or committed to a mental institution" (18 U.S.C. § 922[g]; Appelbaum and Swanson 2010). This statutory language has been further defined by federal regulations (27 C.F.R. § 478.11; McGinty et al. 2014b) and in practice disqualifies individuals who are

- civilly committed to involuntary treatment;
- deemed incompetent to manage their own affairs;
- not able to stand trial for committing a crime because of mental illness; or
- found not guilty of committing a crime by reason of insanity.

These long-standing policies prohibiting owning or possessing firearms were implemented because of the perception that these groups present an elevated risk of "dangerousness." These current broad federal prohibiting categories are problematic, as discussed throughout this volume. Refining these categories to reflect the best available evidence would serve to reduce the morbidity and mortality from gun violence.

For example, as current rates of firearm injury and death indicate (see "Introduction" at the beginning of this book), the federal mental illness prohibitions are not as effective as hoped because of overinclusiveness, difficulty in enforcing prohibitions, and alternate means of access to firearms. At the federal level, these issues reinforce the need for improved background checks and evidence-based criteria for the relief from the prohibition (see Chapter 13, "'Relief From Disabilities': Firearm Rights Restoration for Persons Under Mental Health Prohibitions"). At the state level, these issues lead to the question of whether a different approach based on evidence of heightened risk during a crisis might be more effective in decreasing firearm morbidity and mortality.

Evolving Approach: Firearm Prohibitions Based on Evidence of a Heightened Risk of Dangerous Behavior

In 1994, Congress enacted the Violent Crime Control and Law Enforcement Act (Pub. L. No. 103-322, 108 Stat. 1796), which expanded the categories of individuals prohibited from purchasing or possessing firearms to include individuals subject to a final domestic violence restraining order (18 U.S.C. § 922[g][8]). The Lautenberg Amendment of 1996 further expanded the categories of prohibited persons to those who have been convicted of a domestic violence misdemeanor (18 U.S.C. § 922[g][9]). These policy interventions are based on clear evidence that firearms increase the risk of intimate partner homicide.

Guns are the weapons of choice in domestic violence homicides (Zeoli and Frattaroli 2013). Firearms were used to kill more than two-thirds of spouse and ex-spouse homicide victims between 1990 and 2005. Each year, current or former spouses or dating partners kill approximately 1 in 3 female homicide victims and 1 in 20 male homicide victims. About 60% of these homicides are committed using a firearm (Campbell et al. 2003; Puzone et al. 2000). In addition, abused women are five times more likely to be killed by their abuser if the abuser owns a firearm (Campbell et al. 2003).

The 1994 and 1996 firearm prohibitions related to domestic violence misdemeanors and restraining orders acknowledge the evidence-based potential of fatal firearm violence between intimate partners. Domestic violence restraining orders and the firearm prohibitions that accompany them at both the state and federal levels represent interventions that are intended to prevent violence based on the credible and demonstrable risk of harm at the hands of an intimate partner. In addition, these policy changes acknowledge that restraining orders are an important tool to prevent domestic violence. Obtaining a domestic violence restraining order allows for a civil mechanism to intervene and reduce the risk of violence or de-escalate conflict among intimate partners before additional violence, including firearm violence, occurs.

Research has demonstrated that risk of intimate partner homicide increases when an abuser has access to a firearm (Bailey et al. 1997; Campbell et al. 2003; Kellermann et al. 1993). Therefore, important gun violence prevention policies underlie domestic violence restraining orders. Several states, such as Massachusetts, Illinois, and Wisconsin, go beyond prohibiting purchase and possession and additionally mandate surrender or removal of firearms in conjunction with domestic violence restraining orders (Law Center to Prevent Gun Violence 2014).

Although statutes governing domestic violence restraining orders vary across states, most share similar features. Most states have two levels of domestic violence restraining orders, temporary *ex parte* orders and final orders. In California, for example, temporary *ex parte* protective orders may remain in effect for up to 21 days, whereas final protective orders to prevent further abuse may remain in effect for up to 5 years (Cal. Fam. Code §D.10, Pt. 4. Refs. and Annos. [West]).

Regardless of the state in which the parties reside, victims of domestic violence may petition for a temporary *ex parte* domestic violence restraining order before a hearing for a permanent order of protection is held. A temporary *ex parte* order does not require notice or the presence (hence "*ex parte*") of the accused batterer at the hearing. When seeking this order, the petitioner informs a civil judge of the abusive or violent behavior that forms the grounds for the petition.

On the basis of this evidence, the judge may grant a temporary restraining order, preventing the accused batterer from having any contact with the petitioner. This initial hearing takes place in the absence of the accused batterer to protect the victim, and hopefully assists in removing the victim from imminent danger. Only after the order is granted will law enforcement inform the accused batterer of the restraining order and the restrictions that it imposes. In many states, these restrictions expand on the federal law by prohibiting batterers from purchasing or possessing firearms even when only subject to a temporary *ex parte* domestic violence restraining order (Frattaroli and Vernick 2006).

In all states, victims can also seek a final domestic violence restraining order. At this hearing both the victim and the batterer can be present, and the judge considers evidence from both parties regarding abuse, harassment, or intimate partner violence. If a final restraining order is granted to the victim, federal law prohibits the batterer from purchasing or possessing firearms (18 U.S.C. § 922[g]). Interventions that separate batterers from firearms have largely been held constitutional (Zeoli and Frattaroli 2013).

Furthermore, evidence clearly indicates that these policies save lives by significantly reducing intimate partner homicide (Vigdor and Mercy 2003, 2006; Zeoli and Frattaroli 2013; Zeoli and Webster 2010). Research studies have found that state domestic violence restraining order laws were significantly associated with reductions in domestic violence homicide risk, for both firearm homicide and total domestic homicides, with or without firearms. In a study of large metropolitan cities, researchers found that cities in states that prohibit batterers from purchasing or possessing firearms had 25% fewer intimate partner homicides (Zeoli and Webster 2010).

Similarly, another study has found that laws to restrict firearm purchase for batterers subject to restraining orders are associated with a 10% reduction in rates of intimate homicide of women and a 13% reduction in rates of intimate homicide of women with firearms (Vigdor and Mercy 2006). One study examining the impact of a North Carolina firearm surrender policy found no effect on firearm-related intimate partner violence (Moracco et al. 2006). However, this study differs from the studies that found positive effect because it measured firearm possession by respondents, and whether the removal statute was being implemented is unclear (Zeoli and Frattaroli 2013). Evidence from implementation of a California removal statute suggests that both victims and law enforcement view the measure positively (Wintemute et al. 2014).

Expanded Policy Focus: Gaps in Current Policy Regarding Firearm Suicide

The domestic violence restraining orders and the supporting gun violence prevention policies are directed toward one particular group of individuals at high risk of firearm violence. Another group of individuals, typically suffering from mental illness, are also at high risk of the most statistically frequent type of firearm deaths: suicides. Unlike the overwhelming majority of firearm-related homicides, suicide is commonly associated with serious mental illness, in particular major depression (Bostwick and Pankratz 2000; also see Chapter 2, "Firearms and Suicide in the United States"). However, federal policy prohibiting those disqualified from purchasing or possessing a firearm due to a mental disorder does not adequately address suicidal individuals, because the great majority of individuals who commit suicide do not meet any of the federal government's criteria for mental illness–based firearm prohibitions (Appelbaum and Swanson 2010).

Suicide, as other chapters in this volume discuss, is a serious public health problem that accounts for nearly two-thirds of all gun deaths in the United States (Hoyert and Xu 2012). Specifically, suicide is the tenth overall leading cause of death in the United States, and the second leading cause of death among individuals ages 20–24 (Hoyert and Xu 2012). Notably, more than 50% of the individuals who die from suicide kill themselves with a firearm (Miller et al. 2007).

Research has indicated that access to firearms increases the risk of suicide (Dahlberg et al. 2004; Miller et al. 2007, 2013; Wiebe 2003; Wintemute et al. 1999). Suicide attempts with a firearm are lethal approximately 90% of the time (Miller et al. 2004). Populations with access to more guns, such as those in the military and in rural settings, do not garner much attention in the debates about gun violence prevention policies, despite the fact that they are at higher risk for firearm suicide (Miller et al. 2007).

As reviewed elsewhere in this text, resources for individuals with mental illness in crisis who seek voluntary treatment are limited and difficult to access. As a measure of last resort for those who refuse or cannot access voluntary treatment, concerned others can attempt to involve police and/or emergency medical services to protect their loved ones from harming themselves. Although involuntary commitment laws vary by state, generally the criteria for commitment are narrow, are strictly interpreted, and do not typically include a need for treatment (see Chapter 7, "Mental Illness, Dangerousness, and Involuntary Commitment," and Chapter 11, "Treatment Engagement, Access to Services, and Civil Commitment Reform").

In addition, many families are ambivalent about initiating civil commitment proceedings. The narrow criteria for civil commitment present a significant legal challenge for most families, and both families and the individuals refusing treatment often experience these proceedings as intrusive and adversarial. Families who have made unsuccessful attempts in the past to obtain help through civil commitment proceedings are often unwilling to subject themselves to the emotional stress and consequences associated with the process of civil commitment, which may further agitate and alienate the individual in need of treatment. Under federal law, individuals with serious mental illness who do not meet the commitment criteria and are released after a hearing are still permitted access to firearms.

If a person with acute psychiatric symptoms has not committed a criminal offense, refuses treatment, or does not currently meet the involuntary commitment criteria, in most states no additional options for intervention remain. Except in California, as discussed later in this section, families or intimate partners generally are unable to obtain an order to remove firearms or prevent the purchase of firearms when the harm to their loved ones is self-directed. The question therefore remains: Is it possible to devise and implement a policy intervention that could decrease access to firearms when individuals are at high risk for committing suicide or, much less often but still tragically, violence toward others?

To be clear, we are not suggesting that any one policy will stop the epidemic of firearm-related suicides. Again, as reviewed in other chapters, many different interventions are essential to decreasing suicide rates. Early identification of risk factors, mental health treatment, and community support are upstream solutions that can decrease risk of suicide. However, although these preventive efforts are an important part of public health interventions, policies that address access to lethal means during times of crisis, especially but not exclusively for those at risk of suicide, are also an option that should be available.

Addressing the Gaps in Current Policy: Gun Violence Restraining Orders

The GVRO is an innovative policy intervention that has the potential to fill the violence prevention gap in policies regarding firearm restrictions (Consortium for Risk-Based Firearm Policy 2013). As proposed, the GVRO, just like a domestic violence restraining order, would use the civil court system to intervene to prevent firearm violence from occurring. Specifically, a GVRO would allow family members, intimate partners, or law enforcement officials to petition a court to temporarily prevent access to firearms if they believe that an individual is in crisis, whether or not that individual suffers from a mental illness. Mirroring the current domestic violence restraining order process, the GVRO has two distinct stages: 1) an *ex parte* hearing (again, only the party seeking intervention need be present) for a temporary order and 2) an adversarial hearing where both parties are present for a final order.

Under current federal and most state laws, family members who grow concerned about a person's potential for dangerous behavior have almost no means to limit the individual's ability to purchase or possess firearms. When individuals, with or without mental illness, are in crisis, those closest to them often see warning signs or changes in behavior that indicate increased risk for violent behavior. These warning signs include many common indicators of increasing or high risk of dangerous behavior, from an increase in use of drugs or alcohol to threats or acts of violence (Elbogen and Johnson 2009; McGinty et al. 2014b; Swanson et al. 2013; Van Dorn et al. 2012).

The GVRO, as enacted in California, gives families and law enforcement a tool to limit unchecked access to lethal means of suicide or, less frequently but in some cases, homicide. See Table 12–1 for the types of GVROS established by Assembly Bill No. 1014 and their corresponding burdens of proof.

When a family member files in civil court for an *ex parte* GVRO based on concerns regarding an individual's increased risk of dangerous behavior, the judge will consider evidence demonstrating this risk without the individual in question present (Assem. Bill 1014, 2013–2014 Reg. Sess. [Cal. 2013]). The judge will be asked to consider risk factors that research has shown to be independently associated with violence, such as recent threats or acts of violence (Cook et al. 2005; Wintemute et al. 2001), past incidents of domestic violence (Campbell et al. 2003, 2007; Zeoli and Frattaroli 2013; Zeoli and Webster 2010), or substance abuse (Boles and Miotto 2003; Elbogen and Johnson 2009; Webster and Vernick 2009; Wintemute 2011).

If the judge finds that the individual is at a substantial risk of dangerous behavior to self or others in the near future and should therefore not have access to firearms, the judge can grant an ex parte restraining order that shall last for up to 21 days. It should be noted that this finding requires a lower threshold than that required for civil commitment or involuntary hospitalization, and in no way requires a finding of mental illness. In addition, before the judge can grant the order, he or she must consider whether the GVRO is the least restrictive means available to address the issue. The *ex parte* GVRO will prohibit the purchase and possession of firearms for a short period of time. Upon issuance of any GVRO, the court shall order the restrained person to surrender to the local law enforcement agency all firearms and ammunition in the restrained person's custody or control, or which the restrained person possesses or owns (Assem. Bill 1014, 2013–2014 Reg. Sess. [Cal. 2013]).

These *ex parte* orders are an important preventive measure because they allow the court to address crises requiring immediate and emergent action. However, this process can result in a removal of firearms prior to notice or hearing. To protect the due process rights of the subject of a GVRO, a temporary *ex parte* order must be time-limited and followed by a hearing at which the subject of the order is given a meaningful opportunity to be heard. At the hearing, the petitioner may seek to extend the order. The petitioner will bear the burden of proof during the hearing (Assem. Bill 1014, 2013–2014 Reg. Sess. [Cal. 2013]).

To issue a final order, the judge must decide by clear and convincing evidence that the respondent remains at a substantial risk of dangerous behavior in the near future. Once again the judge is asked to consider whether the GVRO is the least restrictive means available to address the potential risk of violence to self or others. If the judge grants an order, the order's firearm prohibition can be in place for a set length of time, such as 1 year. During this time, respondents will also have the right to restoration through a hearing, wherein they will bear the burden of proof to show by clear and convincing evidence that they are no longer at a substantial risk of dangerous behavior in the near future (Assem. Bill 1014, 2013–2014 Reg. Sess. [Cal. 2013]).

The proposed GVRO policy offers options to reduce the risk of serious injury or death in "real time," before tragic events unfold. Currently, profoundly limited options exist for family members who have reason to believe that their loved one 1) is at an increased risk of dangerous behavior, 2) may attempt to harm self or others, and 3) does not have a serious mental illness. Under these circumstances, all that the concerned others can do, if obtaining a domestic violence restraining order is not an option, is wait for a crime to be committed (18 U.S.C. § 922[g]). Law enforcement is similarly limited in its ability to intervene unless a crime has been committed. By then, it may be too late to prevent firearm violence. This state of affairs is not in the best interest of individuals, families, or communities.

In addition, the GVRO is the least restrictive alternative for ensuring that persons with serious mental illness who are a danger to themselves or others are prevented from having access to firearms. The only legal action available to a family with reason to believe that their loved one is at an increased risk of dangerous behavior due to mental illness and may attempt to commit suicide or harm others, is to attempt to begin civil commitment proceedings. If individuals meet the criteria for commitment—that is, they are found to be both mentally ill and dangerous to self or others—they may be held involuntarily in a psychiatric ward or hospital. When individuals who are involuntarily psychiatrically committed (and not merely temporarily detained) by court order are released from the hospital, they are permanently disqualified under federal law from purchasing or possessing a firearm, although they may be able to have firearm rights restored under state law (see Chapter 13, "'Relief From Disabilities': Firearm Rights Restoration for Persons Under Mental Health Prohibitions").

The proposed GVRO policy is unquestionably less restrictive to the civil liberties of an individual than civil commitment. Unlike a civil commitment, a GVRO merely constrains the right of the individual to purchase and possess firearms for a temporary period of time. Therefore, if the nature of the threat to public safety cannot be mitigated by a civil commitment proceeding, perhaps because mental illness is not the driving cause of the increased risk of dangerous behavior, or if a civil commitment is not medically indicated, even where the person has a mental illness, the GVRO offers an applicable, straightforward, and narrowly tailored option.

Moreover, the GVRO is an approach to addressing firearm violence against self and against others that avoids the stigma associated with being labeled or adjudicated with mental illness. The GVRO emphasizes dangerous behavior, not mental illness. By enacting a policy that centers on considerations of potentially dangerous firearm behaviors, with or without mental illness, policy makers can potentially work to change the negative and erroneous stereotypes that people with mental illness are inherently violent. The GVRO focuses on factors other than mental illness that increase the risk of violence both in the general population and among those with mental illness. Thus, the GVRO will encourage policy makers, law enforcement, the courts, and the public to recognize the importance of risk factors for firearm violence, including access to firearms, instead of simply ascribing firearm violence to individuals with mental illnesses or disorders.

In addition, once GVRO legislation is enacted in a state, public education efforts to inform people of the availability of a GVRO should include information about risk factors for violence other than mental illness. These educational efforts could further decrease stigmatization of individuals with mental illness and increase awareness of other risk factors. Furthermore, removing access to firearms and empowering families who frequently find themselves helpless in the face of a loved one's potentially lethal impulses may help families to more successfully encourage loved ones to seek treatment that could decrease the risk of future violence, especially risk of suicide. Finally, and most importantly, by emphasizing and educating the public about risk factors for firearm violence, which include access to firearms for individuals in crisis, regardless of whether they have mental illness, the GVRO has the potential for decreasing the morbidity and mortality of gun violence.

Evidence Base for the Gun Violence Restraining Order

Although signed into law in California in September 2014, the GVRO will not go into effect there until January 1, 2016, and so has not at the time of this discussion been implemented in any state. Therefore, no direct evaluation or evidence of the policy's effect is yet available, and we recommend that states that enact the GVRO also ensure that evaluation and further research of the policy are undertaken. Nevertheless, the concept of the GVRO is derived from evidence, previously discussed in this chapter (see section "Evolving Approach: Firearm Prohibitions Based on Evidence of a Heightened Risk of Dangerous Behavior"), demonstrating decreased morbidity and mortality following the removal of firearms from individuals subject to domestic violence restraining orders, as well as similar policy initiatives enacted in Indiana and Connecticut that are restricted to use by law enforcement.

Following shootings in Connecticut and Indiana, these state legislatures enacted a law enforcement–driven process that mandates surrender or warranted and warrantless removal of firearms from individuals who are at an increased risk of dangerous behavior (Consortium for Risk-Based Firearm Policy 2013; A.B. 1014, 2013–2014 Reg. Sess. [Cal. 2013]; Conn. Gen. Stat. § 29–38c; Ind. Code Ann. § 35-47-14). These laws differ from a GVRO in that they use the criminal justice system rather than the civil system to provide the legal means to remove firearms.

In Connecticut, a state's attorney or any two police officers can file for a warrant when they believe there is probable cause that an individual 1) poses a risk of imminent injury to self or others and 2) possesses one or more firearms. Law enforcement must also show that "no reasonable alternative to avert the risk of harm exists" (Conn. Gen. Stat. § 29–38c). Connecticut law outlines the definitions of *imminent risk* and *probable cause* without limiting these terms to mental illness. If the state shows probable cause, "a judge may issue a warrant for law enforcement to search for and remove any and all firearms" (Conn. Gen. Stat. § 29–38c). Similar to the California GVRO, Connecticut law mandates that a hearing be scheduled within 14 days to consider whether the guns should be removed for up to 1 year or returned to the owner. At this hearing the state must prove by clear and convincing evidence that the owner remains "a risk of imminent injury to self or others" for the order to be extended (Conn. Gen. Stat. § 29–38c).

Connecticut enacted this law in 1998, and an evaluation of the law's effect from implementation on October 1, 1999, to July 31, 2013, found that 764 warrants had been served (Norko and Baranoski 2014). The majority of the warrants were served after 2010 and were based on behavior posing a threat to self (Norko and Baranoski 2014). Significantly, only 1% of individuals served with warrants were in active psychiatric treatment, and the majority of the individuals served had no history of psychiatric treatment (Norko and Baranoski 2014). This highlights that the imminent danger standard—and the associated broad definitions defining the crisis—allows for intervention to occur during crisis, often before treatment begins. The most current data are limited to an evaluation performed by review of records from the state's Department of Mental Health and Addiction Services; data from the courts on the outcome of the mandatory hearing to consider whether the removal will stand are unavailable (Norko and Baranoski 2014).

Indiana law (Ind. Code Ann. § 35-47-14 et seq.) contains a warrant removal process similar to that in Connecticut. Unique, however, to the Indiana law is a provision that allows law enforcement to remove firearms, without a warrant, from an individual whom they believe to be dangerous. An individual is defined as "dangerous" if "(1) the individual presents an imminent risk of personal injury to the individual or to another individual; or (2) the individual may present a risk of personal injury to the individual or to another individual in the future and the individual: (A) has a mental illness (as defined in IC 12-7-2-130) that may be controlled by medication, and has not demonstrated a pattern of voluntarily and consistently taking the individual's medication while not under supervision; or (B) is the subject of documented evidence that would give rise to a reasonable belief that the individual has a propensity for violent or emotionally unstable conduct" (Ind. Code Ann. § 35-47-14 et seq.). As in Connecticut, this definition of dangerousness may rely on mental illness; however, it also is broadened to include those individuals who have "a propensity for violent or emotionally unstable conduct" (Ind. Code Ann. § 35-47-14 et seq.). Tailoring definitions to include persons who are likely to be dangerous rather than limiting interventions to persons with mental illness is a key component of proposed removal laws such as the GVRO.

As in California's GVRO process described above and in Connecticut, Indiana has established a process and procedures to ensure that a hearing is held to determine whether the removal is necessary and for how long the firearms should be removed. Evaluation of the first 2 years following implementation of the law revealed that only one county, Marion (where Indianapolis is located), had implemented the law (Parker 2010). Furthermore, use in the second year declined due to issues with implementation (Parker 2010). Further education efforts about this policy and evaluation of implementation should be carried out.

Landscape of Second Amendment Litigation

As with any new policy that restricts access to firearms, current jurisprudence requires that a proposed policy such as the GVRO be examined not only for its public health efficacy but also for its constitutional implications. After the Supreme Court's *District of Columbia v. Heller* decision in 2008 (554 U.S. 570, 128 S. Ct. 2783, 171 L. Ed. 2d 637), the central legal question in this examination is whether the GVRO will be in conflict with the right to bear arms in the Second Amendment to the U.S. Constitution.

The U.S. Supreme Court, being the highest court in the judicial branch, ranks above 13 regional circuits (each with a court of appeals) and 94 judicial districts (each with a district court). When the U.S. Supreme Court interprets federal law or the federal constitution, the lower federal and state courts must adhere to its decisions.

In *Heller,* the U.S. Supreme Court struck down the District of Columbia's handgun ban and held for the first time that the Second Amendment protected an individual's right to possess a firearm in the home for self-defense. In striking down the handgun ban, the court asserted that the Second Amendment right need not be connected with service in a militia. This decision precludes legislators from simply banning the sale and possession of firearms in the United States.

The Supreme Court, however, cautioned that the *Heller* decision did not spell the end of all gun violence prevention legislation. In its ruling, the court stated that "the right secured by the Second Amendment is not unlimited" and that "nothing in [the] opinion should be taken to cast doubt on longstanding prohibitions on the possession of firearms by felons and the mentally ill, or laws forbidding the carrying of firearms in sensitive places such as schools and government buildings, or laws imposing conditions and qualifications on the commercial sale of arms" (554 U.S. 570, 128 S. Ct. 2783, 171 L. Ed. 2d 637, 2008).

In 2010, two years after *Heller,* the Supreme Court, in *McDonald v. City of Chicago, Ill.* (561 U.S. 742, 130 S. Ct. 3020, 177 L. Ed. 2d 894), struck down several Chicago city ordinances that effectively banned handgun possession. In this ruling, the Supreme Court held that in addition to the federal government and the District of Columbia, state governments must also adhere to the Second Amendment, but also reasserted the validity of "longstanding regulatory measures."

Neither *Heller* nor *McDonald* precludes federal, state, or local governments from enacting effective, commonsense gun violence prevention legislation. In the wake of *Heller* and *McDonald,* lower courts have routinely upheld laws prohibiting purchase and possession of firearms by any of the following:

- Felons (*United States v. Barton,* 633 F.3d 168, 3d Cir., 2011; *United States v. Rozier,* 598 F.3d 768, 11th Cir., 2010; *United States v. Vongxay,* 594 F.3d 1111, 9th Cir., 2010)
- Persons convicted of misdemeanor domestic violence (*United States v. Booker,* 644 F.3d 12, 1st Cir., 2011; *United States v. Chovan,* 735 F.3d 1127, 9th Cir., 2013; *United States v. Skoien,* 614 F.3d 638, 7th Cir., 2010; *United States v. Smith,* 742 F. Supp. 2d 855, S.D.W. Va., 2010; *United States v. Staten,* 666 F.3d 154, 4th Cir., 2011; *United States v. Tooley,* 717 F. Supp. 2d 580, S.D.W. Va., 2010 [aff'd, 468 F. App'x 357 (4th Cir. 2012)])
- Persons subject to domestic violence restraining orders (*United States v. Bena,* 664 F.3d 1180, 8th Cir., 2011; *United States v. Mahin,* 668 F.3d 119, 4th Cir., 2012; *United States v. Reese,* 627 F.3d 792, 10th Cir., 2010)
- Persons who unlawfully use or are addicted to controlled substances (*United States v. Seay,* 620 F.3d 919, 8th Cir., 2010; *United States v. Yancey,* 621 F.3d 681, 7th Cir., 2010)
- Minors (*Nat'l Rifle Ass'n of Am., Inc. v. Bureau of Alcohol, Tobacco, Firearms and Explosives,* 700 F.3d 185, 5th Cir., 2012 [cert. denied, 134 S. Ct. 1364, 188 L. Ed. 2d 296 (U.S. 2014)]; *United States v. Rene E.,* 583 F.3d 8, 1st Cir., 2009)

Constitutional Analysis of Firearm Prohibitions

Courts use three different levels of scrutiny to evaluate the constitutionality of government actions. All three levels of scrutiny evaluate how closely related a law or regulation is to a government interest. *Rational basis* is the least rigorous level of scrutiny, and most laws are able to meet this test. Rational basis requires a court to uphold a law or regulation so long as it bears a "rational relationship" to a "legitimate governmental interest" (*District of Columbia v. Heller,* 2008).

Intermediate scrutiny, the second level of scrutiny, is more rigorous than rational basis but less rigorous than strict scrutiny. To satisfy intermediate scrutiny, a challenged law or regulation must be substantially related to an important government interest (Shaman 1984).

Strict scrutiny is the most stringent standard of judicial review. Strict scrutiny requires that a law or regulation be narrowly tailored to achieve a compelling government interest. A compelling interest is one that is more significant than the interest required under intermediate scrutiny. Additionally, a narrowly tailored law or regulation is one that is not significantly over- or underinclusive. A law is overinclusive if it significantly restricts that which does not implicate the government interest. It is underinclusive if it fails to restrict that which harms the government interest to about the same degree as does the restricted activity (Volokh 1996). The requirement that a law be narrowly tailored is similar to the "substantially related" requirement in intermediate scrutiny; it simply requires a closer fit. The government must also employ the least restrictive means of achieving the compelling government interest (Volokh 1996).

Courts typically apply strict scrutiny in two contexts: 1) when a fundamental right, such as freedom of speech, is infringed or 2) when a government action applies to a suspect classification, such as race or national origin (16B Am. Jur. 2d Constitutional Law § 862). Courts apply intermediate scrutiny in limited circumstances "when legislation is not facially or constitutionally invidious but nonetheless gives rise to some recurring constitutional difficulties," such as gender discrimination or illegitimacy (16B Am. Jur. 2d Constitutional Law § 861). The *Heller* court noted that "the [rational basis] test could not be used to evaluate the extent to which a legislature may regulate a specific, enumerated right, be it the freedom of speech, the guarantee against double jeopardy, the right to counsel, or the right to keep and bear arms." Neither the *Heller* court nor the *McDonald* court articulated which of the remaining levels of scrutiny—intermediate or strict scrutiny—should apply to future Second Amendment cases, and lower courts were left to determine that for themselves.

In upholding firearm laws and regulations against Second Amendment challenges, lower courts have generally applied intermediate scrutiny. As described earlier in this section, intermediate scrutiny requires that the law or regulation be substantially related to an important government interest. Often courts will look to the evidence base to demonstrate this relationship, as they did in *Heller v. District of Columbia* (670 F.3d 1244, 1252, D.C. Cir., 2011); *Nat'l Rifle Ass'n of Am., Inc. v. Bureau of Alcohol, Tobacco, Firearms and Explosives; United States v. Chester* (628 F.3d 673, 680, 4th Cir., 2010); *United States v. Greeno* (679 F.3d 510, 518, 6th Cir., 2012); and *United States v. Marzzarella* (614 F.3d 85, 89, 3d Cir., 2010).

In *United States v. Reese* (2010), for example, the Tenth Circuit Court held that a law prohibiting possession of firearms by persons subject to final domestic violence restraining orders did not violate the Second Amendment. This court reasoned that this law was substantially related to an important government objective: "to keep firearms out of the hands 'of people who have been judicially determined to pose a credible threat to the physical safety of a family member, or who have been ordered not to use, attempt to use, or threaten to use physical force against an intimate partner or child that would reasonably be expected to cause bodily injury'...because '[s]uch persons undeniably pose a heightened danger of misusing firearms.'" To demonstrate this relationship, the Tenth Circuit Court relied on research studies providing social science evidence that

- "domestic abusers often commit acts that would be charged as felonies if the victim were a stranger, but that are charged as misdemeanors because the victim is a relative (implying that the perpetrators are as dangerous as felons)";
- "[d]omestic assaults with firearms are approximately twelve times more likely to end in the victim's death than are assaults by knives or fists"; and
- the recidivism rate among persons convicted of misdemeanor crimes of domestic violence is high.

The majority of lower courts have required, as did the Tenth Circuit Court in *Reese,* that the law or regulation be substantially related to an important government interest. However, in *Tyler v. Hillsdale Cnty. Sheriff's Dep't, et al.* (No. 13-1876, 2014 WL 7181334, 6th Cir., 2014), the Sixth Circuit Court applied strict scrutiny. To survive strict scrutiny analysis, as described earlier in this section, a law or regulation must be narrowly tailored to achieve a compelling government interest (Winkler 2006). The *Tyler* court held that the challenged prohibition on the possession of firearms by a person "who has been committed to a mental institution," pursuant to 18 U.S.C. § 922[g][4], furthers two compelling interests: "protecting the community from crime" and "preventing suicide" (*Tyler v. Hillsdale Cnty. Sheriff's Dep't, et al.* 2014).

Nevertheless, the court held that the prohibition violates the Second Amendment because it was not narrowly tailored due to the fact that the state in which the respondent resided did not have a restoration process by which he could regain his firearm rights. Implicit in the *Tyler* court's holding is the notion that if a restoration process were available, the commitment prohibition would be constitutional. On April 21, 2015, the Tyler opinion was vacated and the case will be reheard by the entire bench of the Sixth Circuit. For the purpose of this chapter, however, let us assume, arguendo, that the Tyler opinion was not vacated and analyze the GVRO under strict scrutiny as well as intermediate scrutiny because it is possible that a future court may apply strict scrutiny.

The Gun Violence Restraining Order: Constitutional Analysis

Government Interest

The GVRO seeks to ensure that people who have been judicially determined to pose a threat to the physical safety of themselves or others, including family members and the general public, cannot access firearms. Federal courts, if applying an intermediate scrutiny analysis, should therefore conclude, as in *Reese,* that GVRO statutes further this same important government interest of preventing harm in the face of a credible threat. Moreover, because the GVRO is designed to specifically prevent firearm crime and suicide, a court applying a strict scrutiny analysis, similar to that annunciated by the *Tyler* court, should find that the GVRO furthers not only an important government interest but also a compelling government interest.

Relation to the Government Interest in Preventing Crime and Suicide

In determining the relationship between the GVRO policy and the government interest, courts will rely on the social science evidence. For instance, the court in *Reese* relied on social science evidence demonstrating that past acts of dangerous behavior increase the risk of future dangerousness as a basis for concluding that prohibiting persons subject to a domestic violence restraining order from possessing firearms is substantially related to the important government interest in reducing domestic violence. Similarly, in determining whether to issue a GVRO, a judge will consider a respondent's past violence or threats of violence. Again, a robust evidence base supports that acts of violence committed with firearms are more lethal than those committed with other weapons. It also supports that a substantial relationship exists between removing firearms from those most likely to be violent in the future and reducing suicide and violence against family members and the general public.

The broader evidence linking gun violence to risk factors for dangerous behavior is important to bear in mind. The axiom that the best predictor of acts of future violence is a history of past violence is based on an extensive amount of evidence, although a past history of violence is more accurately considered a risk factor for, rather than a predictor of, future violence. Public health research suggests that the attributable risk of homicide due to previous criminal history is very high, at 65.3% (Cook et al. 2005). When individuals convicted of a violent misdemeanor were subsequently denied the ability to purchase a handgun, the relative risk of violent crime and of gun crime significantly decreased in comparison with those not prohibited (Wintemute et al. 2001). Moreover, among a population of individuals with mental illness, a past history of violence is considered the most robust risk factor in the assessment of whether an individual may commit future acts of violence (Swanson et al. 2013; also see Chapter 9, "Structured Violence Risk Assessment"). Similarly, a past history of violence toward self—that is, suicide attempts—is a strong risk factor in the assessment of suicide risk (Kessler et al. 1999; also see Chapter 2, "Firearms and Suicide in the United States," and Chapter 10, "Decreasing Suicide Mortality").

In determining whether to issue a GVRO, a judge will also consider a respondent's alcohol and substance abuse history, which is another significant risk factor for suicide or violence. Alcohol and substance abuse are common throughout the population, and research consistently demonstrates that either chronic or acute alcohol abuse is associated with violence (Auerhahn and Parker 1999; Friedman 1999; Kelleher et al. 1994). Alcohol use has been found to increase the risk of intimate partner violence (Afifi et al. 2012). In one case-controlled study, alcohol or drug abuse in the home was found to increase the risk of homicide for all individuals in the home, highlighting that substance abuse affects not only abusers but also those close to them (Rivara and Mueller 1997). Research also demonstrates that both alcohol use disorders and the acute use of alcohol significantly increase the risk for suicide (*Ezell v. City of Chicago*, 651 F.3d 684, 701–04, 7th Cir., 2011).

The Sixth Circuit Court in *Tyler*, using a strict scrutiny analysis, held that the federal lifetime prohibition incident to a commitment to a mental institution was not narrowly tailored because no restoration process existed by which the plaintiff could regain firearm rights if he was no longer a danger to self or others. However, the GVRO is time-limited and thus a tighter fit with the government interest of preventing crime or suicide. A final GVRO would be in effect for up to 1 year and subject to renewal only following due process, with notice and hearing. Additionally, individuals prohibited from purchasing or possessing firearms under a GVRO would be entitled to one hearing to terminate the GVRO prior to the 1-year time limit and restore firearm rights.

Therefore, because of the strong evidence base and the holding in *Tyler*, courts should have no trouble concluding that the GVRO is narrowly tailored to achieve a compelling government interest and therefore is constitutional under either an intermediate scrutiny or strict scrutiny analysis.

Conclusion

The GVRO is a unique and well-tailored proposal that can decrease the morbidity and mortality of gun violence by removing firearms from those individuals who are in crisis and dangerous, regardless of the cause of the crisis. This policy also has the potential to inform and change community misperceptions about mental illness and violence. The GVRO focuses on and draws attention to factors other than mental illness that are strongly associated with the risk of violence both in the general population and among those with mental illness. Thus, the GVRO will encourage policy makers, law enforcement, the courts, and the broader community to recognize the multiple risk factors associated with violence instead of simply ascribing tragic acts of irrational or interpersonal violence to mental illness or disorder.

Gun violence is a multifaceted epidemic, and no singular policy will curtail the deaths that plague communities and nations. Therefore, additional policy initiatives should be considered alongside the GVRO, such as the following:

- Universal background checks
- Point-of-contact state background check systems
- New prohibitory categories focused on risk of future violence, such as violent misdemeanants and those subject to any domestic violence protective order
- Mandated technological changes to improve gun safety

All these and other interventions have the potential to contribute to decreasing the morbidity and mortality from gun violence in different ways, and as many levels and avenues of intervention as possible should be pursued.

Given the current political climate, however, attempts to enact overarching federal gun violence prevention policies may not survive the dysfunction in our political process. In such a climate, the GVRO is a novel approach for state-level policy that offers hope for an innovative intervention tightly focused on individuals with or without mental illness who are at high risk of committing gun violence. This approach is likely to significantly decrease firearm suicide and may also prove effective in preventing at least some mass shootings without stigmatizing individuals with serious mental illness.

Suggested Interventions

- To decrease the morbidity and mortality from firearms, states should pass laws prohibiting the purchase and possession of firearms for categories of individuals, with or without mental illness, who have been demonstrated by research evidence to present an increased risk of violence.
- States should enact policies to limit access to firearms by individuals, with or without mental illness, during times of personal crisis by enacting and implementing gun violence restraining orders (GVROs).
- Government and private organizations should fund research to continue to identify factors associated with gun violence and to evaluate the efficacy of policies such as GVROs where enacted, as in California, or other interventional policies, such as those in Connecticut and Indiana. This research can provide data that can assist in devising additional interventions to prevent gun violence.

REFERENCES

Afifi TO, Henriksen CA, Asmundson GJ, Sareen J: Victimization and perpetration of intimate partner violence and substance use disorders in a nationally representative sample. J Nerv Ment Dis 200(8):684–691, 2012 22850303

Appelbaum PS, Swanson JW: Law and psychiatry: gun laws and mental illness: how sensible are the current restrictions? Psychiatr Serv 61(7):652–654, 2010 20591996

Auerhahn K, Parker RN: Drugs, alcohol, and homicide, in Studying and Preventing Homicide: Issues and Challenges. Edited by Smith MD, Zahn MA. Thousand Oaks, CA, Sage, 1999, pp 97–114

Bailey JE, Kellermann AL, Somes GW, et al: Risk factors for violent death of women in the home. Arch Intern Med 157(7):777–782, 1997 9125010

Boles SM, Miotto K: Substance abuse and violence: a review of the literature. Aggress Violent Behav 8(2):155–174, 2003

Borges G, Walters EE, Kessler RC: Associations of substance use, abuse, and dependence with subsequent suicidal behavior. Am J Epidemiol 151(8):781–789, 2000 10965975

Bostwick JM, Pankratz VS: Affective disorders and suicide risk: a reexamination. Am J Psychiatry 157(12):1925–1932, 2000 11097952

Campbell JC, Webster D, Koziol-McLain J, et al: Risk factors for femicide in abusive relationships: results from a multisite case control study. Am J Public Health 93(7):1089–1097, 2003 12835191

Campbell JC, Glass N, Sharps PW, et al: Intimate partner homicide: review and implications of research and policy. Trauma Violence Abuse 8(3):246–269, 2007 17596343

Cohen AP, Azrael D, Miller M: Cohen AP, Azrael D, Miller M: Rate of mass shootings has tripled since 2011, Harvard research shows. Mother Jones, October 15, 2014. Available at: http://www.motherjones.com/politics/2014/10/mass-shootings-increasing-harvard-research. Accessed August 3, 2015.

Consortium for Risk-Based Firearm Policy: Guns, Public Health, and Mental Illness: An Evidence-Based Approach for State Policy. Baltimore, MD, Johns Hopkins Center for Gun Policy and Research, 2013. Available at: http://www.jhsph.edu/research/centers-and-institutes/johns-hopkins-center-for-gun-policy-and-research/publications/GPHMI-State.pdf. Accessed August 1, 2014.

Cook PJ, Ludwig J, Braga AA: Criminal records of homicide offenders. JAMA 294(5):598–601, 2005 16077054

Dahlberg LL, Ikeda RM, Kresnow MJ: Guns in the home and risk of a violent death in the home: findings from a national study. Am J Epidemiol 160(10):929–936, 2004 15522849

Elbogen EB, Johnson SC: The intricate link between violence and mental disorder: results from the National Epidemiologic Survey on Alcohol and Related Conditions. Arch Gen Psychiatry 66(2):152–161, 2009 19188537

Frattaroli S, Vernick JS: Separating batterers and guns: a review and analysis of gun removal laws in 50 states. Eval Rev 30(3):296–312, 2006 16679498

Friedman AS: Substance use/abuse as a predictor to illegal and violent behavior: a review of the relevant literature. Aggression and Violent Behavior 3(4):339–355, 1999

Hoyert DL, Xu J: Deaths: preliminary data for 2011. Natl Vital Stat Rep 61(6):1–51, 2012 24984457

Kelleher K, Chaffin M, Hollenberg J, Fischer E: Alcohol and drug disorders among physically abusive and neglectful parents in a community-based sample. Am J Public Health 84(10):1586–1590, 1994 7943475

Kellermann AL, Rivara FP, Rushforth NB, et al: Gun ownership as a risk factor for homicide in the home. N Engl J Med 329(15):1084–1091, 1993 8371731

Kessler RC, Borges G, Walters EE: Prevalence of and risk factors for lifetime suicide attempts in the National Comorbidity Survey. Arch Gen Psychiatry 56(7):617–626, 1999 10401507

Law Center to Prevent Gun Violence: Domestic Violence & Firearms Policy Summary (May 11, 2014). Available at: http://smartgunlaws.org/domestic-violence-firearms-policy-summary/. Accessed August 3, 2015.

McGinty EE, Frattaroli S, Appelbaum PS, et al: Using research evidence to reframe the policy debate around mental illness and guns: process and recommendations. Am J Public Health 104(11):e22–e26, 2014a 25211757

McGinty EE, Webster DW, Barry CL: Gun policy and serious mental illness: priorities for future research and policy. Psychiatr Serv 65(1):50–58, 2014b

Miller M, Azrael D, Hemenway D: The epidemiology of case fatality rates for suicide in the northeast. Ann Emerg Med 43(6):723–730, 2004 15159703

Miller M, Lippmann SJ, Azrael D, et al: Household firearm ownership and rates of suicide across the 50 United States. J Trauma 62(4):1029–1034, discussion 1034–1035, 2007 17426563

Miller M, Barber C, White RA, et al: Firearms and suicide in the United States: is risk independent of underlying suicidal behavior? Am J Epidemiol 178(6):946–955, 2013 23975641

Moracco KE, Clark KA, Espersen C, et al: Preventing Firearms Violence Among Victims of Intimate Partner Violence: An Evaluation of a New North Carolina Law. Washington, DC, U.S. Department of Justice, 2006

Norko MA, Baranoski M: Gun Control Legislation in Connecticut: Effects on Persons With Mental Illness. Conn Law Rev 46(4):1609–1631, 2014

Parker GF: Application of a firearm seizure law aimed at dangerous persons: outcomes from the first two years. Psychiatr Serv 61(5):478–482, 2010 20439368

Puzone CA, Saltzman LE, Kresnow M, et al: National trends in intimate partner homicide, United States 1976–1995. Violence Against Women 6(4):409–426, 2000

Rivara FP, Mueller BA, Somes G, et al: Alcohol and illicit drug abuse and the risk of violent death in the home. JAMA 278(7):569–575, 1997 9268278

Shaman JM: Cracks in the structure: the coming breakdown of the levels of scrutiny. Ohio State Law J 45(1):161–183, 1984

Swanson JW, Robertson AG, Frisman LK, et al: Preventing gun violence involving people with serious mental illness, in Reducing Gun Violence in America: Informing Policy With Evidence and Analysis. Edited by Webster DW, Vernick JS. Baltimore, MD, Johns Hopkins University Press, 2013, pp 33–51

Van Dorn R, Volavka J, Johnson N: Mental disorder and violence: is there a relationship beyond substance use? Soc Psychiatry Psychiatr Epidemiol 47(3):487–503, 2012 21359532

Vigdor ER, Mercy JA: Disarming batterers: the impact of domestic violence firearm laws, in Evaluating Gun Policy: Effects on Crime and Violence. Washington, DC, Brookings Institution Press, 2003, pp 157–201

Vigdor ER, Mercy JA: Do laws restricting access to firearms by domestic violence offenders prevent intimate partner homicide? Eval Rev 30(3):313–346, 2006 16679499

Volokh E: Freedom of speech, permissible tailoring and transcending strict scrutiny. Univ PA Law Rev 144(6):2417–2461, 1996

Webster DW, Vernick JS: Keeping firearms from drug and alcohol abusers. Inj Prev 15(6):425–427, 2009 19959738

Wiebe DJ: Homicide and suicide risks associated with firearms in the home: a national case-control study. Ann Emerg Med 41(6):771–782, 2003 12764330

Winkler A: Fatal in theory and strict in fact: an empirical analysis of strict scrutiny in the federal courts. Vanderbilt Law Rev 59:793–794, 2006

Wintemute GJ: Association between firearm ownership, firearm-related risk and risk reduction behaviours and alcohol-related risk behaviours. Inj Prev 17(6):422–427, 2011 21670071

Wintemute GJ, Parham CA, Beaumont JJ, et al: Mortality among recent purchasers of handguns. N Engl J Med 341(21):1583–1589, 1999 10564689

Wintemute GJ, Wright MA, Drake CM, et al: Subsequent criminal activity among violent misdemeanants who seek to purchase handguns: risk factors and effectiveness of denying handgun purchase. JAMA 285(8):1019–1026, 2001 11209172

Wintemute GJ, Frattaroli S, Claire BE, et al: Identifying armed respondents to domestic violence restraining orders and recovering their firearms: process evaluation of an initiative in California. Am J Public Health 104(2):e113–e118, 2014 24328660

Zeoli AM, Frattaroli S: Evidence for optimism: policies to limit batterers' access to guns, in Reducing Gun Violence in America: Informing Policy With Evidence and Analysis. Edited by Webster DW, Vernick JS. Baltimore, MD, Johns Hopkins University Press, 2013, pp 53–63

Zeoli AM, Webster DW: Effects of domestic violence policies, alcohol taxes and police staffing levels on intimate partner homicide in large U.S. cities. Inj Prev 16(2):90–95, 2010 20363814

13

Relief From Disabilities

Firearm Rights Restoration for Persons Under Mental Health Prohibitions

Liza H. Gold, M.D.
Donna Vanderpool, M.B.A., J.D.

Common Misperceptions

☒ Mental health prohibitions to own or possess firearms are permanent; when people are barred from owning or possessing guns for psychiatric reasons, they cannot regain firearm rights.

☒ Barring people with a history of involuntary psychiatric commitment from possessing firearms makes the public safer.

☒ People whose firearm rights have been suspended for psychiatric reasons are required to undergo a psychiatric evaluation before their rights can be restored.

Evidence-Based Facts

☑ The federal government and 39 states have "relief from disabilities" (RFD) programs that allow individuals who have been barred from owning firearms for mental health reasons to petition to have their firearm rights restored.

- ☑ Individuals with mental illness in the United States are responsible for about 3%–5% of all violence and an even smaller percentage of firearm violence. No evidence supports the belief that prohibiting firearm possession to individuals who meet the current mental health prohibition criteria decreases the incidence of firearm violence or increases public safety.
- ☑ Only a handful of states with RFD programs require risk assessments by a mental health professional as part of the RFD proceedings.

Politicians and advocacy groups, both those who oppose firearm regulation and those who support it, repeatedly insist on the need to keep guns out of the hands of people with mental illness, especially in the wake of tragic mass shootings. All sides agree that denying people with mental illness access to firearms is essential for public safety. The federal government and most states have laws that bar gun ownership by persons who have been involuntarily committed to a psychiatric institution or who, in criminal proceedings, have been adjudicated incompetent to stand trial or not guilty by reason of insanity (see Chapter 6, "Mental Illness and the National Instant Criminal Background Check System").

Many people may therefore be surprised to learn that individuals who have been prohibited from owning firearms on the basis of these mental health criteria may be able to have their gun rights restored. The federal government and the majority of states have "relief from disabilities" (RFD) statutes that provide a legal process through which individuals under mental health firearm prohibitions can petition to regain their gun rights. State RFD programs have proliferated since 2008, and increasing numbers of persons under firearm mental health prohibitions are filing petitions for restoration of gun rights.

Many have questioned the inherent fairness and efficacy of the mental health prohibitory criteria. No matter what one's position is on this subject, logic dictates that if individuals have been prohibited from purchasing or possessing firearms for mental health reasons, the legal restoration process should include a mental health evaluation assessing a petitioner's current mental status and risk of danger to self and others. In fact, the federal government and most states do not require mental health evidence or a mental health risk assessment as part of restoration proceedings.

RFD programs are relatively new and have been far from the spotlight in debates regarding firearm legislation reform. Little medical, psychiatric, or legal literature discussing mental health evaluations or evidentiary requirements in firearm restoration assessments, reports, or testimony is available. In this chapter, we review and discuss mental health RFD statutes and their ethical and legal implications, review the available literature, and suggest an approach to structuring RFD evaluations.

Firearm Legislation and Relief From Mental Health Disabilities

The 1968 Omnibus Crime Control and Safe Streets Act (Pub. L. No. 90-351, 82 Stat. 197) and Gun Control Act (Pub. L. No. 90-618, 82 Stat. 1213, codified at 18 U.S.C. §§ 921–929) prohibited certain categories of individuals from purchasing or possessing firearms, including any individual "who has been adjudicated a mental defective or who has been committed to a mental institution" (Gun Control Act, U.S.C. § 922[g][4] and [d][4]; see Chapter 6, "Mental Illness and the National Instant Criminal Background Check System"). This prohibited category has been defined to include, among others, individuals involuntarily committed to a psychiatric institution and those found incompetent to stand trial or not guilty by reason of insanity in a criminal proceeding (Meaning of Terms, 27 C.F.R. § 478.11, 2012). The National Instant Criminal Background Check System (NICS; see Chapter 6), established by the Brady Handgun Violence Prevention Act of 1993 (18 U.S.C. § 921 et seq.), includes the names of individuals prohibited from purchasing or possessing firearms based on these mental health criteria when this information is supplied by states (U.S. Office of Justice Programs 2014).

State participation in the federal background check system is voluntary and after the Virginia Tech shootings in 2007 was widely acknowledged to be less than ideal. In early 2008, Congress passed the NICS Improvement Amendments Act of 2007 (NIAA; Pub. L. No. 110-180, 121 Stat. 2559, codified at 18 U.S.C. § 922, 2008). This legislation was intended to improve state compliance with NICS and tighten scrutiny and regulation of firearm purchasers, especially those with mental illness (Hickey 2013). However, the NIAA also included a legal framework to restore gun rights to individuals under federal or state restrictions due to mental illness. Given the seemingly contradictory goals of both restricting and restoring access to firearms to those with certain histories of mental illness, we should perhaps not be surprised that the laws pertaining to RFD programs are among the least known and most confusing aspects of firearm regulation.

The NIAA and the Development of RFD Programs

Under the NIAA's provisions, all federal agencies that imposed mental health adjudications or involuntary commitments (such as Veterans Affairs) are required to provide a process for relief from these mental disabilities in regard to possessing firearms. In addition, the NIAA offers financial incentives to states to improve their participation in NICS. The NIAA authorizes the U.S. Department of Justice to provide NICS Act Record Improvement Program (NARIP) grants to improve states' infrastructure for collecting and submitting records to NICS. Eligibility for NARIP grants, the largest source of federal funding for improving state reporting systems (Mayors Against Illegal Guns 2011), requires states to have RFD programs that meet criteria specified in the NIAA. Approval and certification by the Bureau of Alcohol, Tobacco, Firearms and Explosives (ATF) demonstrate that a state program meets the NIAA requirements.

The access to substantial federal grants to improve or create reporting systems proved to be a powerful financial incentive and, as intended, resulted in improvements in states' participation in NICS. Because eligibility depended in part on having a certified RFD program, the NIAA and federal funds also resulted in the proliferation of state RFD programs. Prior to 2008, only a handful of states had RFD programs (Luo 2011); as of January 1, 2015, a total of 27 states had federally approved RFD programs, and at least a dozen more had RFD programs that had not yet been federally approved (U.S. Office of Justice Programs 2014).

Federal Relief From Disabilities

Individuals prohibited from purchasing or possessing firearms because of mental health adjudications or involuntary commitments imposed by federal agencies or authorities have two options for obtaining relief and restoring their firearm rights. They can 1) seek relief from the federal agency that imposed the mental health disability under the agency's NIAA-mandated federal disability relief program or 2) appeal the original federal agency's mental health adjudication or commitment. When relief is granted under a federal program, the event giving rise to the mental health disability is "deemed not to have occurred for purposes of the federal firearm prohibition" as per the NIAA (Pub. L. No. 110-180, 121 Stat. 2559), thereby restoring firearm rights under federal law. However, if the disability is also a prohibition under state law, federal relief may or may not automatically provide relief from the state prohibition (D.V., personal correspondence with various state attorneys general, 2014).

State Programs for Relief From Disabilities

A state RFD program that meets NIAA criteria must contain, at a minimum, provisions for

1. Application for relief from the *federal* prohibition on the purchase and possession of firearms
    a. through a *state* procedure
    b. with due process;

2. A judicial appeal of a denial of the initial petition; and
3. Updating records by removing the person's name from state and federal firearm prohibition databases if relief is granted.

The U.S. Department of Justice also recommends, but does not require, that the state have a written procedure, such as a state law, regulation, or administrative order, to address the NIAA's requirement for updating the NICS database when rights are restored (U.S. Department of Justice, Bureau of Alcohol, Tobacco, Firearms and Explosives 2013).

Not all states have a codified RFD program. Those that do have wide variation in RFD statutes as a result of the NIAA's lack of specificity in regard to criteria for restoration and the political issues that complicate any proposed firearm regulations. Even ATF-approved state RFD programs differ significantly. For example, states may allow petitions to be heard by courts, an existing board, a new board created to hear RFD petitions, or a state agency. State evidentiary standards also differ. Some states require a preponderance of the evidence, others require clear and convincing evidence, and still others do not specify a standard of proof. In addition, whether restoration of firearm rights and RFD legal proceedings are available to those who have been adjudicated incompetent to stand trial or not guilty by reason of insanity remains unclear and undecided by case law.

Moreover, not all states that have mental health prohibitions require an RFD hearing for firearm rights to be restored. For example, California, which has some of the strictest firearm regulations in the United States, provides for automatic termination of mental health prohibitions after a specified period of time. However, California also allows those who wish to restore their gun rights to petition for relief prior to the statutory time limit (Cal. Welf. and Inst. Code § 8103 [f][3]). Other states require an RFD hearing for restoration of firearm rights. In Maine, for example, individuals under mental health prohibitions must petition for relief but are only allowed to do so after a minimum 5-year period of prohibition (15 M.R.S.A. § 393[4-A]).

Relief From Firearms Disabilities Statutes and Mental Health Evidence

Hearings for restoration of firearm rights based on mental health prohibitions lack standard requirements for mental health records, current mental health evaluations, or violence and suicide risk assessments. The need for a current mental health evaluation, including risk assessment, seems self-evident in an administrative or court proceeding to determine whether gun rights should be restored to an individual whose gun rights have been suspended due to a mental health prohibition. Nevertheless, federal RFD programs and the great majority of states with RFD statutes do not require mental health evidence beyond access to medical records. When mental health evidence is required, states generally provide little statutory guidance regarding the specifics of the required evidence.

Almost all states with RFD programs require that relief be based on the findings, as per the NIAA, that restoration is "not contrary to the public interest and does not present a danger to public safety" (NIAA, § 101[c)[2][A][iii], referring to 18 U.S.C. § 925[c]). Also as per the NIAA, the court must consider the following evidence in coming to these findings:

1. circumstances regarding the firearms disabilities imposed by 18 U.S.C § 922(g)(4);
2. applicant's record, which must include, *at a minimum,* the applicant's mental health *and* criminal history records; and
3. applicant's reputation, developed, at a minimum, through character witness statements, testimony, and other character evidence. (U.S. Department of Justice, Bureau of Alcohol, Tobacco, Firearms and Explosives 2013)

Beyond these general criteria, guidance as to how federal authorities and states are to fulfill these requirements is minimal.

Almost all states with RFD statutes require that the court review "medical records," to be submitted with the petition for relief. Despite this requirement, most state statutes only vaguely indicate the specific type or types of medical records that are to be submitted. Some states, such as Oregon, provide the petitioner with the option of providing current treatment records or a letter from the current treatment provider, containing diagnosis, medications, history of compliance, and any other relevant information (Or. Admin. R. 859-300-0050, 2009), in addition to all mental health records pertaining to the disqualifying mental health determination (Britton and Bloom 2015). Other states, such as New York, require that extensive and specific records accompany the applicant's petition (New York Office of Mental Health 2012; see also Fisher et al. 2015).

Of the 39 states we identified as having RFD programs, only 13 have statutes that indicate a role for some form of mental health evidence beyond the applicant's medical records. Among these states, specifications for evaluations and documentation vary considerably in regard to the required qualifications of the professional providing the evidence, the time frame within which the documentation or assessment must be provided relative to the filing of the petition for relief, and the issues to be addressed and documented (Table 13–1).

Oregon is the only state that specifies that an applicant must have an independent forensic mental health assessment, including an opinion and a basis for that opinion, of the petitioner's risk of interpersonal violence and self-harm. Only 6 of the 13 states explicitly require a mental health evaluation. Six states also have statutes that incorporate an explicit reference to a risk assessment, defined for purposes of this discussion as a mental health assessment of level of risk of

TABLE 13–1. States with statutory mental health evidence requirements (other than mental health records)

State and statute	Federally approved	Risk assessment[a] specifically required	Type of professional specified	Evidence specifications	Time limits
Delaware DE ST 11 § 1448A	Yes	Yes	Medical doctor or psychiatrist	"A certificate of a medical doctor or psychiatrist licensed in this State that the person is no longer suffering from a mental disorder which interferes with or handicaps the person from handling deadly weapons." *and* "Board shall have the authority to require that the petitioner undergo a clinical evaluation and **risk assessment.**"	No
Georgia GA ST § 16-11-129 *Optional*	No	**Yes for danger to others;** No for danger to self	Superintendent of any mental hospital or treatment center	"Court may require any such person to sign a waiver authorizing the superintendent of any mental hospital or treatment center to make to the judge **a recommendation regarding whether such person is a threat to the safety of others.**"	No
Hawaii HI ST § 134-6.5	Yes	No	No	"Medical documentation that the petitioner is no longer adversely affected by the condition that resulted in the petitioner's adjudication or commitment and is **not likely to act in a manner dangerous to public safety.**"	No

TABLE 13–1. States with statutory mental health evidence requirements (other than mental health records) *(continued)*

State and statute	Federally approved	Risk assessment[a] specifically required	Type of professional specified	Evidence specifications	Time limits
Indiana IN ST § 33-23-15-2	Yes	No	Psychiatrist or psychologist	"A recent mental health evaluation by a psychiatrist or psychologist licensed to practice in Indiana."	No
Maine ME ST 15 § 393	No	No	Independent psychologist or psychiatrist	"Report of an independent psychologist licensed to practice in this State specifically addressing…that the circumstances that led to the involuntary commitment to a hospital have changed, that the applicant is **not likely to act in a manner dangerous to public safety** and that granting the application for relief will not be contrary to the public interest."	No
Maryland MD ST Pub Saf § 5-133.3	Yes	**Yes**	Board-certified psychiatrist or psychologist	"Form stating: i) the length of time the applicant has not had symptoms that cause the applicant to be a danger to the applicant or others…; ii) the length of time that the applicant has been compliant with the treatment plan for the applicant's mental illness…; iii) **an opinion as to whether the applicant, because of mental illness, would be a danger to the applicant if allowed to possess a firearm and a statement of reasons for the opinion**; and iv) **an opinion as to whether the applicant, because of mental illness, would be a danger to another person or poses a risk to public safety if allowed to possess a firearm.**"	Form must be completed within 30 days of submission of application

TABLE 13–1. States with statutory mental health evidence requirements (other than mental health records) *(continued)*

State and statute	Federally approved	Risk assessment[a] specifically required	Type of professional specified	Evidence specifications	Time limits
Minnesota MN ST § 624.713 *Optional*	No	No	Medical doctor or clinical psychologist	"The court may consider evidence from a licensed medical doctor or clinical psychologist that the person is no longer suffering from the disease or condition that caused the disability or that the disease or condition has been successfully treated for a period of three consecutive years."	No
New York NY ST Ment. Hyg. § 7.09 NY ADC 14 NYCRR 543.5 *Optional*	Yes	**Yes**	Qualified psychiatrist, defined as board certified or board eligible	"The applicant may provide a psychiatric evaluation performed no earlier than 90 calendar days from the date the request for the certificate of relief was submitted to the Office, conducted by a qualified psychiatrist. The evaluation should include an opinion, and basis for that opinion, as to whether or not the applicant's record and reputation are such that the applicant **will or will not be likely to act in a manner dangerous to public safety** and whether or not the granting of relief would be contrary to public interest." *and* "The Office reserves the right to request that the applicant undergo a clinical evaluation and **risk assessment.**"	Psychiatric evaluation must have been performed no earlier than 90 days prior to filing application

TABLE 13–1. States with statutory mental health evidence requirements (other than mental health records) *(continued)*

State and statute	Federally approved	Risk assessment[a] specifically required	Type of professional specified	Evidence specifications	Time limits
Oregon OR ST § 166.274 OR ADC § 859-300-0050	Yes	**Yes**	1. Licensed psychiatrist or psychologist, but not petitioner's current or previous provider	1. "An independent forensic mental health assessment performed no more than 90 calendar days prior to submission of the petition for relief.…This assessment may not be performed by petitioner's current or previous mental health provider. The assessment shall be performed by a licensed psychiatrist or psychologist. **The assessment shall include, at a minimum, an opinion and a basis for that opinion, of petitioner's interpersonal violence and self-harm risk.**"	Independent forensic mental health assessment must have been performed no more than 90 days prior to submission of petition
			2. Letter from current mental health practitioner	2. "Records may also include a letter from petitioner's current treating mental health practitioner, if any. The letter may contain the petitioner's current medical health diagnosis, a list of psychiatric medicines and dosage, if any, the petitioner is currently prescribed, history of compliance with the medication, and any other information the practitioner deems relevant to petitioner possessing a firearm."	

TABLE 13–1. States with statutory mental health evidence requirements (other than mental health records) *(continued)*

State and statute	Federally approved	Risk assessment[a] specifically required	Type of professional specified	Evidence specifications	Time limits
Rhode Island RI ST § 11-47-63	No	**Yes**	Medical doctor or psychiatrist	"Certificate of a medical doctor or psychiatrist licensed in this state certifying that the person is no longer suffering from a mental disorder which interferes or handicaps the person from handling deadly weapons." *and* "Board shall have the authority to require that the petitioner undergo a clinical evaluation and **risk assessment.**"	No
South Carolina SC ST § 23-31-1030	Yes	**Yes**	Department of Mental Health or physician licensed in South Carolina specializing in mental health	"Current evaluation [documented on form] presented by the petitioner conducted by the Department of Mental Health or a physician licensed in this State specializing in mental health specifically addressing whether **due to mental defectiveness or mental illness the petitioner poses a threat to the safety of the public or himself or herself.**"	No

TABLE 13–1. States with statutory mental health evidence requirements (other than mental health records) *(continued)*

State and statute	Federally approved	Risk assessment[a] specifically required	Type of professional specified	Evidence specifications	Time limits
Utah UT ST § 76-10-532	Yes	No	Licensed psychiatrist	"Mental health evaluation…which shall include a statement regarding: (i) the nature of the commitment, finding, or adjudication that resulted in the restriction on the petitioner's ability to purchase or possess a dangerous weapon; (ii) the petitioner's previous and current mental health treatment; (iii) the petitioner's previous violent behavior, if any; (iv) the petitioner's current mental health medications and medication management; (v) the length of time the petitioner has been stable; (vi) external factors that may influence the petitioner's stability; (vii) the ability of the petitioner to maintain stability with or without medication; and (viii) **whether the petitioner is dangerous to public safety.**"	Evaluation must have been within 30 days prior to filing of petition
West Virginia WV ST § 61-7A-5	Yes	No	Licensed psychologist or psychiatrist	"Certificate of mental health examination by a licensed psychologist or psychiatrist occurring within thirty days prior to filing of the petition which supports that the petitioner is competent and **not likely to act in a manner dangerous to public safety.**"	Mental health examination must have been within 30 days prior to filing

Note. **Boldface** text highlights statutory language that specifies an element or elements of risk assessment required as part of mental health evidence.
[a]Defined as dangerous to self or others.

danger to self or others. Of these 6, only Maryland, Oregon, and South Carolina specify evaluation of risk of harm to self as a consideration.

Relief From Disabilities Hearings: What's Happening on the Ground?

Although increasing numbers of people under federal and/or state mental health–based firearm restrictions are filing petitions for restoration of gun rights (Luo 2011), many states' RFD programs are so new that many courts or administrative agencies are just beginning to hear these cases on a regular basis. Very little information is available regarding how these hearings are actually conducted, whether and how mental health evidence affects the outcomes of the hearings, and how a mental health RFD evaluation might be structured. A literature search for information about the RFD legal process and psychiatric evaluation practices identified only one published study from California (Simpson and Sharma 2008) and two reviews of actual practices, one in Oregon (Britton and Bloom 2015) and the other in New York State (Fisher et al. 2015).

Simpson and Sharma (2008) provide the only systematic review of the use of mental health evidence in relief hearings. Their study, examining cases heard in 2005 and 2006, comes out of the practices of one court in California, a state that has had an RFD statute since 1990. Although California's RFD statute does not require that an individual petitioning for relief be evaluated by a mental health clinician or any health care professional, the Los Angeles County court hearing these cases made an informal decision to have a forensic psychiatrist evaluate all petitioners (Simpson 2007b).

The forensic psychiatrists conducting the RFD evaluations addressed the specific question under California law of whether or not the individual would be able to use firearms in a safe and lawful manner. The evaluating psychiatrists interpreted this language as encompassing the risk of suicide and homicide, as well as additional potential risks regarding unintentional injury to self or others. Simpson and Sharma (2008) described the RFD evaluation as "similar to other types of risk or dangerousness assessments performed for the court system including determinations regarding civil commitment or suitability for probation" (p. 973).

The RFD psychiatric evaluation consisted of a review of records from the involuntary admission resulting in the state firearm prohibition, and an evaluation utilizing unaided clinical judgment in the determination of risk (see Chapter 9, "Structured Violence Risk Assessment"). This included a forensic psychiatric interview with the petitioner and, if deemed necessary, contact with collateral sources such as family members or current treatment providers (Simpson and Sharma 2008). If any doubt remained about the level of risk after the clinical interview, the examiners recommended that the petition be denied, unless contact with collateral sources allowed examiners to conclude that the risk was low. In many cases, the court heard testimony, often including that of the forensic psychiatrist (Simpson and Sharma 2008).

The authors examined the demographic and psychiatric features of a sample of 57 relief petitions in regard to the outcome. In the 40 of 41 cases in which the petitions had not been withdrawn or automatically denied, the judge ruled in accordance with the forensic psychiatrist's recommendation. No demographic factors were significantly associated with petition outcome. The only psychiatric factor significantly correlated with examiner recommendation was involuntary psychiatric detention beyond the 72-hour hold on California's 14-day hold (Simpson and Sharma 2008).

While acknowledging the study's multiple limitations, Simpson and Sharma (2008) suggested that the involvement of a forensic mental health professional and mental health evidence might have enhanced the decision-making process. This belief was based on their finding that individuals with a greater burden of mental illness, as demonstrated by progression from a 72-hour to a 14-day hold, were less likely to have their firearm prohibitions lifted. The authors concluded, "It would be reasonable to assume that expert input and testimony in such proceedings would be likely to reduce the chance of errors, i.e., the unnecessary denial of petitions made by individuals at low risk and the granting of petitions made by individuals who appear safe but in fact pose a higher risk" (Simpson and Sharma 2008, p. 973).

In Oregon, as described by Britton and Bloom (2015), the firearm restoration process is conducted through an administrative agency, the Psychiatric Security Review Board. Prior to 2009, Oregon had a restoration process, but it only provided relief for state, not federal, imposition of firearm restrictions for individuals with mental disabilities. Oregon revised its restoration process to allow both federal and state relief through the state process, as required by the NIAA for ATF certification and, therefore, eligibility for NARIP grants. Oregon's new relief policy received ATF certification in 2009, and between 2009 and 2014, the state used NARIP grants to upgrade its reporting systems and to revise and partially fund the RFD program (Britton and Bloom 2015).

Oregon has some of the most specific and stringent evidentiary requirements among states with RFD programs. The petitioner must provide certified copies of the following (Britton and Bloom 2015):

- All mental health records pertaining to the disqualifying mental health determination;
- All court records related to the circumstances surrounding the firearm prohibitor;
- The petitioner's FBI criminal history, including juvenile adjudications; and

- An independent forensic psychiatric assessment performed by a nontreating psychiatrist or psychologist no more than 90 days prior to the submission of the petition for relief.

Britton and Bloom (2015) reported that at the time of their review, although the Oregon Psychiatric Security Review Board had received dozens of requests for relief applications, the Board had received only two incomplete petitions and had conducted only three relief hearings. All three petitioners had been civilly committed, had little or no criminal history, and were granted restoration of firearm rights. The authors speculated that the relative ease with which a firearm can be purchased in the United States without a background check was at least one reason why Oregon has received so few relief petitions.

Britton and Bloom (2015) also endorsed the value of a forensic psychiatric evaluation in relief proceedings: "A robust relief process that includes a current psychiatric evaluation and consideration of a petitioner's mental health and criminal history can provide an opportunity for all citizens to receive fair consideration of restoration of their firearm privileges, while at the same time recognizing any public safety concerns" (p. 330). Although they did not describe the specifics of such an evaluation, they stated their opinion that "at a minimum, a relief authority should have a complete picture of a person's psychiatric history and current mental status and a risk assessment in order to effectively make a decision."

Fisher et al. (2015) provide a detailed description of the forensic psychiatric evaluations conducted in many of the restoration hearings in New York State. As in Oregon, New York uses an administrative process for consideration of relief petitions. New York's Office of Mental Health (OMH) created an RFD program in 2010, and New York is another one of the few states to provide specific guidance regarding the psychiatric evidence to be considered. Many of New York's evidentiary requirements are identical or similar to those of Oregon, as listed above.

Unlike Oregon, New York does not require independent psychiatric examinations as part of the evidence to be considered. However, following the initiation of the disability relief program, OMH recruited forensic psychiatry fellowship training programs to provide clinical evaluations and risk assessments (Fisher et al. 2015). OMH frequently requests psychiatric evaluations for RFD petitioners (L.H.G., personal communication with P. Appelbaum, January 22, 2015).

Fisher et al. (2015) also note that RFD evaluations have no guidelines with which to help structure an evaluator's psychiatric examination and little empirical data regarding psychiatric factors involved in an assessment of safety in managing firearms. In the absence of guidance, Fisher and colleagues describe choosing to use a structured professional judgment approach to risk assessment in RFD evaluations (see Chapter 9). "The forensic psychiatric assessment is grounded in the fundamentals of forensic psychiatric practice: record review, psychiatric interview, and clinical judgment (supplemented with a structured clinical assessment tool)" (Fisher et al. 2015, p. 340).

Two forensic psychiatry fellows, supervised by senior forensic psychiatrists, conduct the RFD examinations. Examiners synthesize the information obtained from the record and the clinical interview, and come to a clinical determination of risk of dangerous behavior. Their opinions are based on risk factors associated with the petitioner's past dangerous behavior and the extent to which these factors have been mitigated (Fisher et al. 2015). The examiners prepare a report, including the opinion, required by regulation, as to whether or not the applicant's "record and reputation are such that the applicant will or will not be likely to act in a manner dangerous to public safety and whether or not the granting of relief would be contrary to public interest" (p. 337). An OMH-appointed committee reviews this report as well as other evidence presented.

Fisher et al. (2015) conclude that the clinical risk assessment is "an essential component of the petition review process" (p. 343) but also stress that the committee makes the ultimate determination regarding restoration of firearm rights. These authors state that at least one advantage of requiring forensic mental health evaluations in RFD hearings "may be a greater likelihood that restoration proceedings will pay appropriate attention to the sometimes significant risk of suicide" (p. 343)

The only additional information regarding RFD hearings and mental health evidence comes from a report in the *New York Times* of a 2009–2010 investigation of RFD hearings conducted across the country (Luo 2011). A team of investigators found that like California, most states use the court system to adjudicate RFD petitions and use little, if any, documentation or evidence other than the petitioner's affidavit. The investigators concluded that across the country, judicial determinations in gun rights restoration hearings "are marked by vague standards and few specific requirements" (Luo 2011).

The judicial process for RFD petitioners in the Commonwealth of Virginia, for example, is typical of the process in many states. Hearings in Virginia are held in each jurisdiction's general district court, which also adjudicates small claims and traffic infractions. Virginia has a federally certified RFD program, and its statutes are typical in regard to the evidence to be considered. These vaguely specify only that "treatment records" be considered in coming to the findings that the petitioner "will not likely act in a manner dangerous to public safety" and that "the granting of the relief would not be contrary to the public interest" (Virginia Code Ann. § 18.2-308.1:3).

One legal review of Virginia's firearm laws in relation to individuals with mental illness concluded, "Virginia's firearm rights restoration proceeding affords adequate procedural safeguards to keep at-risk individuals from lawfully possessing firearms in Virginia" (Luther 2014, pp. 357–358). In contrast, the *New York Times* investigators described Virginia's RFD hearings as "often relatively brief, sometimes perfunctory," and noted that "judges had wide latitude in handling the petitions" (Luo 2011). The investigators reported that "in case after case...judges made decisions without important information about an applicant's mental health" (Luo 2011). When the investigators provided one Virginia judge with detailed information regarding a successful petitioner's mental health history of four involuntary commitments over the previous 5 years as well as substance use history, the judge said he might have made a different decision had he been aware of this information (Luo 2011).

The *New York Times* report concluded that in Virginia, "[d]octors' declarations clearly influenced judges" (Luo 2011). However, whereas some Virginia judges insisted on seeing a doctor's note, others did not. When medical evidence was reviewed, the *New York Times* investigators (Luo 2011) reported the following:

- The doctors providing documentation were often general practitioners, not mental health professionals;
- The documentation provided was usually a short note consisting of only a few sentences;
- All medical documentation was provided by the petitioner's treating physician at the request of the petitioner, leading the report to conclude that treating doctors might feel pressured to comply with their patients' requests; and
- None of the Virginia physicians who wrote letters on behalf of their patients when contacted reported conducting a risk assessment of the patient.

Dangerousness, Risk Assessment, and Relief From Disability Evaluations

The term *dangerousness* continues to be used in legal terminology, as in the NIAA and state RFD statutes or regulations. Nevertheless, mental health professionals have come to rely on evaluations of *level of risk* when the question of future violence or suicide arises (see Chapter 9, "Structured Violence Risk Assessment," and Chapter 10, "Decreasing Suicide Mortality"). Heilbrun (2009) observed, "'Unelaborated legal standards'—particularly the use of the words 'dangerous' and 'dangerousness'—were a substantial reason why medical and behavioral science moved from using these terms to using 'risk assessment'" (p. 42).

That said, multiple issues complicate risk assessment methodology for purposes of evaluations related to restoration of firearm rights. First, the mistaken assumption that people with serious mental illness pose a high risk of violence toward others underlies the required legal findings in most state RFD statutes. Mental health firearm prohibitions were not enacted to prevent people from committing suicide with firearms; concerns regarding suicide are for the most part absent from RFD statutes. Nevertheless, suicidal ideation or suicide attempts are among the most common reasons for involuntary psychiatric commitments that trigger the prohibitions (Britton and Bloom 2015). Courts and administrative agencies whose primary concern is preventing the infrequent occurrence of a person with mental illness committing firearm violence against others might easily overlook the significantly higher risk of suicide associated with mental illness and access to firearms. RFD risk assessments therefore need to both include and emphasize suicide risk assessment as well as violence risk assessment.

Second, restoration evaluations are another example of the imperfect fit between the fields of law and behavioral science. The most useful risk assessments are usually conducted in response to questions that are clear, specific, and clinically focused (Buchanan et al. 2012). Less than a handful of state RFD statutes could be said to meet this description. In addition, risk assessments conducted for purposes such as restoration of firearm rights result in opinions regarding level of risk, not a yes-or-no determination. The courts or administrative agencies, however, are tasked with providing a yes-or-no determination, and often ask mental health professionals to provide a yes-or-no answer (Fisher et al. 2015). Thus, communication of mental health opinions regarding restoration of firearm rights needs to be clear, especially in regard to the authority of the court or administrative agency in making the ultimate determination regarding restoration and the limitations of the mental health opinions provided.

Third, specific data are not available regarding the factors necessary to conclude that individuals with a history of involuntary commitment do or do not pose a danger to the public, or more likely themselves, if access to firearms is restored or denied. Absent hard data, general principles of risk assessment must be adapted, as far as possible, to the specific legal and clinical circumstances associated with RFD hearings (Buchanan et al. 2012; Heilbrun 2009). Such adaptations impose additional complexities, because the data underlying risk assessment methodology are based on specific clinical and forensic populations. Conclusions in RFD evaluations are therefore necessarily extrapolated from risk assessment data that may have varying degrees of relevance to RFD populations in general and to any single case specifically.

In addition, risk assessment methodology is based on repeated evaluations of level of risk over time, including evaluation of treatment interventions, their efficacy, and whether they mitigate risk. People's mental states change, as do their circumstances (Buchanan et al. 2012; Simon 2012). However, RFD evaluations are likely to be based on a single clinical interview. The validity and reliability of a single risk assessment decrease over time. RFD evaluations based on a single assessment are therefore essentially evaluations of short-term level of risk (Buchanan et al. 2012). This limitation should be explicitly acknowledged, as should the limited ability to balance level of risk with evidence of factors or interventions that can mitigate future risk (Buchanan et al. 2012).

Opinions based on a single assessment will therefore also require adaptation of risk assessment methodology. For example, clinicians may have to weigh risk factors associated with past history and patterns of behavior more heavily than assessments performed in circumstances that include ongoing access and repeated evaluation. Patterns of past behavior are therefore relevant and sometimes critical (Buchanan et al. 2012). In the absence of reliable information regarding past history, examiners may not be able to reach an opinion with a degree of certainty and may need to request access to additional information.

No professional guidelines for suicide or violence risk assessment in civil psychiatric contexts have been adopted, and no specific evaluation for RFD has been formally proposed. In the absence of such guidelines, psychiatrists and psychologists must recognize and communicate limitations while adapting the best available methodology to the task at hand. This is consistent with current clinical and forensic practice under circumstances in which access to an evaluee is limited and specific data are limited or absent. Psychiatrists and psychologists should also be prepared to evaluate and change methodology when data indicating the need to do so become available.

In RFD evaluations, the application of best practices in suicide and violence risk assessments suggests the need for systematic review of empirically validated risk factors for suicide and violence, considered in conjunction with the petitioner's specific and unique clinical circumstances. RFD risk assessments also should include, as far as possible, consideration of whether and how level of risk based on empirically identified risk factors and clinical circumstances may change with access to firearms, particularly in light of the evidence for the additional risk and lethality associated with firearms and suicide (see Chapter 2, "Firearms and Suicide in the United States").

RFD Risk Assessments, Firearms, and Physician Training

Assuming that courts and administrative agencies accept the logic of including current mental health risk assessments as a standard element of the evidence considered in RFD hearings, such assessments should preferably be provided by appropriately trained mental health professionals. Unfortunately, finding such professionals can be challenging. New York State's solution to this problem offers one model for involving forensically trained clinicians (see Fisher et al. 2015). However, the option of accessing a postgraduate forensic mental health training program may not be available to every administrative agency or court.

Performing assessments of risk of violence (Simon and Tardiff 2008) and suicide (Accreditation Council for Graduate Medical Education 2014; Cramer et al. 2013; Hung et al. 2012; Simon 2012; Wortzel et al. 2013) is a core competency for mental health professionals. Unfortunately, the few studies available suggest than many psychiatrists and psychologists receive little formal training in violence risk assessment, particularly in civil psychiatric contexts (McNiel et al. 2008; Teo et al. 2012; Tolman 2001; Tolman and Mullendore 2003; Wong et al. 2012). Similarly, many mental health professionals for whom suicide risk assessment is a required competency also lack basic skills and adequate training (Cramer et al. 2013; Hung et al. 2012; Jacobson et al. 2012; Melton and Coverdale 2009; Schmitz et al. 2012; Silverman 2014).

As a result, the use of unaided clinical judgment, the least reliable methodology for violence risk assessment (Buchanan 2008; Monahan 2008; Tolman and Rotzien 2007), is common among mental health professionals and non–mental health professionals alike. Even among forensically trained mental health professionals, use of an unstructured clinical judgment approach in risk assessment is often standard practice (Monahan 2008; Tolman 2001; Tolman and Mullendore 2003). Years of clinical experience, absent adequate training in risk assessment, do not necessarily result in better judgment or improved competence in either suicide risk assessment (Silverman 2014) or violence risk assessment (McNiel et al. 2008; Teo et al. 2012).

Many mental health professionals are also ill prepared to consider levels of risk associated with firearms. Indeed, regardless of medical specialty, no physician training programs or standards exist for the assessment of competency to carry firearms. Aside from several articles discussing older adults with dementia and related physical and mental competence to own firearms (Greene et al. 2007; Mertens and Sorenson 2012), the extant literature on medical training regarding firearms typically indicates there is none available and calls for formal physician training (see, e.g., Coverdale et al. 2010; Khubchandani et al. 2009).

Only one brief article, published in 1968 (Rotenberg and Sadoff 1968), could be found that directly addressed elements of competency to possess firearms. These authors suggested three "preliminary empirical criteria" (p. 842), which centered on identifying individuals who should *not* be considered competent to possess firearms:

1. Individuals who are psychotic
2. Individuals with a history of poor impulse control
3. Individuals with drug and alcohol addictions

The authors stated, "A person free of any of the above conditions should be competent to buy firearms provided he gives an acceptable reason for owning a gun" (p. 842). They also suggested that a gun owner who acquired any of these criteria "should be given a psychiatric examination to determine his competency to retain a gun" (p. 842).

In the only study to date of physicians' roles in assessing competency to carry firearms, a group of clinicians examined physicians' beliefs in regard to assessing competency in safely carrying concealed weapons. The researchers also looked at related issues associated with patients' requests to provide such documentation (Goldstein et al. 2013, 2015; Pierson et al. 2014). Goldstein et al. (2015) started examining these issues after they began receiving letters from county sheriffs asking whether the permit applicant (i.e., the patient) suffered from "any physical or mental infirmity that prevents the safe handling of a handgun" related to a patient's application for a concealed weapon permit.

The authors sent out 600 surveys and had a response rate of 40%; of the respondents, 35% were family physicians, 38% were psychiatrists, and 27% were internists. Physicians were asked about eight specific psychiatric or psychological conditions or use of psychiatric medications, and nine specific physical conditions. More than one-third of physicians were unsure whether a patient was competent to carry in 12 of the 17 conditions queried; more than one-third of the respondents were unsure about competence to carry in six of the eight mental conditions (Goldstein et al. 2015).

Pierson et al. (2014) noted, in their publication regarding results of a similar and overlapping study, that among physicians who were asked to sign competency permits, 79% agreed to certify competency, although 47% did not feel comfortable assessing mental capability to carry concealed weapons. Fifty-nine percent reported concerns that refusing to sign a competency certificate would cause problems in the doctor-patient relationship. Notably, "physicians' beliefs about their capability to assess the physical competence of patients to carry concealed weapons were not significantly related to their actual signing of those permits" (Pierson et al. 2014, p. 2453).

Goldstein et al. (2015) indicated that continued physician involvement in issues of competence to carry a firearm (in this case a concealed weapon) requires action to "improve physician comfort with the process" (p. 244). They noted that recent research has "reinforce[d] the need for clinicians and provider professional organizations to develop continuing medical education about state and federal laws, firearm safety counseling, and data collection related to these processes" (p. 244). They also emphasized the need for research to determine factors that affect competency to carry a concealed weapon in order to develop effective guidelines for such evaluations.

Goldstein et al. (2013) observed that in the absence of training or comprehensive standards, "physicians may choose whether to sign off on such permits guided as much by their own views about gun ownership as by any standard" (p. 2252). Candilis et al. (2015) raised similar concerns regarding firearms and mental health evaluations:

> It is not difficult to imagine that those with a certain political outlook will be more willing to minimize dangerousness and craft evaluations that allow patients to retain their weapons, while those with a different politics will be more hesitant to allow gun ownership. (p. 2252)

Goldstein et al. (2015) did in fact find that the only consistent predictor for physicians' beliefs regarding competency to carry a concealed weapon was physician male gender and personal ownership of a gun. This finding and the others reviewed in this section support the general observation that in the absence of guidelines, standards, and training, many physicians' opinions, including those of mental health professionals, may be influenced more by personal or political values or the desire to avoid disrupting the patient-physician relationship than by an understanding of the increased risks of suicide or homicide conferred by access to a firearm.

The concerns expressed by Goldstein et al. (2013, 2015) and supported by Pierson et al. (2014) are timely and valid. The need for appropriate physician training and guidance is supported by the finding that in North Carolina over a 5-year period, despite a physician's endorsement of the ability to safely carry a concealed weapon, more than 2,400 concealed carry permit holders were convicted of crimes, including 900 drunk-driving offenses and 200 felonies (Webster et al. 2012). Many of the physicians surveyed recognized this need: 84% of physician respondents felt that medical assessments for competency to carry a concealed weapon should be performed by physicians specifically trained in making such assessments (Pierson et al. 2014).

RFD Mental Health Evaluations

Recommendations

Finding suitably trained and qualified professionals to conduct RFD evaluations is only one challenge facing courts and administrative agencies should they seek to include mental health evaluations as evidence. RFD hearings also present a significant policy challenge, created by the need to find a balance between personal and public safety and the right to possess firearms as mediated by a legal process for relief from mental health disabilities. Finding this balance requires development of "workable models of judicial authority informed by clinical expertise" (Swanson 2013, p. 1234).

Some general recommendations regarding the nature of the clinical expertise needed in RFD mental health evaluations have been offered. As discussed above, Rotenberg and Sadoff (1968) offered the earliest comments on this subject, stating that an evaluation of competency to possess firearms "serves as a consultation to the appropriate legal and administrative authority which makes the final determination," and that "on recovery from the condition rendering him incompetent, an individual should be reexamined before his gun is returned" (p. 842). Appelbaum et al. (2013) commented, "Whether, and when, to restore gun rights to a person with a mental disorder is an important determination that should be made in a separate proceeding informed by appropriate expert opinion about a person's recovery and the likelihood of relapse." As the American Psychiatric Association (2014) noted, "The process for restoring an individual's right to purchase or possess a firearm following a disqualification relating to mental disorder should be based on adequate clinical assessment, with decision-making responsibility ultimately resting with an administrative authority or court" (p. 2).

The Consortium for Risk-Based Firearm Policy, a multidisciplinary group of legal, medical, mental health, and public health professionals, has offered specific recommendations outlining what it considers to be the minimum requirements for mental health RFD evaluations and their evidentiary role in RFD hearings. This group has proposed model language for state (Consortium for Risk-Based Firearm Policy 2013b) and federal (Consortium for Risk-Based Firearm Policy 2013a) restoration statutes based on the need to balance the interests of the individual and those of public safety. Notably, the Sandy Hook Advisory Commission in its final report cited and agreed with the Consortium's recommendations regarding mental health evaluations and legal process in restoration of gun rights (Sandy Hook Advisory Commission 2015, p. 70).

The Consortium's proposals were also derived from evidence-based analysis. For example, the consortium suggests a 1-year minimum waiting period after discharge from an involuntary commitment before a petition for relief can be filed, specifically to address the increased risk of suicide during the time period following an inpatient discharge (see, e.g., Bickley et al. 2013; Dougall et al. 2014). This waiting period offers clinicians the additional benefit of being able to assess the petitioner's clinical status over the previous year, including compliance with treatment and ability to maintain abstinence from substance abuse, if relevant, and subsequent legal or criminal history, if any.

The Consortium's model language suggests that state RFD statutes include a requirement for evaluation of the petitioner by a psychiatrist or licensed clinical psychologist with a doctoral degree. Records and information concerning the person's mental health and treatment history should accompany the mental health opinions. Information provided and reviewed should include adherence to recommended treatment, history of suicide and prior violence, history of use of firearms and other weapons, history of use of alcohol and other drugs, and history of criminal justice involvement.

After personal examination of the petitioner and review of the documentary evidence, the mental health examiner should be able to attest to the following (Consortium for Risk-Based Firearm Policy 2013b):

1. The petitioner no longer manifests the symptoms of mental disorder that necessitated the involuntary commitment or symptoms that otherwise significantly elevate the risk of harm to self or others.

2. The petitioner appears to have adhered consistently to recommended treatment, if any, for a substantial period of time preceding the filing of the petition and intends to continue treatment, if necessary.
3. If ongoing treatment is necessary, adherence to treatment is likely to minimize the risk that the petitioner will relapse so as to present a danger to self or others in the foreseeable future.

States should be statutorily allowed to request an independent clinical evaluation even if the applicant provides this mental health documentation.

The Consortium emphasizes that a court or other administrative authority should make the ultimate determination of whether or not to grant the petition for relief after considering the mental health evidence as well as other evidence. The Consortium suggests that the judicial or administrative findings for granting relief mirror the three professional mental health findings listed above. In addition, as per the NIAA, the court or administrative agency should also find that "granting the relief would be compatible with the public interest" (Consortium for Risk-Based Firearm Policy 2013b, p. 13).

A Model for RFD Evaluations

General Principles

Consistent with recommendations from the Consortium for Risk-Based Firearm Policy (2013b) and the American Psychiatric Association (2014), we recommend that RFD proceedings routinely include as evidence review of mental health evaluations, including suicide and violence risk assessments. These evaluations should encompass best practices in forensic and clinical mental health evaluation and risk assessment, with a focus on risk factors associated with access to firearms.

The best available methodology for violence risk assessment (Buchanan et al. 2012; Conroy and Murrie 2007; Heilbrun 2009) (also see Chapter 9, "Structured Violence Risk Assessment") as well as suicide risk assessment (Silverman 2014; Simon 2012) (see also Chapter 10, "Decreasing Suicide Mortality") is widely considered to be the use of clinical judgment structured by risk assessment tools. In the absence of data providing direct support for a risk assessment approach relative to restoring firearm rights, adapting best practices as a first step to structuring a new type of evaluation seems most reasonable. In addition, many of the risk factors evaluated in violence and suicide risk assessments overlap with considerations of risk of harm to self or others if access to a firearm is restored. Fisher et al.'s (2015) description of the RFD evaluations conducted in New York State is an instructive example of the utilization of this approach.

In addition, we recommend that mental health evaluators be court-appointed independent psychiatrists or psychologists who have appropriate training in conducting risk assessments. The use of court-appointed independent evaluators offers multiple advantages. Independent mental health evaluators are not subject to the dual agency pressures and conflicts that arise when patients ask their treating clinicians to provide documentation for restoration of firearms. Courts would also be able to maintain qualification standards, ensuring that evaluators have the requisite expertise to perform the evaluations. Finally, as we discuss below (see "Liability Issues in Relief From Disability Evaluations"), court-appointed mental health professionals are generally protected from lawsuits by quasi-judicial immunity, even if not explicitly so protected by state statutes.

In jurisdictions where access to qualified mental health professionals is limited, we recommend that a treating clinician offering opinions regarding restoration of firearms for a patient be required to meet the Consortium's minimum standards for conducting an RFD evaluation. These include a review of specific documentary evidence, a personal evaluation, and formulation of the relevant mental health opinions. If the mental health evidence provided by the petitioner does not meet these minimum requirements, courts or administrative agencies should attempt to obtain an independent forensic mental health evaluation.

We also support the recommendations of the Consortium for Risk-Based Firearm Policy (2013b) and the American Psychiatric Association (2014) that a court or administrative agency make the ultimate determination of whether or not to restore firearm rights based on consideration of all relevant evidence. This determination should include and rely on, but not be limited to, the mental health evidence presented. The court or administrative agency may have to consider a variety of issues in addition to the petitioner's mental health in attempting to balance an individual's firearm rights against public safety concerns, which include concerns regarding suicide.

Structuring the RFD Evaluation

Heilbrun (2009) identified 10 principles underlying "best practices" in violence risk assessment when evaluating the functional legal capacities in question in a forensic evaluation. These can be adapted to include overlapping best practices in suicide risk assessment. This adaptation results in eight principles relevant to risk assessment in regard to restoration of firearm rights and that can be utilized to structure clinical RFD evaluations (Table 13–2).

1. Identification of the task. Mental health risk assessments in RFD evaluations should provide the court with information and opinions regarding the petitioner's current mental state, level of risk of suicide or violence toward others should firearm rights be restored, and the nexus between these opinions. As in assessments of other types of competencies, this task is best approached by focusing on the petitioner's functional capacities rather than a specific diagnosis or the ultimate legal question of whether the petitioner should or should not

TABLE 13–2. Principles of risk assessment in relief from disability evaluations

Principles of risk assessment	Implications for relief from disability evaluations
1. Identification of the task	Advise court of level of risk associated with access to firearms and interventions that may increase or decrease level of risk.
2. Specification of context	Remind court that petitioners live in their communities.
3. Specification of outcome	Advise court that primary consideration is suicide; violence toward others is also possible, although generally less likely.
4. Identification of the population	Identify specific basis of firearm prohibition. This population will typically be individuals with a history of involuntary psychiatric commitment. The nexus between the circumstances of the involuntary commitment and firearms, if any, and the reason(s) why the individual is seeking to regain access to firearms should be clearly identified.
5. Identification of risk factors and protective factors	Describe both risk and protective factors for the petitioner, in particular in regard to firearms.
6. Individualization of assessment	Describe factors or circumstances unique to petitioner and their relevance to the question of risk of suicide or violence toward others if access to firearms is restored.
7. Formulation of risk assessment	Focus assessments on circumstances and history unique to petitioner as well as general associated risk and protective factors should access to firearms be restored. Utilize structured or semi-structured clinical judgment methodology to determine level of risk.
8. Communication of risk	Provide written report, using terms of relative risk (low, moderate, high); describing different levels of risk under different circumstances, if any, should access to firearms be restored; and suggesting length of time over which assessment is likely to be accurate.

Source. Adapted from Heilbrun 2009.

have firearm rights restored. In the event that a range of potential outcomes can be identified, evaluators should provide opinions regarding these different outcomes and the circumstances associated with them (Heilbrun 2009).

Mental health professionals providing RFD evaluations in states where statutes require responses to specific questions will have to include these in their opinions. In these cases, if the legal question posed does not translate clearly into a mental health concept, we recommend that evaluators clarify the nature of their opinions when providing a response. For example, Delaware's RFD statutes require "certification" that the petitioner "is no longer suffering from a mental disorder which interferes with or handicaps the person from handling deadly weapons" (DE ST 11 § 1448A). This question assumes that an evaluator can provide a straightforward yes-or-no answer, and the evaluator's response may need to be parsed to provide reasonable opinions.

State statutes often require that medical or mental health evidence address the question of "dangerousness" (see Fisher et al. 2015). Hawaii, for example, requires "medical documentation that the petitioner is no longer adversely affected by the condition that resulted in the petitioner's adjudication or commitment and is not likely to act in a manner dangerous to public safety" (HI ST § 134-6.5). A comprehensive mental health evaluation can address the first part of the evidentiary requirement with a psychiatric opinion. In contrast, broader considerations regarding public safety are not properly mental health questions, and a psychiatric risk assessment may not provide a satisfactory answer.

In these cases, evaluators should provide all the necessary supporting information using a risk assessment model. They should then note the distinction between the advisory role of the evaluator and the decision-making authority of the court before opining on whether restoration of firearms is "contrary to the public interest" and does or does not "present a danger to public safety." This resolution offers several advantages, including acknowledgment of the limits of the use of risk assessment methods and the clear delineation between medical opinions, legal opinions, and the court or administrative agency's decision-making authority.

2. Specification of context. RFD petitioners presumably are living independently in their communities, alone or with others. Therefore, situational factors relevant to access to firearms should be considered, such as plans for safe storage of firearms in the event of a crisis or whether domestic conflict is an issue. Routine firearm safety practices and storage should also be considered. For example, an individual with cognitive impairments who may not remember to keep firearms safely stored but who lives with small children might unintentionally pose an increased risk of harm to others.

3. Specification of outcome. Clinicians should assume that the outcome of restoring access to firearms could be death or serious injury to the petitioner or others. Heilbrun (2009) suggests that evaluators estimate the base rate of outcomes of the decision as part of risk assessment. No data are yet available that inform the incidence of firearm suicide or violence toward others after restoration of firearm rights. As RFD proceedings become increasingly common, hopefully such studies will be undertaken. That said, clinicians should be knowledgeable regarding the risk associated with access to firearms by individuals with or without mental illness. This knowledge includes the evidence discussed throughout this volume that access to or living in a home with firearms is an independent factor that increases the risk of suicide as well as injury or death of others in the home.

4. Identification of the population. Individuals undergoing RFD assessments typically have a history of involuntary civil commitment to psychiatric treatment. As discussed in Chapter 7, "Mental Illness, Dangerousness, and Involuntary Commitment," involuntary commitment generally requires a judicial finding that an individual is dangerous to self or others due to mental illness. Not all individuals who have been involuntarily committed will have had similar degrees of risk relative to firearms, and for many, meeting criteria for involuntary commitment will have had nothing to do with firearms. Thus, identifying mental illness and involuntary commitment only as the bases for firearms prohibition is not sufficient identification of the petitioner in an RFD evaluation.

In addition to having a history of mental illness and involuntary psychiatric commitment, RFD petitioners have self-selected as a population motivated to go through a legal or administrative process to regain firearms. These circumstances require that evaluators clearly identify the basis of the involuntary commitment beyond, for example, simply listing a psychiatric diagnosis. Evaluators should determine whether or not the petitioner has a history of a suicidal behavior, suicide attempts, or violence toward others and the role, if any, of firearms in these events. If evaluators have not already identified the reason(s) for a petitioner's interest in regaining legal access to firearms, they should do so as part of this step in the RFD evaluation. A petitioner's reason for wanting firearm rights restored might not be psychiatrically significant, but it might just as easily be a factor that increases risk for suicide or violence.

5. Identification of risk factors and protective factors. Review of "static" or fixed and "dynamic" or changing risk factors that increase or decrease risk of violence or suicide is a standard part of risk assessment. Use of structured or semi-structured clinical judgment methodology is recommended. Research has provided evidence that identifies a number of demographic, historical, and clinical factors associated with violence toward others (see Chapter 9, "Structured Violence Risk Assessment") and with suicide (see Chapter 10, "Decreasing Suicide Mortality"), as well as factors that mitigate those risks. In many cases, research has been able to identify the strength or weakness of various factors' association with suicide or violence. For example, the risk of suicide or violence is significantly increased in individuals with a history of mental illness, a history of substance use, suicidal or violent behavior, and access to firearms.

The index of suspicion, particularly in regard to suicide, should be relatively high in firearm restoration evaluations, due to the lethality of firearms and the increased risk of suicide associated with access to firearms. In addition, a considerable proportion of petitioners will have at least two significant risk factors for suicide—a history of mental illness and a history of suicidal ideation or attempts; the combination of these circumstances is often the precipitant for involuntary commitment. Data regarding access to weapons and history of use of weapons are important to include in suicide risk assessments.

A smaller proportion of RFD petitioners have a history of mental illness and violence toward others that resulted in involuntary commitment. Although mental illness is only weakly linked to violence, a history of violent behavior is strongly associated with risk of future violence. A review of criminal history, if any, both prior to commitment and since discharge, and particularly whether weapons were used in the perpetration of violent crime, is essential, as these may identify risk factors more strongly associated with potential future violence toward others.

Protective factors that mitigate risk of suicide or violence toward others should also be explored in detail. For example, a history of treatment compliance, abstinence from substance use, and strong social connections are all factors that can mitigate the risk of violence or suicide, even if serious mental illness is present. Use of structured professional judgment methodology for violence risk assessment and suicide risk assessment ensures that relevant risk factors are reviewed, allowing evaluators to assess these factors both on the basis of the evidence relating to increase or decrease risk and their own clinical experience and judgment.

6. Individualization of assessment. All petitioners will have a set of unique circumstances associated with their past history, current mental status, and functioning. RFD risk assessments should not be based on generalizations associated with any specific psychiatric diagnosis, any single risk factor, or any single protective factor. Evidence-based risk factors should be assessed in the context of each person's specific social, family, and employment circumstances in order for evaluators to assess overall level of risk.

7. Formulation of risk assessment. Evaluators should use as many sources of information as indicated in addition to the structured or semi-structured clinical judgment methodology to identify risk and mitigating factors and determine level of risk. Use of multiple sources of information will assist in focusing assessments on circumstances and history unique to petitioner as well as the evidence-based general data associated empirically identified risk and protective factors should access to firearms be restored. We recommend that RFD mental health evaluators be certain to review of relevant records and additional collateral information, if necessary. All these sources of data, in addition to the clinical interview, will form the bases of evaluators' opinions.

Review of records. Records reviewed should include the petitioner's other inpatient and outpatient mental health and treatment history, substance use history, and criminal records. Many of the historical or clinical issues relevant to the RFD proceedings, such as the circumstances resulting in involuntary commitment, adherence to recommended treatment, clinical course since discharge, and involvement with the criminal justice system, can be obtained from review of these records.

As discussed above, the records of and circumstances around the involuntary commitment that precipitated the mental health prohibition also should be reviewed specifically in regard to the nexus between the involuntary commitment and access to firearms and the current presence or absence of risk factors associated with the involuntary commitment. In cases where cognitive impairment is suspected, review of medical records may also be necessary. Narrative letters or statements from treatment providers should also be reviewed if provided, but these alone do not constitute sufficient evidence upon which to base opinions.

Collateral information. If evaluators still have questions regarding elements of the petitioner's history essential or relevant to a risk assessment for firearm restoration, they should if possible obtain information from collateral sources. Evaluators may also wish to contact third parties to verify information provided by the petitioner or to determine a family member's or friend's level of comfort with restoration of firearm rights to the petitioner. Individuals who may have important and relevant information include treating mental and medical health providers, spouses or life partners, parents, siblings, and concerned others, such as friends or clergy. If any of these individuals voice concerns regarding the petitioner regaining access to firearms, these should be taken very seriously, and the petitioner should be questioned directly about these concerns.

Evaluators should obtain consent for contacting third parties from petitioners. In some jurisdictions, it may be possible for the court or administrative agency to issue an order allowing such contact. Nevertheless, if petitioners refuse to give consent, this should be noted in the evaluation and considered as a factor that potentially indicates increased risk.

Clinical evaluation. After a review of records, evaluators should conduct a standard clinical forensic psychiatric evaluation (see Glancy et al. 2015). The clinical interview should address the questions listed in Table 13–3. Determining why the petitioner is seeking to have firearm rights restored at this time is one of the most important considerations in the RFD evaluation. Evaluators should assess the petitioner's current mental status and whether the petitioner demonstrates clinical evidence of ongoing or active symptoms of mental illness. Clinicians should also determine whether the symptoms associated with the past suicidal or violent behavior, if any, have been addressed through mental health and non–mental health interventions. Adequate control of symptoms may be evident in changes in the petitioner's functioning over time (Fisher et al. 2015), such as the ability to maintain employment or stable relationships.

Regardless of petitioners' psychiatric diagnosis, issues related to their judgment, impulsivity, and irritability, as well as anger management and other emotional coping skills, are highly significant in a risk assessment in which the outcome will be regaining access to firearms. Circumstances that impair judgment and increase impulsivity, when combined with access to a firearm, increase the risk of suicide and violence toward others. Circumstances that indicate good emotional coping skills, including the ability to seek help when needed, high frustration tolerance, and unimpaired insight and judgment, decrease risks of harm associated with access to a firearm. Continued legal problems due to substance use or violent behavior may indicate increased future risk of violence or suicide if access to firearms is restored.

As is common in some forensic examinations, individuals petitioning for restoration of firearm rights may be inclined to minimize problematic behaviors, past history, or current symptoms. Therefore, an assessment of a petitioner's understanding of past suicidal or violent behavior is crucial (Fisher et al. 2015). This requires discussion of the events that precipitated the firearm prohibition and the role, if any, that firearms played. Does the petitioner believe he or she presented a risk of firearm violence to self or others? If so, what has decreased this risk (other than loss of legal access to firearms)?

The petitioner's level of insight and understanding may be indicated by comparing his or her account of events with the accounts contained in the records or accounts obtained from third parties. Lack of congruence between records or third-party accounts and a petitioner's self-report can indicate lack of insight, which might increase risk for both suicide and violence toward others. Alternatively, an incongruent account may indicate an attempt at manipulation, which again should raise suspicions regarding the reasons the individual wants firearm rights restored.

If a petitioner is able to verbalize an understanding that reflects reasonable insight and judgment, as corroborated by the records, third-party accounts, and the petitioner's presentation, evaluators should determine the concrete steps taken, if any, to mitigate risk factors. For example, evidence of decrease in depressive symptoms due to ongoing treatment may mitigate future risk of suicide. Evaluators should also confirm the petitioner's report of mitigating interven-

TABLE 13–3. Relief from disability mental health evaluation

1. Why is the petitioner seeking restoration of firearm rights at this time?
2. What was the nature of the event that resulted in a mental health firearm prohibition?
   a. Were firearms involved? If so, how?
   b. Were any other weapons involved?
   c. Was substance use involved?
3. Did the event that resulted in the prohibition also result in increased risk of suicide or violence toward others?
   a. Were firearms involved? If so, how?
   b. Were any other weapons involved?
   c. Was substance use involved?
4. What psychosocial factors, if any, contributed to the prohibiting event? Have these been mitigated through non–mental health interventions?
5. Was the precipitating event related to a mental health disorder?
   a. What were the symptoms?
   b. What was (or is) the diagnosis?
6. Was this event unique or did it represent one episode in a pattern of behavior that indicates heightened risk of suicide or violence?
7. Was treatment recommended, and if so, is ongoing adherence to treatment necessary to
   a. reduce the risk of relapse?
   b. reduce the risk of suicide or violence?
8. Has the petitioner consistently adhered to treatment, if recommended, for the time period between the prohibiting event and filing of the petition?
   a. If so, what factors have supported treatment compliance?
   b. If not, what factors have contributed to treatment noncompliance?
9. Does the petitioner intend to continue treatment if recommended?
10. If applicable, has the petitioner adhered to recommended treatment in the past, prior to the event precipitating firearm prohibition?
11. Does the petitioner currently have active symptoms of the mental disorder? Describe current symptoms.
    a. Has the petitioner had periods of abstinence?
    b. What factors or circumstances have supported ability to abstain from substance use?
    c. What factors or circumstances have contributed to relapses?

TABLE 13–3. Relief from disability mental health evaluation *(continued)*

12. Does the petitioner currently have any symptoms that elevate the risk of harm to self or others?
13. Has the petitioner had any involvement with the criminal justice system since the event that precipitated the firearm prohibition? If so, did this involve
    a. violent behavior?
    b. substance use?
    c. use of a weapon of any kind?
14. Is the petitioner's level of risk likely to increase or decrease in the foreseeable future
    a. due to mental health factors?
    b. due to psychosocial circumstances?
    c. due to substance use?
    d. due to treatment adherence or nonadherence?
15. Will access to firearms increase or decrease the current level of risk to self or others due to mental illness under reasonably foreseeable future circumstances (possibly based on evaluation of established past patterns of behavior and coping skills)?
16. What factors, other than mental illness or access to firearms, may increase or decrease current level of risk to self or others?

Source. Adapted in part from Consortium for Risk-Based Firearm Policy 2013a and 2013b.

tions by comparing the petitioner's account with documentary evidence and with third parties, if necessary.

Finally, RFD evaluations should be certain to adhere to standard professional ethics (American Academy of Psychiatry and the Law 2005; American Psychological Association 2013). Evaluators should do the following:

1. Advise evaluees of the limits of confidentiality, while respecting confidentiality when possible.
2. Be aware of relevant literature.
3. Conduct an appropriately thorough assessment, gathering all available relevant information.
4. Approach risk assessment with objectivity and honesty.
5. Maintain an appropriate degree of modesty regarding the level of accuracy that can be reasonably expected of assessments of violence and suicide risk. (Buchanan et al. 2012; Glancy et al. 2015)

8. Communication of risk. The written RFD report is the primary method of communication of risk and should reflect best practices (see, e.g., Buchanan and Norko 2011). Reports should include the opinions discussed above and the bases of opinions—that is, the relevant data obtained from medical and legal records; clinical evaluation, risk assessment, and mental status examination; and corroborating third-party information when relevant. The evaluators should tailor the opinions as narrowly as possible, bearing in mind that the purpose of the evaluation is to establish the nexus, if any, between past and present psychiatric status and risk if access to firearms is restored.

Level of risk of harm to self or others if firearm access is restored should be communicated using relative terms, such as *low, moderate,* and *high,* and should include an estimate of how long this assessment is likely to be reasonably accurate. In addition, combinations of circumstances and risk factors that would result in changes in or different levels of risk should be described. Examiners should indicate if they are lacking enough information to come to opinions regarding current levels of risk and should specify what additional information might allow formulation of reasonable opinions. If offering opinions that address the ultimate issue, such as dangerousness or public safety, evaluators should clearly distinguish between the evaluator's advisory role and the court's or administrative agency's authority to make the final determination.

Ethical Concerns in Relief From Disability Evaluations

Candilis et al. (2015) observed that psychiatrists are increasingly serving as "gatekeepers of gun ownership." The absence of guidelines for RFD evaluations, the gaps in mental health training in suicide and violence risk assessment, and the lack of research data upon which to base RFD evaluations and assess their validity have been discussed. Ethical issues have been presented regarding the role of mental health professionals in firearm-related evaluations and whether courts should routinely consider requiring mental health evidence in RFD hearings.

Regardless of the absence of data specifically addressing the functional abilities associated with competency to safely possess and use firearms, mental health professionals are already providing RFD evaluations for courts and administrative agencies (Britton and Bloom 2015; Fisher et al. 2015; Simpson 2007b). Legislation that implies or requires a need for mental health evaluations or documentation for a specific legal issue, as do the increasing number of state RFD programs, inevitably leads courts and patients to request such evaluations and documentation. Thus, developing best practices, standards for evaluation, and professional guidelines for RFD evaluations, and indeed for all types of clinical and forensic firearm-related evaluations, will hopefully provide guidance to those professionals already conducting RFD evaluations. In addition, providing a model for evaluation can facilitate clinical training and increase the number of mental health professionals qualified to perform these evaluations.

Although ethical practice requires careful delineation of the current limits of the knowledge base, it also requires effective use of scientific reasoning as new areas of application present themselves (Buchanan et al. 2012; Heilbrun 2009; Tolman and Rotzien 2007). As RFD hearings continue to increase in frequency, the need for data on which to structure such evaluations can lead to collaborative mental health and legal research to assess outcomes and establish standards that can be used in mental health training programs. Data that would be helpful include

- Results from studies of the implementation of firearm restoration processes in different states
- Outcomes of hearings with and without mental health evidence
- Results from studies of the incidence of firearm violence or suicide following either judicial denial or restoration of firearm rights
- Identification of the most relevant risk factors in relation to outcomes
- Types of mental health evidence presented and their relative weight in the hearings

Such data would also help address the ethical problems that arise due to the influence of personal and political biases. The combination of a small evidence base and the lack of legal, psychiatric, or psychological guidance on a politically charged and socially divisive mental health evaluation, such as evaluation for restoration of firearm rights, can result in the increased influence of an evaluator's political and social opinions on the evaluation's conclusions (Simpson 2007a). Unstructured and uninformed assessments are particularly vulnerable to the influence of such biases (Heilbrun 2009).

More structured clinical risk assessment allows both increased specificity and decreased reliance on one's own values (Heilbrun 2009). Almost all risk factors for violence and suicide are affected by factors other than mental illness, including culture, age, gender, and others (Lim and Bell 2008; Skeem et al. 2005). Clinicians have a responsibility not to stereotype patients with higher or lower levels of risk when the data do not support that linkage (Lim and Bell 2008). Use of even preliminary standards or guidelines that help structure evaluations can help reduce the influence of evaluators' personal values on their professional opinions.

RFD evaluations and hearings also offer an opportunity to educate courts and the public regarding suicide, access to firearms, and the relationship between mental illness and firearm violence. The role of the risk evaluator as a neutral party and educator for courts on risk issues has been characterized as one of the defining characteristics of forensic clinicians (Tolman and Rotzien 2007). RFD statutes and other firearm regulations related to mental illness focus on the relatively small risk those with mental illness pose to public safety and tend to ignore the more common occurrence and higher risk of firearm suicide. As Swanson (2013) observed, a rule that denies a firearm to a formerly involuntarily committed patient who had threatened another's life but that does not deny a firearm to a similar patient who had threatened his or her own life "is a rule that lacks reason and fairness" (p. 134).

Most RFD statutes reflect institutional stigmatization of individuals with mental illness, in that they are based on negative stereotypes regarding the danger to others posed by individuals with mental illness. RFD risk assessments offer an opportunity to help the courts avoid stigma-related errors of commission and omission (Simpson 2007a). Individuals who still pose a significant risk to themselves may have their rights restored because courts are less likely to consider risk of suicide; individuals who never posed a substantial risk to themselves or others may be denied their firearm rights based simply on stigmatizing and erroneous beliefs that those with a diagnosis of mental illness are inherently dangerous to others.

Liability Issues in Relief From Disability Evaluations

Independent medical evaluations of nonpatients generally represent a low liability risk, even when assessing "dangerousness." The low risk of professional liability is due largely to the fact that a treatment relationship does not exist between the evaluee and the examining clinician (Vanderpool 2011a, 2011b). RFD evaluations, as a type of independent medical evaluation, fall into this category of low-liability-risk forensic activity.

However, for RFD evaluations, as for other types of independent medical evaluations, liability risks increase if mental health professionals combine treatment and forensic roles and provide the assessments for their own patients (Vanderpool 2011a, 2011b). The ethical and practical conflicts of attempting to fulfill dual roles simultaneously (Strasburger et al. 1997) have already been noted in firearm-related assessments (Goldstein et al. 2013; Luo 2011; Pierson et al. 2014). Both increased liability and dual agency conflicts suggest that mental health professionals should, if possible, avoid occupying dual roles in RFD assessments. If patients request RFD or other firearm-related evaluations or documentation, treating clinicians should consider referral to or consultation with a forensic clinician.

Ideally, all RFD evaluations would be conducted by court-appointed independent mental health professionals (Consortium for Risk-Based Firearm Policy 2013b). In addition to the advantages previously discussed in this chapter, court-appointed evaluators are protected from liability by quasi-judicial immunity (*LaLonda v. Eissner,* 405 Mass. 207, 539 N.E.2d 538, 1989). Even if quasi-judicial immunity is not provided, general witness immunity, under which RFD evaluators have immunity from lawsuits based on testimony or opinions in judicial proceedings, may be available. Alternatively, legislatures could explicitly provide immunity to professionals providing RFD evaluations. Currently, only Maryland specifically provides immunity for health care professionals providing opinions and certifications in restoration hearings (Maryland Code § 5-133.3).

That said, other significant issues relative to providing RFD evaluations beyond issues of liability and immunity have yet to be resolved. Being asked to provide medical or psychiatric opinions regarding the risk of restoring firearm rights to an individual with a history of mental illness and/or suicidal or violent behavior—an evaluation currently without specific training, guidelines, or standards—is likely to raise understandable anxiety in mental health professionals, even absent liability concerns. For example, Fisher et al. (2015) observe that although RFD evaluators are indemnified from damage claims in New York State, "they are not immune from other harms, such as adverse publicity or negative career impact" (p. 344). Concerns regarding negative publicity and damage to reputations are not misplaced, considering that suicide or homicide, although statistically rare events, are potential outcomes of RFD hearings. In a social climate in which a single bad outcome could be widely publicized, even forensically trained clinicians might be reluctant to perform RFD evaluations.

Conclusion

In 2007, Simpson called for the development of guidelines for RFD evaluations (Simpson 2007a). Unfortunately, little attention has been given to developing standards, guidelines, or training for firearm-related mental health evaluations in general and RFD evaluations in particular. Almost 10 years later, as noted by Fisher et al. (2015, p. 344), "[t]he evolution of procedures for restoration is still relatively young, and several years after the NICS Improvement Act, these procedures vary considerably." Nevertheless, on the basis of the scant evidence available, mental health professionals' evaluations and opinions, when requested, do influence judges' decisions in RFD proceedings (Luo 2011; Simpson 2007a).

Mental health clinicians should approach RFD evaluations with caution. Just as suspension of firearm rights based on mental health prohibitions has not decreased the incidence of mass shootings, restoring firearm rights to individuals with such prohibitions is not likely to result in more mass shootings or even a statistically significant increase in firearm violence toward others. The greater concern is that those who petition to have firearm rights restored are much more likely to have histories of suicidal ideation or suicide attempts and to be at increased risk to themselves. Individuals with serious mental illness much more commonly use firearms to commit suicide than to commit violence against others.

Until more specific data regarding relevant risk factors for and outcomes of RFD hearings become available, mental health professionals who perform RFD evaluations should use best practices in suicide and violence risk assessment, while making clear that collective data are not available. Evaluations and reports should be designed to provide the court with information regarding what an individual's risk factors are in regard to suicide and violence and how access to firearms increases or decreases risk. Courts' decisions to restore firearm rights should be based on individualized assessment of risk factors rather than on stereotypes regarding individuals with mental illness and political beliefs and bias regarding regulation of firearms.

Suggested Interventions

- State statutes should require independent psychiatric or psychological evaluations of RFD petitioners, similar to those of Oregon, and should specify that these evaluations include violence and suicide risk assessment. Absent such statutes, courts and administrative agencies that hear RFD petitions should consider adopting policies requiring mental health risk assessments as part of the evidence to be considered in RFD hearings.
- Postgraduate training programs and professional organizations should work toward developing standards for teaching and training in suicide and violence risk assessment, and institute formal instruction based on these standards.
- Postgraduate training programs and professional organizations should develop standardized and systematic training in risk assessments involving civilians and firearms, because requests for firearm-related mental health evaluations, including RFD evaluations, continue to increase.
- As RFD hearings and evaluations become more common, research should be undertaken to study outcomes in regard to suicide and violence and to identify relevant risk and protective factors specific to restoration of firearm rights after a mental health–based prohibition.

References

Accreditation Council for Graduate Medical Education: ACGME Program Requirements for Graduate Medical Education in Psychiatry. Chicago, IL, Accreditation Council for Graduate Medical Education, 2014. Available at: http://www.acgme.org/acgmeweb/Portals/0/PFAssets/ProgramRequirements/400_psychiatry_07012014.pdf. Accessed August 22, 2015.

American Academy of Psychiatry and the Law: Ethics Guidelines for the Practice of Forensic Psychiatry. Bloomfield, CT, American Academy of Psychiatry and the Law, May 2005. Available at: http://aapl.org/ethics.htm. Accessed January 15, 2014.

American Psychiatric Association: Position Statement on Firearm Access, Acts of Violence, and the Relationship to Mental Illness and Mental Health Services. Arlington, VA, American Psychiatric Association, 2014. Available at: http://www.psychiatry.org/File%20Library/Learn/Archives/Position-2014-Firearm-Access.pdf. Accessed January 9, 2015.

American Psychological Association: Specialty guidelines for forensic psychology. Am Psychol 68(1):7–19, 2013 23025747

Appelbaum PS, Bonnie RJ, Swanson JW: Don't arm people in a mental health crisis. The Hill (blog), June 13, 2013

Bickley H, Hunt IM, Windfuhr K, et al: Suicide within two weeks of discharge from psychiatric inpatient care: a case-control study. Psychiatr Serv 64(7):653–659, 2013 23545716

Britton J, Bloom JD: Oregon's gun relief program for adjudicated mentally ill persons: the Psychiatric Security Review Board. Behav Sci Law 33(2–3):323–333, 2015 25728522

Buchanan A: Risk of violence by psychiatric patients: beyond the "actuarial versus clinical" assessment debate. Psychiatr Serv 59(2):184–190, 2008 18245161

Buchanan A, Norko MA (eds): The Psychiatric Report. Cambridge, UK, Cambridge University Press, 2011

Buchanan A, Binder R, Norko M, et al: Resource document on psychiatric violence risk assessment. Am J Psychiatry 169(3 suppl):1–10, 2012

Candilis PJ, Khurana G, Leong GB, et al: Informed consent at gunpoint: when psychiatry affects gun ownership. Behav Sci Law 33(2–3):346–355, 2015 25640524

Conroy MA, Murrie DC: Forensic Assessment of Violence Risk: A Guide for Risk Assessment and Risk Management. New York, Wiley, 2007

Consortium for Risk-Based Firearm Policy: Guns, Public Health, and Mental Illness: An Evidence-Based Approach for Federal Policy. Baltimore, MD, Johns Hopkins Center for Gun Policy and Research, 2013a

Consortium for Risk-Based Firearm Policy. Guns, Public Health, and Mental Illness: An Evidence-Based Approach for State Policy. Baltimore, MD, Johns Hopkins Center for Gun Policy and Research, 2013b

Coverdale JH, Roberts LW, Balon R: The public health priority to address the accessibility and safety of firearms: recommendations for training. Acad Psychiatry 34(6):405–408, 2010 21041461

Cramer RJ, Johnson SM, McLaughlin J, et al: Suicide risk assessment training for psychology doctoral programs: core competencies and a framework for training. Train Educ Prof Psychol 7(1):1–11, 2013 24672588

Dougall N, Lambert P, Maxwell M, et al: Deaths by suicide and their relationship with general and psychiatric hospital discharge: 30-year record linkage study. Br J Psychiatry 204:267–273, 2014 24482439

Fisher CE, Cohen ZE, Hoge SK, et al: Restoration of firearm rights in New York. Behav Sci Law 33(2–3):334–345, 2015 25711715

Glancy GD, Ash P, Bath EP, et al: AAPL Practice Guideline for the Forensic Assessment. J Am Acad Psychiatry Law 43 (2 suppl):S3–S53, 2015 26054704

Goldstein AO, Barnhouse KK, Viera AJ, et al: Assessing competency for concealed-weapons permits—the physician's role. N Engl J Med 368(24):2251–2253, 2013 23593979

Goldstein AO, Viera AJ, Pierson J, et al: Physician beliefs about physical and mental competency of patients applying for concealed weapon permits. Behav Sci Law 33(2–3):238–245, 2015 25708569

Greene E, Bornstein BH, Dietrich H: Granny, (don't) get your gun: competency issues in gun ownership by older adults. Behav Sci Law 25(3):405–423, 2007 17559168

Heilbrun K: Evaluation for Risk of Violence in Adults (Best Practices in Forensic Mental Health Assessment). New York, Oxford University Press, 2009

Hickey JD: Gun prohibitions for people with mental illness—what should the policy be? Developments in Mental Health Law 32(3):1–12, 2013

Hung EK, Binder RL, Fordwood SR, et al: A method for evaluating competency in assessment and management of suicide risk. Acad Psychiatry 36(1):23–28, 2012 22362432

Jacobson JM, Osteen P, Jones A, et al: Evaluation of the recognizing and responding to suicide risk training. Suicide Life Threat Behav 42(5):471–485, 2012 22924960

Khubchandani J, Price JH, Dake JA: Firearm injury prevention training in preventive medicine residency programs. J Community Health 34(4):295–300, 2009 19326195

Lim KF, Bell CC: Cultural competence in violence risk assessment, in Textbook of Violence Assessment and Management. Edited by Simon RI, Tardiff K. Washington, DC, American Psychiatric Publishing, 2008, pp 35–57

Luo M: Some with histories of mental illness petition to get their rights back. New York Times, July 2, 2011. Available at: http:/www.nytimes.com/2011/07/03/us/03guns.html. Accessed August 22, 2015.

Luther R: Mental health and gun rights in Virginia: a view from the battlefield. N Engl J Crim Civ Confine 40:345–358, 2014

Mayors Against Illegal Guns: Fatal Gaps: How Missing Records in the Federal Background Check System Put Guns in the Hands of Killers. New York, Everytown for Gun Safety, 2011. Available at: http://3gbwir1ummda16xrhf4do9d21bsx.wpengine.netdna-cdn.com/wp-content/uploads/2014/04/Fatal-Gaps-Report.pdf. Accessed March 27, 2015.

McNiel DE, Chamberlain JR, Weaver CM, et al: Impact of clinical training on violence risk assessment. Am J Psychiatry 165(2):195–200, 2008 18245189

Melton BB, Coverdale JH: What do we teach psychiatric residents about suicide? A national survey of chief residents. Acad Psychiatry 33(1):47–50, 2009 19349444

Mertens B, Sorenson SB: Current considerations about the elderly and firearms. Am J Public Health 102(3):396–400, 2012 22390501

Monahan J: Structured risk assessment of violence, in Textbook of Violence Assessment and Management. Edited by Simon RI, Tardiff K. Washington, DC, American Psychiatric Publishing, 2008, pp 17–33

New York Office of Mental Health: Certification of Relief Request Pursuant to Mental Hygiene Law, Section 7.09(j) and Part 543 of Title 14 NYCRR. Albany, New York Office of Mental Health, 2012. Available at: https://www.omh.ny.gov/omhweb/nics/requirements.html. Accessed August 22, 2015.

Pierson J, Viera AJ, Barnhouse KK, et al: Physician attitudes and experience with permit applications for concealed weapons. N Engl J Med 370(25):2453–2454, 2014 24941197

Rotenberg LA, Sadoff RL: Who should have a gun? Some preliminary psychiatric thoughts. Am J Psychiatry 125(6):841–843, 1968 5698456

Sandy Hook Advisory Commission: Final Report of the Sandy Hook Advisory Commission. Hartford, CT, Sandy Hook Advisory Commission, 2015

Schmitz WM Jr, Allen MH, Feldman BN, et al: Preventing suicide through improved training in suicide risk assessment and care: an American Association of Suicidology Task Force report addressing serious gaps in U.S. mental health training. Suicide Life Threat Behav 42(3):292–304, 2012 22494118

Silverman MM: Suicide risk assessment and suicide risk formulation: essential components of the therapeutic risk management model. J Psychiatr Pract 20(5):373–378, 2014 25226200

Simon RI: Suicide risk assessment: gateway to treatment and management, in The American Psychiatric Publishing Textbook of Suicide Assessment and Management, 2nd Edition. Edited by Simon RI, Hales RE. Washington, DC, American Psychiatric Publishing, 2012, pp 3–28

Simon RI, Tardiff K: Preface, in Textbook of Violence Assessment and Management. Edited by Simon RI, Tardiff K. Washington, DC, American Psychiatric Publishing, 2008, xxi–xxii

Simpson JR: Bad risk? An overview of laws prohibiting possession of firearms by individuals with a history of treatment for mental illness. J Am Acad Psychiatry Law 35(3):330–338, 2007a 17872555

Simpson JR: Issues related to possession of firearms by individuals with mental illness: an overview using California as an example. J Psychiatr Pract 13(2):109–114, 2007b 17414687

Simpson JR, Sharma KK: Mental health weapons prohibition: demographic and psychiatric factors in petitions for relief. J Forensic Sci 53(4):971–974, 2008 18503522

Skeem J, Schubert C, Stowman S, et al: Gender and risk assessment accuracy: underestimating women's violence potential. Law Hum Behav 29(2):173–186, 2005 15912722

Strasburger LH, Gutheil TG, Brodsky A: On wearing two hats: role conflict in serving as both psychotherapist and expert witness. Am J Psychiatry 154(4):448–456, 1997 9090330

Swanson J: Mental illness and new gun law reforms: the promise and peril of crisis-driven policy. JAMA 309(12):1233–1234, 2013 23392291

Teo AR, Holley SR, Leary M, et al: The relationship between level of training and accuracy of violence risk assessment. Psychiatr Serv 63(11):1089–1094, 2012 22948947

Tolman AO: Clinical training and the duty to protect. Behav Sci Law 19(3):387–404, 2001 11443699

Tolman A, Mullendore K: Risk evaluations for the courts: is service quality a function of specialization? Prof Psychol Res Pr 34(3):225–232, 2003

Tolman AO, Rotzien AL: Conducting risk evaluations for future violence: ethical practice is possible. Prof Psychol Res Pr 38(1):71–79, 2007

U.S. Department of Justice, Bureau of Alcohol, Tobacco, Firearms and Explosives: Certification of Qualifying State Relief From Disabilities Program, OMB No. 1140-0094. Washington, DC, U.S. Department of Justice, January 2013. Available at: https://www.atf.gov/files/forms/download/atf-f-3210-12.pdf. Accessed December 20, 2014.

U.S. Office of Justice Programs: Bureau of Justice Statistics: State Profiles. Washington, DC, Bureau of Justice Statistics, 2014. Available at: http://www.bjs.gov/index.cfm?ty=tp&tid=491. Accessed December 20, 2014.

Vanderpool DL: Legal and ethical issues in providing mental health disability evaluations, in Clinical Guide to Mental Disability Evaluations. Edited by Gold LH, Vanderpool DL. New York, Springer Science + Business Media, 2011a, pp 37–74

Vanderpool DL: Risks of harm to the forensic expert: the legal perspective, in Ethical Issues in Forensic Psychiatry: Minimizing Harm. Edited by Sadoff RL, Baird JA, Bertoglia SM, et al. London, Wiley-Blackwell, 2011b, pp 198–211

Webster DW, Vernick JS, McGinty EE, et al: The Case for Gun Policy Reforms in America. Baltimore, MD, Johns Hopkins Bloomberg School of Public Health, 2012

Wong L, Morgan A, Wilkie T, et al: Quality of resident violence risk assessments in psychiatric emergency settings. Can J Psychiatry 57(6):375–380, 2012 22682575

Wortzel HS, Matarazzo B, Homaifar B: A model for therapeutic risk management of the suicidal patient. J Psychiatr Pract 19(4):323–326, 2013 23852108

14

Decreasing Gun Violence

Social and Public Health Interventions

Shannon Frattaroli, Ph.D., M.P.H.
Shani A. L. Buggs, M.P.H.

Common Misperceptions

- ☒ Teaching children to be safe around guns effectively prevents unintentional gun deaths among children.
- ☒ Guns are inherently dangerous, and efforts to make guns safer will not reduce the number of gun deaths and injuries.
- ☒ With so many guns in civilian hands, interventions to control access to people identified as dangerous are futile.
- ☒ Only law-abiding citizens are affected by gun policies because criminals do not abide by gun laws.
- ☒ Gun policy is so polarizing that any effort to make changes at the policy level is futile.

Evidence-Based Facts

- ☑ Although teaching children how to be safe around guns may seem like a commonsense strategy to reduce unintentional gun deaths among children, evidence suggests that such efforts are unlikely to accomplish that goal without intensive intervention, including the use of multiple skill-based training sessions in which children practice gun avoidance in real-life settings. Whether the effects of such training are maintained over the span of childhood is unknown.
- ☑ Gun design matters, and embracing innovation and technology with the potential to reduce the gun injuries and deaths that occur as a result of unauthorized access to guns is one way forward in the ongoing discussion about strategies to reduce the current toll of gun-related morbidity and mortality. Changing the characteristics of the injury-causing consumer product builds on a long line of successful consumer product–focused interventions in the field of injury prevention, including motor vehicles (seat belts and airbags), prescription medications (child-resistant bottles), children's sleepwear (flame-resistant standards), and toys (warnings about a choking hazard).
- ☑ Laws designed to prevent people at high risk of committing gun violence from legally purchasing guns can affect their access to guns and are associated with reductions in gun violence where these laws are in place.
- ☑ Although it is true that law-abiding people will comply with the law, people who commit crimes are also affected by policies that govern gun purchases and possession. This is evidenced by evaluations of laws that require a permit to purchase guns and prohibit the purchase and possession of guns by violent misdemeanants and respondents to domestic violence restraining orders.
- ☑ Polling data suggest that when the dialogue about gun policy moves beyond broad statements to specific policies, broad support exists for many gun violence prevention policies.

The national dialogue about guns is informed by different beliefs. Public debate about important issues such as the role of guns in society is essential to democracy. Beliefs about guns and gun policy may be influenced by experiences and knowledge about the risks and benefits associated with guns in civil society. New knowledge, rooted in evidence provided by research, has the potential to alter beliefs commonly held by individuals and shared by larger communities.

In this chapter, we review some common beliefs about gun violence prevention strategies in the context of available evidence, as well as ways to reduce gun violence that have proven effective for other public health problems.

A Public Health Approach

We use the five common misperceptions that introduce this chapter as the building blocks for our discussion. A public health approach serves as the foundation for the discussion. This approach consists of defining the problem, identifying risk and protective factors, developing and evaluating preventive interventions, and implementing effective policies and programs (Violence Prevention Alliance 2014). One core aspect of a public health approach to gun violence is the definition of the problem. A public health perspective encompasses all gun injuries in defining the scope of the problem. Gun assaults and homicides are part of a public health definition of gun violence. Self-harm injuries that too often result in completed suicide are also included in the definition, as are unintentional gun injuries that occur when, for instance, a child finds a gun and unintentionally shoots a playmate.

This definition of gun violence reveals a problem much larger than its individual parts but also may lead to solutions that are responsive to particular types of gun injuries that fall within this definition. The prominence of firearm suicide, which makes up about 60% of all gun deaths in the United States (62% in 2012) and 51% of all suicides, is striking (Centers for Disease Control and Prevention 2012a). As discussed in multiple chapters of this book, the link between mental illness and violence is strongest and most relevant to intervention strategies relating to suicide (not assault or homicide).

Further examination of the epidemiology of gun suicide highlights the high case fatality rate associated with suicide attempts using guns in comparison to all other means. In 2012, for every five people who killed themselves with a gun, roughly one person survived an attempt (case fatality rate, 83%) (Table 14–1). In contrast, for every one person who committed suicide by a means other than guns, 24 people survived (case fatality rate, 4%) (Centers for Disease Control and Prevention 2012b). Similarly, the case fatality rate for gun assaults, although lower than that for gun suicide attempts, is higher than that for assaults by all other means. Seventeen percent of gun assaults result in fatalities, compared with a fatality rate of less than 1% in non-gun assaults (Centers for Disease Control and Prevention 2012a). More people survive unintentionally inflicted gunshot injuries than injuries resulting from intentional shootings; however, when compared with all other types of unintentional injuries, the lethality of gun-related injuries is high.

The lethal nature of guns, as reflected in the high case fatality rate of gun injuries, brings to light a second characteristic of a public health approach to gun

TABLE 14–1. Case fatality rates by injury type in the United States, 2012

	Intentional—suicide			Intentional—homicide			Unintentional		
	Gun	Non-gun	Total	Gun	Non-gun	Total	Gun	Non-gun	Total
Deaths	20,666	19,934	40,600	12,093	5,145	17,238	548	127,244	127,792
Attempts	4,086	479,510	483,596	59,948	1,761,991	1,821,939	17,362	29,420,131	29,437,493
Case fatality rate	83%	4%	8%	17%	<1%	1%	3%	<1%	<1%

Source. Centers for Disease Control and Prevention 2012a.

violence: the emphasis on prevention. Primary prevention strategies, which are intended to be used to intervene before a violent event has occurred, typically address risk factors associated with gun violence (e.g., poor access to quality education, housing, and employment opportunities; ready access to a gun) or enhance protective factors that reduce gun violence risk (e.g., financial and employment stability, effective stress coping and conflict management skills). Secondary prevention strategies are interventions developed in response to violence that has already occurred (e.g., prohibiting people convicted of felony crimes from purchasing and possessing guns) (Cohen et al. 2010). In this chapter, we review strategies intended to decrease deaths and injuries that result from gun violence, as well as those that complement the criminal justice response that typically focuses on ensuring that perpetrators are identified and brought to justice after a gun crime occurs.

A third characteristic of a public health approach to gun violence involves recognizing the larger context in which gun violence occurs and incorporating that context into intervention strategies. This emphasis on context is represented in the ecological model commonly used in public health to depict the different settings that influence health. The Institute of Medicine (2003) defines an ecological model as "a model of health that emphasizes the linkages and relationships among multiple factors affecting health" (p. 5) and includes factors at the individual, family, institutional, community, and policy levels (Figure 14–1). Intervention strategies that reduce gun violence risk at any of these levels then lend themselves to the fourth characteristic of a public health approach: the implementation of sound, feasible, and cost-effective policies and programs that will effectively reduce gun violence.

As a field, public health draws from many disciplines to promote health and reduce the burden of injury and disease through intervention opportunities at each of the five levels represented in Figure 14–1. At its best, this multidisciplinary orientation results in interventions that complement the contributions of related fields by using a more "upstream" approach to tackle the problem.

The ecological model is an appropriate framework for addressing the issue of gun violence. The most common approach to gun violence currently is one in which it is viewed as a criminal justice issue, with the target being postincident identification of the person who pulled the trigger. The criminal justice response is a valuable use of resources and is central to our system of justice. However, a broader conceptualization of the problem, which also examines the system that led to an operable gun in the hand of an individual who used that gun to harm others or himself or herself, provides the opportunity to design and implement new potential interventions to address the problem.

The opportunities available through this broader frame are well illustrated by the Haddon matrix, a tool used in the field of injury prevention (Baker et al. 1992). The Haddon matrix includes these upstream opportunities by consider-

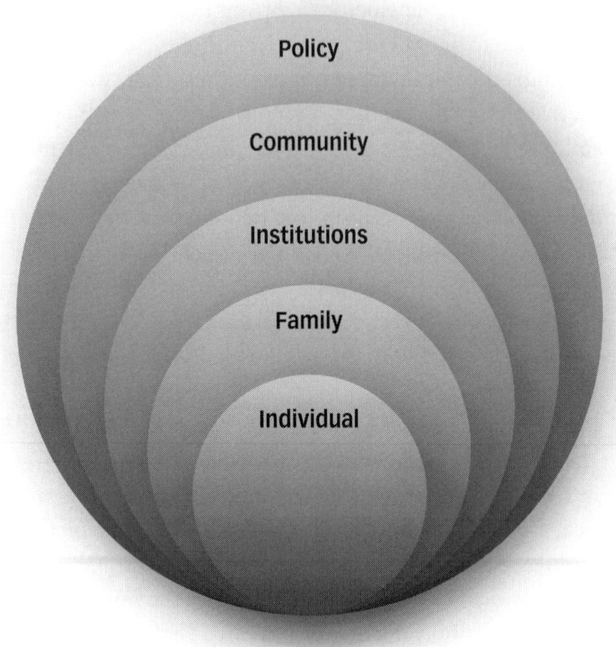

FIGURE 14–1. Ecological model.

ing the people involved (host), the gun as the injury-causing product (agent), and the environment in which the injury occurred (Runyan 1998). The inclusion of injury-causing products and the environments in which injuries occur expands the potential intervention targets from dangerous or at-risk individuals to include dangerous products and dangerous environments.

An example of the efficacy of such an approach is found in the success of motor vehicle–related death reduction. Public health interventions to address motor vehicle deaths include education about the risks and corresponding solutions (e.g., seat belt use), complemented by policy interventions (e.g., state seat belt laws) that mandate behaviors and establish enforcement mechanisms to reinforce the desired, injury-reducing behaviors. This type of multipronged approach is important to understanding how reductions in the rate of motor vehicle deaths have been realized. In 1983, an estimated 14% of people "buckled up" in the United States (National Highway Traffic Safety Administration 2008). That number did not change significantly until states passed laws requiring seat belt use. By 2012, all states, with the exception of New Hampshire, had mandatory seat belt laws in effect, and 86% of people were in compliance with the law (National Highway

Traffic Safety Administration 2014). The combination of information about a problem, a solution, and a policy to realize that solution provides both the message and the means to achieve the public health goal.

Importantly, products and environments may be more amenable to intervention than individuals, and a product-focused strategy can have wide-reaching impacts. For example, the regulatory decision to require child-resistant caps on prescription medications is associated with a significant decline in child poisoning deaths (Walton 1982). As a result of the modified design of prescription bottles to make the contents less accessible to children, generations of children have been and will continue to be protected by the change in prescription medication packaging. Notably, this intervention did not rely on educational interventions to teach millions of children not to ingest prescription medications or to train caregivers to store their prescriptions to make them inaccessible to children.

Intervening to alter the agent of injury or disease is a hallmark of public health and injury prevention, and this strategy has led to notable progress in areas such as motor vehicle safety (e.g., creation of airbags and shatterproof windshields) and home fire safety (e.g., development of fire and building codes, use of smoke alarms and residential sprinkler systems) (Baker et al. 1992). Although product change can yield impressive declines in morbidity and mortality, changing the agent of injury is not always feasible. Limitations of technology, political or public opposition, and cost are some of the most significant barriers to realizing design changes in injury-causing products. If practitioners and policy-makers systematically consider opportunities for intervention using tools such as an ecological framework and the Haddon matrix, a full assessment of available options is possible.

Interventions to Reduce Gun Morbidity and Mortality

Individual-Level Approaches

Attention to individual risk is an important part of the discussion about gun violence. In previous chapters in Part II, "Moving Forward," discussions of clinical options for intervening with the subset of people diagnosed with a mental illness and engaged in violent risky behaviors emphasized the role of risk assessment and clinical interventions, such as counseling patients and families to remove firearms during mental health crises. The authors of these chapters provide a comprehensive and insightful review of therapeutic approaches to gun violence prevention at the individual level, and we do not repeat those findings here. Rather, we review individual-level interventions that do not use therapeutic techniques.

Interventions aimed at reducing unintentional gun injuries are among the more common individual-level approaches discussed in the literature. Most of these interventions involve efforts to teach children and youth how to be safe around guns. This focus on children is due to the vulnerability they face when it comes to gun injury. According to Leventhal et al. (2014), approximately 7,000 children are hospitalized every year in the United States because of gun injuries. In 2012, gun-related injuries constituted 32% of pediatric trauma deaths between ages 0 and 19 years (Centers for Disease Control and Prevention 2014).

Educational efforts designed to prevent the unintentional gun injuries that occur when a child finds and fires a gun have been the subject of several evaluations over the past two decades and provide some empirical insight regarding the value of this approach. Unintentional gun deaths among children have declined 78% in the past 20 years and 34% in the past decade (Centers for Disease Control and Prevention 2012a); competing explanations for the reason behind this decline have been suggested. Proponents of one educational program developed by the National Rifle Association point to their program as the reason for the decline (National Rifle Association of America 2015); others cite the declining prevalence of households with guns (Frattaroli et al. 2002) or increases in safe storage of guns (Hepburn et al. 2006). Still others question whether the statistical declines are real in light of evidence that some coroners and medical examiners underreport these types of deaths (Schaechter et al. 2003). Given the attention to gun safety programs for children and their relevance to understanding trends in unintentional gun deaths, we review the available evidence here.

Educational interventions are responsive to the common belief that teaching children to be safe around guns effectively prevents unintentional gun deaths among children. Educational programs vary in terms of the venue in which they are delivered, the time devoted to the topic, and the background and skills of the trainer. However, the content generally focuses on conveying to children that guns are dangerous and that if they find a gun or know where one is, they should not touch it. If effective, teaching children to be safe around guns would meet the goal of reducing the number of children who find a gun and then accidentally shoot themselves, their siblings, or playmates.

Although such programs appear promising, the evidence challenges the assumption that such training is in fact effective in changing children's behavior. Attempts to educate children about how to be safe around guns may produce knowledge gains, as demonstrated by pre- and posttraining questionnaires used in some of the studies (Liller et al. 2003). Nevertheless, gun safety training and education interventions fail to yield the desired behavior change when children discover guns in simulated home environments (Hardy 2002). For example, in one study, children randomly assigned to receive an educational intervention using a structured gun safety curriculum were then asked to play in a room filled with toys. Hidden among the toys were a toy gun and a disabled real gun. Researchers observing the children noted no difference in gun-play behaviors between the children who received the educational intervention and those who did not (Hardy 2002). This general finding has been replicated in different populations, also in a simulated environment, without producing the desired behavior change (Hardy 2002; Himle et al. 2004).

Training approaches that move beyond verbal instruction about safe gun handling and incorporate behavioral skills training (BST)—in which children practice the desired behaviors and use in situ (real-world) training to further emphasize the desired behaviors—have shown positive impacts on knowledge and behaviors (Gatheridge et al. 2004; Himle et al. 2004; Miltenberger 2008). In these studies, children whose behaviors are unchanged following BST receive additional BST combined with instruction at the point of the behavioral failure. Specifically, when a child fails to practice the desired behaviors in a real-life setting, instructors intervene to again model the gun avoidance behaviors. This intensive approach sometimes requires multiple in situ interventions to demonstrate the desired effect at follow-up (Gatheridge et al. 2004; Himle et al. 2004). Thus, although teaching children how to be safe around guns may seem like a commonsense strategy to reduce unintentional gun deaths among children, the evidence suggests that such efforts are unlikely to accomplish that goal without the use of multiple, skill-based training sessions in which children practice gun avoidance in real-life settings. In addition, whether these effects are maintained over the span of childhood is unknown.

Family-Level Approaches

Complementary approaches to educational efforts directed only at children are interventions to promote safe storage among gun-owning parents. Educational messages to "lock your guns" through clinical (Grossman et al. 2005; Oatis et al. 1999) and media (Sidman et al. 2005) campaigns also have been tested, without a measurable change in self-reported safe storage behaviors. In a study by Brent et al. (2000), clinicians encouraged gun removal among parents of suicidal adolescents, but the authors noted that only 27% of participants reported that they removed guns from their homes. In addition, 17% of non-gun-owning parents reported acquiring a gun during the 2-year follow-up. The study authors concluded that parents who sought help for their child in crisis were often noncompliant with gun removal recommendations and therefore "more efficacious interventions to reduce access to guns in the homes of at-risk youth are needed" (p. 1220).

Although messages regarding safe storage and gun removal were relatively ineffective motivations for either action, initiatives that combine "lock your guns" messages with easy access to locking products (gun locks, safes, cables) are promising. Evaluations of community campaigns in Alaska and North Carolina demonstrated observed use of gun safes at follow-up (Horn et al. 2003) and self-reported increases in gun locking among participants (Coyne-Beasley et al. 2001), respectively. The Alaska study demonstrated high uptake of gun safes provided and installed free of charge by the intervention team; researchers observed that 86% of homes were using locked safes when the researchers returned 3 months after distributing the safety products. However, at 3-month follow-up, only 30% of the participants were using the free trigger locks provided (Horn et al. 2003). The North Carolina study measured self-reported gun-locking increases after the intervention, which included gun safety education and free gun locks. Notably, on measures of safe storage and removing guns from the home, larger effects were found among participants who had children than among those without children (Coyne-Beasley et al. 2001).

The potential efficacy of such interventions for families with children is further supported by results from a pediatric clinic–based counseling program that included distribution of a free gun lock. Self-reported survey data demonstrated significant improvements in the intervention group compared with the control group on self-reported measures of gun storage at 1-month follow-up (Carbone et al. 2005). Results from a cluster-randomized trial involving 24 pediatric practices from 41 U.S. states, Canada, and Puerto Rico demonstrated a significant change in self-reported safe firearm storage among parents receiving a violence prevention counseling intervention that included information about safe firearm storage and provided free gun cable locks, compared with a control group (Barkin et al. 2008). The brief intervention occurred during well-child visits and assessed readiness to change firearm storage behaviors using motivational interviewing techniques; this allowed clinicians to tailor the messages to families.

Community and clinic-based studies, therefore, offer optimistic findings that safe storage practices can be achieved through interventions that combine education with product distribution. Such interventions rely on the continued supply of products and maintenance of the behaviors by both the messenger and the recipients of the safe storage messages. We note that these studies do not measure the effects of these interventions on gun deaths and, with the exception of the Alaska study, rely instead on self-reports that may be affected by social desirability bias. Observational studies of safe storage practices and accounting for the impact of these interventions on rates of firearm injury and death among children are logical next steps in this line of research.

Unfortunately, to date, many educational interventions aimed at teaching children to be safe around guns have fallen short of the desired behavior change, although the more intensive efforts show promise. Efforts to encourage parents to store guns safely have yielded mixed results, with favorable evidence in support of messages about safe storage combined with access to the tools to accomplish that task. This evidence is consistent with findings in other areas of injury prevention (e.g., fire and burn prevention, fall prevention, poison storage) that show improvements in safety behaviors when educational interventions are tailored and combined with access to safety products (e.g., smoke alarms, safety gates for stairs, ipecac syrup) that facilitate compliance with the desired behaviors (Gielen et al. 2002; Kendrick et al. 2009).

At the family level, approaches that build on the idea that social norms can be powerful motivators for adopting desired behaviors are being applied to encourage parent-to-parent dialogue about gun storage in homes where children play (Frattaroli et al. 2012; Hemenway and Miller 2013). The Asking Saves Kids (ASK) campaign, a collaboration between the American Academy of Pediatrics and the Brady Center to Prevent Gun Violence, promotes the idea that parents should ask other parents if there is an unlocked gun in the home where their children play (http://askingsaveskids.org). Campaign developers reason that by asking, parents will establish a norm that promotes discussion of guns in the home and the importance of safe storage when children are present.

An evaluation of the ASK campaign did not demonstrate a significant effect on parents' asking behaviors, although the modest, nonsignificant differences between the intervention and control communities indicated that the intended attitudes addressed and the intentions to ask were higher among the intervention group (Johnson et al. 2012). The authors cite the small sample as one explanation for the lack of statistically significant findings. Nevertheless, the success of social norms campaigns to address other public health issues within focused intervention communities (e.g., binge drinking and tobacco use specifically on college campuses) (Perkins 2003) suggests that additional, more rigorous examinations of ASK and other efforts focused on family interactions around firearm storage are needed to assess the value of such an approach to gun violence prevention.

Institution-Level Approaches

Guns are dangerous products. When used as designed, they have the potential to injure and kill. The dangerous quality of firearms is one reason behind Congress's decision to exclude firearms from the Consumer Product Safety Commission's oversight (Teret and Draisin 2014). (The Consumer Product Safety Commission is the federal agency charged with overseeing the safety of products manufactured for consumer use.) This dangerous quality underlies the second common belief that we address in this chapter: guns are inherently dangerous, and efforts to make guns safer will not reduce the number of gun deaths and injuries.

Based on experiences with other consumer products such as cars and medication packaging, as discussed above (see "A Public Health Approach"), optimism about gains that can be made through safer gun design is justified. Gun design changes may be particularly effective at reducing gun-related morbidity and mortality associated with individuals prohibited from purchasing and possessing guns because of age, past criminal convictions, or other disqualifying criteria. These risk factors are discussed in Chapter 1, "Gun Violence and Serious Mental Illness," which also provides a review of the available evidence.

Considering gun design as a strategy for reducing unintentional gun deaths is not a new idea. Gun manufacturer Smith & Wesson produced a childproof gun for decades before ending its production to help supply the U.S. military's demand for guns during World War II (Teret and Draisin 2014). The Smith & Wesson gun was designed so that a child's hand could not simultaneously grip the gun and pull the trigger. Several other gun designs that restrict access by certain users have been developed since Smith & Wesson stopped production of its childproof model, but more recent advances demonstrate the feasibility and promise of personalized guns.

Guns that fire only for an authorized user are in development and available for sale outside the United States (Armatix 2014; Smart Tech Challenges Foundation 2014; Teret and Draisin 2014). Sales of such guns would likely limit the numbers of guns stolen each year in the United States (an average of 232,400 were stolen per year from 2005 to 2010; Langton 2012) and reduce access to guns by the hundreds of young people who are too young to buy the guns they use to commit suicide (Centers for Disease Control and Prevention 2011, 2012a). Such guns would also decrease the chances that a young child would discover a gun and unintentionally shoot himself or herself, a sibling, or a playmate (Wintemute et al. 1987).

Interventions that focus on gun design, embracing innovation and technology options with the potential to reduce the gun injuries and deaths that occur as a result of unauthorized access to guns, could make a significant difference in firearm morbidity and mortality. This focus on changing the characteristics of the injury-causing consumer product builds on a long line of successful consumer product–focused interventions in the field of injury prevention, including motor vehicles (seat belts and airbags), medications (child-resistant bottles), children's sleepwear (flame-resistant standards), and toys (warnings about a choking hazard) (Hemenway 2009). As personalized gun technology becomes increasingly available, efforts to monitor the impact on gun injuries and deaths, whether self-inflicted, accidental, or intentional, will be critical to assessing the potential of gun design to reduce current levels of gun mortality and morbidity.

Community-Level Approaches

Community-level interventions involving broad coalitions of government and nongovernment stakeholders have demonstrated promising results in addressing the approximately 40% of gun deaths (11,068 in 2011) classified as homicides (Centers for Disease Control and Prevention 2012a). In 1996, a comprehensive initiative involving law enforcement (including local police, prosecutors, judges, parole and probation officers, and the federal Bureau of Alcohol, Tobacco, Firearms and Explosives), faith-based organizations, and street outreach workers organized to field Operation Ceasefire: Boston Gun Project (National Institute of Justice 2001). The initiative focused attention on the most violent groups in specific Boston communities. By communicating that violence would not be tolerated and bringing a coordinated, aggressive law enforcement response when the groups within those specific communities did engage in violence, the project brought about reductions in shootings and killings.

An evaluation of the Boston program's effects on youth violence revealed impressive declines in key outcomes (63% decrease in youth homicide; 25% decrease in gun assaults; and 32% reduction in reported gunshots) (National Institute of Justice 2001). Several other cities have replicated the Boston program, with similar positive results (Office of Juvenile Justice and Delinquency Prevention 1999). Boston revised the initiative in 2007, and a second, more rigorous evaluation concluded that shootings in the communities where interventions were implemented were 31% lower than in a matched comparison group (Braga et al. 2013). The difference was statistically significant and lends further support to deterrence strategies aimed at groups responsible for much of the violence in communities where rates of gun violence exceed the national average (Braga et al. 2013).

Outreach to those most involved with perpetrating violence in communities is the foundation of several community-based initiatives that use gang organizations (Office of Juvenile Justice and Delinquency Prevention 2008), shootings (Skogan et al. 2008; Webster et al. 2013), and youth development (Frattaroli et al. 2010) as opportunities to intervene with youth to reduce their reliance on violence and guns for solving conflicts. These programs vary somewhat on the basis of their provision of counseling and support services, as well as the populations on which they focus, but share the basic approach of employing community residents as street outreach workers to connect with the youth who are engaging in violence or at risk of violence.

Published evaluations are available of the Cure Violence program in Chicago (Skogan et al. 2008) and replications in Baltimore (Webster et al. 2013; Whitehill et al. 2013) as well as of the United Teen Equality Center's street outreach worker program in Lowell, Massachusetts (Frattaroli et al. 2010; Pollack et al. 2011). These reports provide useful insights into the implementation of the programs (Frattaroli et al. 2010; Skogan et al. 2008; Whitehill et al. 2013); youth perceptions of the programs and their impacts (Pollack et al. 2011); and the association between these programs and shootings and homicides in the specific communities in which the programs have been implemented (Skogan et al. 2008; Webster et al. 2013). An evaluation of the Chicago program found statistically significant reductions in shootings and homicides in four of the seven neighborhoods examined (Skogan et al. 2008). Although an evaluation of a similar program in Pittsburgh demonstrated no effect (Wilson and Chermak 2011), the Baltimore replication study showed a statistically significant reduction in homicides and/or shootings in three of the four intervention communities (Webster et al. 2013). Although the outcome evaluations have yielded mixed results, the negative findings most often implicate implementation challenges as opposed to problems with the underlying approach (Webster et al. 2013).

The original CeaseFire initiative in Chicago (now known as Cure Violence) is based on the idea that violence can be effectively addressed using the same general approach as that used to reverse disease epidemics. The "essential elements" of the Cure Violence model borrowed from epidemic control include "1) interrupting transmission of the disease [violence], 2) reducing the risk of the highest risk, and 3) changing community norms" (Cure Violence 2014). Although adapting a disease epidemic orientation to gun violence may not be an obvious approach, this strategy has resulted in the creation of a viable model for intervention associated with 16%–34% reductions in the number of people shot or killed in four of the seven communities evaluated (Skogan et al. 2008).

Overall, the use of outreach workers to connect with youth at risk for violence is viewed with optimism, as demonstrated by numerous replications in the United States and abroad, and is recognized as a viable strategy for preventing violence at the community level (David-Ferdon and Simon 2014). Research that continues to monitor and inform these community interventions in order to assess the long-term effects on gun violence, identify strategies for achieving program scale-up, and inform best practices is important to maximizing the impact of this approach.

Policy-Level Approaches

Policy interventions intended to reduce gun violence through local, state, and federal laws offer another opportunity to reduce current levels of gun death and injury. Perhaps one of the most sensitive areas of the highly polarized debate regarding firearms involves legislation and regulation of firearms. However, policy interventions are a critical element of a broad public health–based model for effecting change that lead to reductions in mortality and morbidity (as demonstrated, e.g., by seat belts laws and drunk-driving laws). A robust evidence base demonstrates that firearm policies directed toward individuals at high risk of committing gun violence toward themselves or others can be effective in reducing gun-related morbidity and mortality.

Interventions Intended to Reduce Gun Purchases by People at High Risk of Committing Violence

Controlling firearm access by individuals at elevated risk of violence because of past violent behavior is complicated by the large number of guns in civilian hands. Accurate statistical estimates of civilian gun ownership in the United States are difficult to obtain because no central or national firearm registry exists. However, the Small Arms Survey, an international group based in Switzerland, estimates that approximately 270 million guns are in private possession in the United States, the highest number of civilian-owned firearms in any country and the highest rate of firearm ownership in the world (89/100 residents) (Small Arms Survey 2011). The high prevalence of firearms in the United States has often led to the dismissal of policy attempts to restrict access to firearms because of the common belief that with so many guns in civilian hands, interventions to control access to people identified as dangerous are futile.

Contrary to these beliefs, laws designed to prevent people at high risk of committing gun violence from legally purchasing guns can affect their access to guns and are associated with reductions in gun violence where these laws are in place. Examples of the relationship between firearm policies and access to firearms are found in the associations between licensing laws in Missouri and lower gun homicide rates (Webster et al. 2014) and California's law prohibiting violent misdemeanants from purchasing and possessing guns and fewer gun crimes (Wintemute et al. 2001).

In 2007, Missouri repealed its gun owner licensing law. Gun homicides in the state increased by 25% in the postrepeal period, while the rates in the surrounding states and the nation declined (Webster et al. 2014). Similarly, people convicted of violent misdemeanors who were then able to legally buy a gun in California were documented to be at a higher risk of subsequent arrest for gun crimes and/or violent crimes compared to violent misdemeanants whose gun purchase application was denied following a California law to prohibit those with such criminal records from purchasing and possessing firearms (Wintemute et al. 2001). Interestingly, a comparable elevated risk was not found for non-gun, nonviolent crimes, suggesting a specific effect of gun access on risk for violence.

Perhaps the clearest evidence of efficacy of gun purchase and possession prohibitions is demonstrated by the laws that focus on intimate partner violence (Zeoli and Frattaroli 2013). In the United States, intimate partners were responsible for 14% of all homicides in 2007 (Catalano et al. 2009), and over half of intimate partner homicides are committed with guns (Cooper and Smith 2011). Women make up 70% of the victims in intimate partner homicides (Catalano et al. 2009). In a 12-city study comparing abused women who were murdered by their partners or ex-partners with abused women who were still alive, gun access and/or ownership was found to increase the risk of homicide by 5.4 times, even after controlling for other relevant factors such as prior abuse history (Campbell et al. 2003). Given this increased risk of lethal violence associated with guns in violent intimate relationships, serious consideration of how to effectively prohibit intimate partner abusers from owning and accessing guns is a logical focus for intervention policy.

Gun-specific intimate partner violence strategies often address respondents to domestic violence restraining orders (DVROs). Since 1994, federal law has prohibited respondents to DVROs, issued after a hearing in which the respondent was present, from purchasing and possessing guns. About half of U.S. states have a law that mirrors the federal prohibition (Frattaroli and Vernick 2006), and at least 19 states extend the prohibition beyond federal law to include respondents to *ex parte* DVROs, often referred to as temporary restraining orders, which can be issued in the absence of the respondent (Zeoli and Frattaroli 2013).

Although the common belief that people who commit crimes will circumvent laws prohibiting firearm access has led some to criticize the efficacy of legally barring ownership of guns from violent intimate partners, evidence demonstrates the value of such an approach. Evaluations of state policies prohibiting respondents to DVROs from purchasing and possessing guns conclude that such laws are associated with reductions in both intimate partner gun homicides and intimate partner homicides overall (including non-gun homicides) (Vigdor and Mercy 2006; Zeoli and Webster 2010). These studies demonstrate consistent and significant reductions in homicide associated with the law. At the state level, the evaluation findings reveal a 7% overall decline in intimate partner homicide (Vigdor and Mercy 2006); at the city level, a 19% decline in intimate partner homicide and a 25% reduction in intimate partner homicides committed with guns were noted (Zeoli and Webster 2010).

Interventions Aimed at Reducing Illegal Possession

The impressive declines demonstrated by evaluations of state laws prohibiting DVRO respondents from purchasing and possessing guns are largely thought to be associated with the prohibition on purchase rather than possession, because the available evidence suggests that the prohibition on possession is not widely implemented (State of California, Office of the Attorney General Web site [oag.ca.gov]; Frattaroli and Teret 2006; Zeoli and Frattaroli 2013). Attention to the implementation of the possession provision would likely yield additional decreases in the incidence of intimate partner violence homicide. Small-scale efforts to realize these laws have demonstrated the efficacy of removing guns from DVRO respondents (Wintemute et al. 2014).

One demonstration project in two California counties involved a commitment by local law enforcement to implement the possession prohibition and resulted in guns being removed from 23% and 51% of respondents identified as in possession of a gun at the time the court issued a DVRO (Wintemute et al. 2014). Failure to recover firearms from these prohibited people most often occurred because the order was never served or the respondent denied possessing firearms (Wintemute et al. 2014). Importantly, a sample of petitioners surveyed after law enforcement removed respondents' guns reported no retaliation associated with gun removal and generally described the gun removal provision favorably (Vittes et al. 2013). No data have yet been collected to indicate whether these efforts resulted in a decreased incidence of gun violence. Research to evaluate the long-term impacts of such efforts on intimate partner violence and gun-involved intimate partner violence is needed.

Another California initiative to remove guns from prohibited possessors is also of interest. California's Armed and Prohibited Persons System (APPS) uses data to identify people who legally purchased firearms and then subsequently became prohibited (State of California, Office of the Attorney General 2014). Through APPS, law enforcement agencies identify people prohibited from having firearms who are likely in possession and, in accordance with the law, remove their guns. In 2011, the APPS program yielded 1,209 firearms and 155,731 rounds of ammunition from Californians prohibited from possessing guns (State of California Office of the Attorney General Web site [https://oag.ca.gov]). Although we are unaware of any evaluations of California's APPS program, we include it here as an intervention that should be examined.

Evidence from community-level law enforcement interventions demonstrates how law enforcement impacts illegal gun carrying in communities, further challenging the popular belief that only law-abiding citizens are affected by gun policies because criminals do not abide by gun laws. For example, increasing the number of gun-carrying suppression units, or police patrol units trained to identify people carrying guns illegally in gun violence "hot spots," leads to decreased criminal gun use. In Kansas City, Missouri, "hot spot" policing resulted in a 49% decline in gun-related crime. Importantly, no corresponding increase was found in gun-related crime in nearby or demographically similar areas (Sherman and Rogan 1995). More recently, in high-crime areas of Pittsburgh, Pennsylvania, the use of gun-carrying suppression units was associated with a 71% decrease in intentional gunshot injuries treated in local hospitals (Cohen and Ludwig 2003). This law enforcement initiative is an example of how data about high-risk environments (high prevalence of gun violence) and dangerous behaviors (illegal gun carrying) can be used to intervene before gun violence occurs.

Attention to the unregulated private gun market that is responsible for an estimated 40% of gun sales in the United States (Cook and Ludwig 1997) is also needed. This source of firearms is important for addressing the ready access to guns that underlies the common belief, listed at the beginning of this chapter, that the ubiquitous nature of guns in the United States renders ineffective any efforts to control the supply of guns to prohibited people. Seventeen states and the District of Columbia have expanded their regulatory authority to include some or all private gun sales (Law Center to Prevent Gun Violence 2013). For example, Maryland requires anyone who buys a regulated firearm (defined by the state to include all handguns and a small subset of long guns) to undergo a background check prior to completing the sale. Such background checks can be completed by the state police or through licensed firearm dealers who process private-seller transactions using the same system for conducting background checks of purchasers who buy guns from retail locations (Department of Maryland State Police 2014). By requiring gun buyers on the private market to undergo the same background checks as those who purchase from licensed firearm dealers, prohibited purchasers (those at increased risk of committing gun violence) are further limited in their ability to access guns.

Strategies like the Maryland law are consistent with the upstream focus of a public health approach to gun violence described at the beginning of this chapter (see "A Public Health Approach"). Whether these laws are being implemented and enforced is not known. We are not aware of any demonstration projects involving implementation of state private-sale policies or any evaluations of the effects of these private-sector sales policies on violence outcomes. Intervention research to establish the efficacy of these laws and evaluation research to measure their effectiveness would inform the current debate surrounding universal background check proposals at the federal level.

Nevertheless, the belief that efforts to limit access to illegal guns are futile is difficult to support in light of mounting evidence. In addition to the evaluations of licensing laws and purchase and possession prohibitions for violent, nonfelony offenders, an ethnographic study of Chicago's underground illegal gun markets revealed that guns can be difficult to access by people who cannot or do not want to buy from a federally licensed firearm dealer. Specifically, the study revealed that waiting times for guns are common in illegal markets, that purchasers cannot always obtain a gun, and that guns purchased on the street are costly relative to those available in gun stores (Cook et al. 2007). An important aspect of these findings is that the city of Chicago and the state of Illinois both regulate gun sales more extensively than most states. Furthermore, Chicago has long invested in law enforcement units that target the sources of guns used in crime and illegal gun trafficking (Chicago Police Department, Bureau of Investigative Services 2007; Office of Juvenile Justice and Delinquency Prevention 1999). The legal market interventions, combined with the enforcement focus, appear to have increased the price of dealing illegal guns in Chicago by decreasing the available supply (Cook et al. 2007).

Law enforcement agencies play a crucial role in violence prevention efforts and in the implementation of laws designed to keep firearms out of the hands of individuals at high risk of committing violence. Such strategies are vulnerable to criticism by those who subscribe to the common beliefs that guns are everywhere, that no policy will prevent people who want to commit gun crimes from obtaining guns, and that only law-abiding people comply with the law. Although it is true that law-abiding people, by definition, will comply with the law, people who commit crimes are also affected by policies that govern gun purchase and possession.

Preventing People Who Behave Dangerously From Accessing Guns

The policy initiatives reviewed thus far use past violent behavior and, to a lesser extent, serious mental illness as indicators of risk for future violence. Arguably these indicators establish a high bar for behaviors that lead to a gun purchase and possession prohibition. The two main disqualifiers at issue are 1) a response from a law enforcement agency that results in a charge and a conviction and 2) intervention by mental health professionals and involuntary treatment for an extended period of time. The sequences of events are generally understood to occur only after a history of dangerous behaviors that may (or may not) have included interactions with law enforcement, mental health professionals, or both.

From a public health perspective, if the current indicators of risk are preceded by more upstream behaviors with the potential to identify individuals engaging in dangerous behaviors before those behaviors manifest in a way that precipitates a law enforcement or mental health response, those earlier behaviors should be viewed as an opportunity for intervention. Some precedent for such laws exists, with efforts more broadly focused on law enforcement's authority to remove guns from people, with or without mental illness, who pose a risk of violence. As of 2014, three states had laws authorizing law enforcement to remove firearms from individuals whom they determine are at risk for harming themselves and/or others: Connecticut (Conn. Gen. Stat. § 29–38c, Seizure of Firearms of Person Posing Risk of Imminent Personal Injury to Self or Others, 1999), Indiana (Ind. Code Ann. § 35-47-14, Proceedings for the Seizure and Retention of a Firearm, 2001), and Texas (Tex. H.S. Code Ann. § 573.001, Apprehension by Peace Officer Without Warrant, 2001). The precise definitions for what constitutes risk and corresponding due process provisions vary among the states, as detailed elsewhere (Consortium for Risk-Based Firearm Policy 2013).

The data available regarding these laws are limited, but efficacy is demonstrable in Connecticut and Indiana, where the laws have been in place, respectively, since 1999 and 2006. During the first 10 years that Connecticut's policy was in effect, judges issued 274 warrants that resulted in the removal of more than 2,000 guns from people determined to be at imminent risk of perpetrating violence (Rose and Cummings 2009). In the first 2 years that Indiana's law was in effect (2006 and 2007), one Indianapolis county court processed 133 cases in which law enforcement removed firearms; most (65%) of these cases were in response to suicide threats (Parker 2010). These laws offer law enforcement an additional tool to use when responding to complaints about someone behaving dangerously. The authority to respond, assess, and take action to remove a gun offers a tangible strategy for de-escalating a dangerous situation and allowing officers to focus on the cause underlying the crisis that prompted their intervention.

Recognizing this potential, in May 2014, following the mass shooting in Isla Vista, California, several state senators introduced a bill to create a gun violence restraining order (GVRO) (see Chapter 13, “Relief From Disabilities: Firearm Rights Restoration for Persons Under Mental Health Prohibition”). Modeled after the DVRO systems in place in all 50 states and the District of Columbia, the GVRO will provide family members and intimate partners with a mechanism to petition the court to issue a restraining order that will temporarily prohibit the respondent from purchasing and possessing firearms when the court determines the respondent is a danger to self or others (Calif. AB-1014, Gun Violence Restraining Orders, 2014). Governor Brown signed the bill into law on September 30, 2014. As a result, California has become the first state to implement a GVRO law.

The GVRO provides a more upstream opportunity for family members and intimate partners to intervene when they notice that a loved one is in crisis and the family or individual is unable to engage the needed resources. Law enforcement is also empowered under the terms of California's GVRO to petition the court when someone is at risk of harming self or someone else. Several of the recent mass shootings in the United States demonstrate that early signs of crisis were evident, and in many cases family members intervened before the shootings occurred. Media coverage of these events described parents who removed guns, alerted law enforcement, and encouraged their children to seek treatment. However, these efforts were ultimately insufficient to prevent violence. The GVRO provides another tool for family members and intimate partners, who often are the first responders when an individual is in crisis.

Public Opinion and the Role of Advocacy

Whether the effective and promising policy recommendations reviewed in this chapter are feasible given the divisive nature of gun policy in this country is an important consideration. Although policy interventions have the potential to effect sweeping changes, that potential will remain unrealized unless the political will to pursue policy change becomes a factor. The popular belief on this matter—that gun policy is so polarizing that any effort to make changes at the policy level is futile—may reflect the absence of any significant federal legislation in recent decades and the tendency of the media to depict all gun policy as simply a “gun rights” versus “gun control” ideological debate.

No shortage exists of media attention about the strong feelings held by many in the United States about gun ownership and the equally strong opinions held by proponents of stronger prevention policies. Nevertheless, polling data suggest that when the dialogue moves beyond broad statements about gun control to specific policies, the level of agreement is higher than media portrayals suggest (Barry et al. 2013). One of the highest levels of public support for reform policies was recorded in 2013 after the shooting at Sandy Hook Elementary School (Newtown, Connecticut), in response to a question about requiring background checks for all gun sales. Eighty-nine percent of all respondents indicated they favored such a policy, including 90% of people who do not own guns, 83% of gun owners, and 74% of self-described National Rifle Association members (Barry et al. 2013).

Similarly, although federal policy on gun violence prevention has been virtually absent in the twenty-first century, activity in state legislatures on the issue has been quite robust (Zeoli and Frattaroli 2013). In the face of multiple mass shootings, a number of organizations have emerged, many with an explicit focus on enacting policy interventions designed to regulate gun sales and access to guns in ways that protect both legal gun owners and potential victims of gun violence. Importantly, from our perspective, efforts to inform new gun policy decisions with evidence about their effectiveness are needed, and resources are increasingly available to inform stakeholders who are committed to reducing gun morbidity and mortality (Consortium for Risk-Based Firearm Policy 2013; Webster and Vernick 2013).

Suggested Interventions

The various stakeholders highlighted in this chapter that influence and deliver public health interventions to decrease gun violence are vital voices in the discussion about guns and the lives lost to gun violence in the United States. In this chapter, we organized these stakeholders' contributions using the public health ecological framework to highlight the different levels of opportunity for intervention. Our recommendations build on this approach.

- At the individual and family levels, interventions that encourage and facilitate safe gun storage are most promising and should be pursued based on the available evidence and evaluated.
- Guns that can be fired only by an authorized user are being developed and are available for sale to a limited extent outside the United States. Support is needed to bring these designs to the U.S. market and to help people understand the potential of these guns to reduce gun death and injury.
- Community-level interventions that use outreach by trained community members to intervene when violence is imminent have been demonstrated, when properly implemented, to be effective in reducing shootings. Current efforts should continue to be supported, and new sites for replication should be pursued.

- Evidence-based gun violence prevention policy interventions should be adopted and implemented, and promising policy interventions should be enacted, implemented, and evaluated.
- Investments in public health programs, policy, and research are needed in order to realize potential significant and sustained reductions in gun violence.

References

Armatix: 21st Century Intelligent Systems [Web site], 2014. Available at: http://www.armatix.us/?L=7. Accessed October 14, 2014.

Baker SP, O'Neill B, Ginsburg MJ, et al: The Injury Fact Book, 2nd Edition. New York, Oxford University Press, 1992

Barkin SL, Finch SA, Ip EH, et al: Is office-based counseling about media use, timeouts, and firearm storage effective? Results from a cluster-randomized, controlled trial. Pediatrics 122(1):e15–e25, 2008 18595960

Barry CL, McGinty EE, Vernick JS, et al: After Newtown—public opinion on gun policy and mental illness. N Engl J Med 368(12):1077–1081, 2013 23356490

Braga AA, Hureau DM, Papachristos AV: Deterring gang-involved gun violence: measuring the impact of Baltimore's Operation Ceasefire on street gang behavior. J Quant Criminol 30(1):113–139, 2013

Brent DA, Baugher M, Birmaher B, et al: Compliance with recommendations to remove firearms in families participating in a clinical trial for adolescent depression. J Am Acad Child Adolesc Psychiatry 39(10):1220–1226, 2000 11026174

Campbell JC, Webster D, Koziol-McLain J, et al: Risk factors for femicide in abusive relationships: results from a multisite case control study. Am J Public Health 93(7):1089–1097, 2003 12835191

Carbone PS, Clemens CJ, Ball TM: Effectiveness of gun-safety counseling and a gun lock giveaway in a Hispanic community. Arch Pediatr Adolesc Med 159(11):1049–1054, 2005 16275796

Catalano S, Smith E, Snyder H, et al: Female Victims of Violence. Washington, DC, Bureau of Justice Statistics, 2009

Centers for Disease Control and Prevention, National Center for Injury Prevention and Control: Web-based Injury Statistics Query and Reporting System (WISQARS), Fatal Injury Report, 2011. Available at: www.cdc.gov/injury/wisqars/index.html. Accessed August 10, 2015,

Centers for Disease Control and Prevention: Injury Prevention & Control: Data & Statistics (WISQARS). Fatal Injury Data. Atlanta, GA, Centers for Disease Control and Prevention, 2012a. Available at: http://www.cdc.gov/injury/wisqars/fatal.html. Accessed November 30, 2014.

Centers for Disease Control and Prevention: Injury Prevention & Control: Data & Statistics (WISQARS). Nonfatal Injury Data. Atlanta, GA, Centers for Disease Control and Prevention, 2012b. Available at: http://www.cdc.gov/injury/wisqars/nonfatal.html. Accessed November 30, 2014.

Centers for Disease Control and Prevention: About Underlying Cause of Death, 1999–2013 (CDC WONDER). Atlanta, GA, Centers for Disease Control and Prevention, 2014. Available at: http://wonder.cdc.gov/ucd-icd10.html. Accessed November 30, 2014.

Chicago Police Department, Bureau of Investigative Services: Trafficking: Case Studies of Five Trafficked Guns in Chicago. Chicago, IL, Chicago Police Department Reproduction and Graphic Arts Section, October 2007. Available at: https://portal.chicagopolice.org/portal/page/portal/ClearPath/News/Department%20Publications/Guns-CaseStudies.pdf. Accessed November 12, 2014.

Cohen J, Ludwig J: Policing crime guns, in Evaluating Gun Policy: Effects on Crime and Violence. Edited by Cook PJ, Ludwig J. Washington, DC, Brookings Institution Press, 2003, pp 217–239

Cohen L, Chavez V, Chehimi S (eds): Prevention Is Primary: Strategies for Community Well Being, 2nd Edition. San Francisco, CA, Jossey-Bass, 2010

Consortium for Risk-Based Firearm Policy: Guns, Public Health, and Mental Illness: An Evidence-Based Approach for State Policy. Baltimore, MD, Johns Hopkins Center for Gun Policy and Research, 2013. Available at: http://www.jhsph.edu/research/centers-and-institutes/johns-hopkins-center-for-gun-policy-and-research/publications/GPHMI-State.pdf. Accessed October 16, 2014.

Cook PJ, Ludwig J: Guns in America: National Survey on Private Ownership and Use of Firearms. Washington, DC, National Institute of Justice, Office of Justice Programs, 1997

Cook PJ, Ludwig J, Venkatesh S, et al: Underground gun markets. Economic Journal 117:F558–F588, 2007

Cooper A, Smith EL: Homicide Trends in the United States, 1980–2008. Washington, DC, Bureau of Justice Statistics, 2011. Available at: http://bjs.ojp.usdoj.gov/content/pub/pdf/htus8008.pdf. Accessed November 11, 2014.

Coyne-Beasley T, Schoenbach VJ, Johnson RM: "Love our kids, lock your guns": a community-based firearm safety counseling and gun lock distribution program. Arch Pediatr Adolesc Med 155(6):659–664, 2001 11386952

Cure Violence: The Cure Violence Health Model. Available at: http://cureviolence.org/the-model/essential-elements/. Accessed October 20, 2014.

David-Ferdon C, Simon TR: Preventing Youth Violence: Opportunities for Action. Atlanta, GA, Centers for Disease Control and Prevention, National Center for Injury Prevention and Control, 2014

Department of Maryland State Police: Regulated Firearm Purchases. Baltimore, MD, Department of Maryland State Police, 2014. Available at: https://www.mdsp.org/Organization/SupportServicesBureau/LicensingDivision/MainLicensingPage/LicensingandRegistration/Firearms/RegulatedFirearmPurchases.aspx. Accessed October 14, 2014.

Frattaroli S, Teret SP: Understanding and informing policy implementation: a case study of the domestic violence provisions of the Maryland Gun Violence Act. Eval Rev 30(3):347–360, 2006 16679500

Frattaroli S, Vernick JS: Separating batterers and guns: a review and analysis of gun removal laws in 50 states. Eval Rev 30(3):296–312, 2006 16679498

Frattaroli S, Webster DW, Teret SP: Unintentional gun injuries, firearm design, and prevention: what we know, what we need to know, and what can be done. J Urban Health 79(1):49–59, 2002 11937615

Frattaroli S, Pollack KM, Jonsberg K, et al: Streetworkers, youth violence prevention, and peacemaking in Lowell, Massachusetts: lessons and voices from the community. Prog Community Health Partnersh 4(3):171–179, 2010 20729607

Frattaroli S, Vittes K, Johnson SB, et al: Firearm injuries, in Injury Prevention for Children and Adolescents: Integration of Research, Practice and Advocacy, 2nd Edition. Washington, DC, American Public Health Association, 2012

Gatheridge BJ, Miltenberger RG, Huneke DF, et al: Comparison of two programs to teach firearm injury prevention skills to 6- and 7-year-old children. Pediatrics 114(3):e294–e299, 2004 15342889

Gielen AC, McDonald EM, Wilson MEH, et al: Effects of improved access to safety counseling, products, and home visits on parents' safety practices: results of a randomized trial. Arch Pediatr Adolesc Med 156(1):33–40, 2002 11772188

Grossman DC, Mueller BA, Riedy C, et al: Gun storage practices and risk of youth suicide and unintentional firearm injuries. JAMA 293(6):707–714, 2005 15701912

Hardy MS: Teaching firearm safety to children: failure of a program. J Dev Behav Pediatr 23(2):71–76, 2002 11943968

Hemenway D: While We Were Sleeping: Success Stories in Injury and Violence Prevention. Oakland, University of California Press, 2009

Hemenway D, Miller M: Public health approach to the prevention of gun violence. N Engl J Med 368(21):2033–2035, 2013 23581254

Hepburn L, Azrael D, Miller M, et al: The effect of child access prevention laws on unintentional child firearm fatalities, 1979–2000. J Trauma 61(2):423–428, 2006 16917460

Himle MB, Miltenberger RG, Flessner C, et al: Teaching safety skills to children to prevent gun play. J Appl Behav Anal 37(1):1–9, 2004 15154211

Horn A, Grossman DC, Jones W, et al: Community based program to improve firearm storage practices in rural Alaska. Inj Prev 9(3):231–234, 2003 12966011

Institute of Medicine, Board on Health Promotion and Disease Prevention, Committee on Educating Public Health Professionals for the 21st Century: Who Will Keep the Public Healthy? Educating Public Health Professionals for the 21st Century. Edited by Gebbie K, Rosenstock L, Hernandez LM. Washington, DC, National Academies Press, 2003

Johnson RM, Lintz J, Gross D, et al: Evaluation of the ASK campaign in two Midwestern cities. International Scholarly Research Notices 2012:1–6, 2012

Kendrick D, Smith S, Sutton AJ, et al: The effect of education and home safety equipment on childhood thermal injury prevention: meta-analysis and meta-regression. Inj Prev 15(3):197–204, 2009 19494100

Langton L: Firearms Stolen During Household Burglaries and Other Property Crimes, 2005–2010 (NCJ 239436). Washington, DC, Bureau of Justice Statistics, 2012. Available at: http://www.bjs.gov/content/pub/pdf/fshbopc0510.pdf. Accessed October 21, 2014.

Law Center to Prevent Gun Violence: Universal Background Checks & the Private Sale Loophole Policy Summary. San Francisco, CA, Law Center to Prevent Gun Violence, 2013. Available at: http://smartgunlaws.org/universal-gun-background-checks-policy-summary/. Accessed August 10, 2015.

Leventhal JM, Gaither JR, Sege R: Hospitalizations due to firearm injuries in children and adolescents. Pediatrics 133(2):219–225, 2014 24470651

Liller KD, Perrin K, Nearns J, et al: Evaluation of the "Respect Not Risk" firearm safety lesson for 3rd-graders. J Sch Nurs 19(6):338–343, 2003 14622039

Miltenberger RG: Teaching safety skills to children: prevention of firearm injury as an exemplar of best practice in assessment, training, and generalization of safety skills. Behav Anal Pract 1(1):30–36, 2008 22477677

National Highway Traffic Safety Administration: How States Achieve High Seat Belt Use Rates. Washington, DC, U.S. Department of Transportation, August 2008. Available at: http://www-nrd.nhtsa.dot.gov/Pubs/810962.pdf. Accessed October 18, 2014.

National Highway Traffic Safety Administration: Traffic Safety Facts: Seat Belt Use in 2013—Overall Results. U.S. Department of Transportation, January 2014. Available at: http://www-nrd.nhtsa.dot.gov/Pubs/811875.pdf. Accessed November 18, 2014.

National Institute of Justice: Reducing Gun Violence: The Boston Gun Project's Operation Ceasefire. Washington, DC, U.S. Department of Justice, 2001

National Rifle Association of America: Eddie Eagle GunSafe Program, 2015. Available at: https://eddieeagle.nra.org/. Accessed August 10, 2015.

Oatis PJ, Fenn Buderer NM, Cummings P, et al: Pediatric practice based evaluation of the Steps to Prevent Firearm Injury program. Inj Prev 5(1):48–52, 1999 10323570

Office of Juvenile Justice and Delinquency Prevention: Promising Strategies to Reduce Gun Violence. Washington, DC, U.S. Department of Justice, 1999. Available at: http://www.ojjdp.gov/pubs/gun_violence/173950.pdf. Accessed October 15, 2014.

Office of Juvenile Justice and Delinquency Prevention: Best Practices to Address Community Gang Problems: OJJDP's Comprehensive Gang Model. Washington, DC, U.S. Department of Justice, 2008. Available at: https://www.ncjrs.gov/pdffiles1/ojjdp/222799.pdf. Accessed October 15, 2014.

Parker GF: Application of a firearm seizure law aimed at dangerous persons: outcomes from the first two years. Psychiatr Serv 61(5):478–482, 2010 20439368

Perkins HW (ed): The Social Norms Approach to Preventing School and College Age Substance Abuse: A Handbook for Educators, Counselors, and Clinicians. San Francisco, CA, Jossey-Bass, 2003

Pollack KM, Frattaroli S, Whitehill JM, et al: Youth perspectives on street outreach workers: results from a community-based survey. J Community Health 36(3):469–476, 2011 21080041

Rose V, Cummings L: Gun Seizure Law: OLR Research Report. Hartford, Connecticut General Assembly, 2009. Available at: http://www.cga.ct.gov/2009/rpt/2009-R-0306.htm. Accessed October 26, 2014.

Runyan CW: Using the Haddon matrix: introducing the third dimension. Inj Prev 4(4):302–307, 1998 9887425

Schaechter J, Duran I, De Marchena J, et al: Are "accidental" gun deaths as rare as they seem? A comparison of medical examiner manner of death coding with an intent-based classification approach. Pediatrics 111(4 Pt 1):741–744, 2003 12671106

Sherman L, Rogan D: Effects of gun seizures on gun violence: "hot spots" patrol in Kansas City. Justice Q 12(4):755–781, 1995

Sidman EA, Grossman DC, Koepsell TD, et al: Evaluation of a community-based handgun safe-storage campaign. Pediatrics 115(6):e654–e661, 2005 15930192

Skogan WG, Hartnett SM, Bump N, et al: Evaluation of CeaseFire—Chicago. Rockville, MD, National Institute of Justice, 2008

Small Arms Survey: Small Arms Survey 2011: States of Security. Geneva, Cambridge University Press, 2011

Smart Tech Challenges Foundation [Web site], 2014. Available at: https://smarttechfoundation.org. Accessed October 18, 2014.

State of California, Office of the Attorney General: Armed and Prohibited Persons System Fact Sheet, 2014. Available at: https://oag.ca.gov/system/files/attachments/press_releases/n2521_apps_fact_sheet.pdf. Accessed October 16, 2014.

Teret SP, Draisin NA: Personalized guns: using technology to address gun violence. Abell Report 27(2):1–8, 2014

Vigdor ER, Mercy JA: Do laws restricting access to firearms by domestic violence offenders prevent intimate partner homicide? Eval Rev 30(3):313–346, 2006 16679499

Violence Prevention Alliance: The Public Health Approach. Geneva, World Health Organization, 2014. Available at: http://www.who.int/violenceprevention/approach/public_health/en/. Accessed October 18, 2014.

Vittes KA, Webster DW, Frattaroli S, et al: Removing guns from batterers: findings from a pilot survey of domestic violence restraining order recipients in California. Violence Against Women 19(5):602–616, 2013 23759665

Walton WW: An evaluation of the Poison Prevention Packaging Act. Pediatrics 69(3):363–370, 1982 7063294

Webster DW, Vernick JS (eds): Reducing Gun Violence in America: Informing Policy With Evidence and Analysis. Baltimore, MD, Johns Hopkins University Press, 2013

Webster DW, Whitehill JM, Vernick JS, et al: Effects of Baltimore's Safe Streets program on gun violence: a replication of Chicago's CeaseFire program. J Urban Health 90(1):27–40, 2013 22696175

Webster D, Crifasi CK, Vernick JS: Effects of the repeal of Missouri's handgun purchaser licensing law on homicides. J Urban Health 91(2):293–302, 2014 24604521

Whitehill JM, Webster DW, Frattaroli S, et al: Interrupting violence: how the CeaseFire program prevents imminent gun violence through conflict mediation. J Urban Health 91(1):84–95, 2013 23440488

Wilson JM, Chermak S: Community-driven violence reduction programs: examining Pittsburgh's One Vision One Life. Criminol Public Policy 10(4):993–1027, 2011

Wintemute GJ, Teret SP, Kraus JF, et al: When children shoot children: 88 unintended deaths in California. JAMA 257(22):3107–3109, 1987 3586229

Wintemute GJ, Wright MA, Drake CM, et al: Subsequent criminal activity among violent misdemeanants who seek to purchase handguns: risk factors and effectiveness of denying handgun purchase. JAMA 285(8):1019–1026, 2001 11209172

Wintemute GJ, Frattaroli S, Wright MA, et al: Identifying armed respondents to domestic violence restraining orders and recovering their firearms: process evaluation of an initiative in California. Am J Public Health 104(2):e113–e118, 2014

Zeoli AM, Frattaroli S: Evidence for optimism: policies to limit batterers' access to guns, in Reducing Gun Violence in America. Edited by Webster DW, Vernick JS. Baltimore, MD, Johns Hopkins University Press, 2013

Zeoli AM, Webster DW: Effects of domestic violence policies, alcohol taxes and police staffing levels on intimate partner homicide in large U.S. cities. Inj Prev 16(2):90–95, 2010 20363814

APPENDIX

Resources

This list of resources is provided for readers who want to obtain additional information or access research, education, or treatment resources. The list is not exhaustive but it does provide starting places for those who may be looking for assistance for themselves or loved ones, those who wish to learn more, or those who are interested in engaging in or supporting public health initiatives. Organizations that also engage in political advocacy regarding firearms are so noted.

Mental Health: Accessing Treatment or Engaging in Mental Health Advocacy

Individuals seeking immediate treatment should consider beginning by contacting their state and/or county departments of mental health or departments of behavioral health.

General

American Psychiatric Association (APA)

www.psychiatry.org

Bazelon Center for Mental Health Law

www.bazelon.org

This national nonprofit organization is intended to protect and advance the rights of adults and children who have mental disabilities.

Centers for Disease Control and Prevention (CDC) Mental Health Web Site

www.cdc.gov/mentalhealth/index.htm

This Web site offers basic public health information, including statistics, publications, and reports, regarding mental health disorders and issues. Importantly, this page includes a General Resources link (www.cdc.gov/mentalhealth/gen-resources.htm) that provides access to Web sites of national organizations that provide information and resources on specific mental disorders.

MentalHealth.gov

www.mentalhealth.gov/basics/index.html

This Web site provides information on and access to resources for multiple mental health issues (e.g., stigma, accessing treatment) for individuals, families, treatment providers, educators, and communities.

National Alliance on Mental Illness (NAMI)

www.nami.org

This national nonprofit organization provides information regarding access to mental health resources, advocacy, and support for individuals with mental illness and their families. NAMI also provides information to combat the stigma associated with mental illness in the article "Misconceptions About Mental Illness" (www.nami.org/Content/Microsites88/NAMI_Olmsted_County/Discussion_Groups115/Discussion/Test_Page_Ignore1/Ways_You_Can_Help/Misconceptions.doc).

National Institute of Mental Health (NIMH)

www.nimh.nih.gov/index.shtml

NIMH offers extensive information about specific mental health disorders on its health and education page (www.nimh.nih.gov/health/index.shtml); it also offers information about its public outreach activities (www.nimh.nih.gov/outreach/index.shtml) and research priorities and funding (www.nimh.nih.gov/research-priorities/index.shtml).

Substance Abuse and Mental Health Services Administration (SAMHSA)

www.samhsa.gov

SAMHSA is the agency within the U.S. Department of Health and Human Services that leads public health efforts to advance the behavioral health of the nation. SAMHSA seeks to reduce the impact of substance abuse and mental illness, and to provide information regarding treatment resources in communities across the United States.

Treatment Advocacy Center

www.treatmentadvocacycenter.org

This national nonprofit organization is dedicated to eliminating barriers to the timely and effective treatment of severe mental illness; promoting laws, policies, and practices for the delivery of psychiatric care; and supporting the development of innovative treatments for and research into the causes of severe and persistent psychiatric illnesses, such as schizophrenia and bipolar disorder. The Treatment Advocacy Center also provides resources to combat the stigma of mental illness at "Stigma and Serious Mental Illness: What Is the Relationship?" (www.treatmentadvocacycenter.org/about-us/our-blog/69-no-state/2622-stigma-and-serious-mental-illness-what-is-the-relationship).

U.S. Department of Health and Human Services (DHHS)

www.hhs.gov/healthcare/facts/index.html

DHHS is the U.S. government's principal agency for protecting the health of all Americans and providing essential human services, especially for those who are least able to help themselves. Its Web site provides information to assist in accessing the following:

a. Health care insurance through Medicare (www.medicare.gov) and Medicaid (www.medicaid.gov), and opportunities for obtaining health insurance under the Affordable Care Act (www.healthcare.gov)
b. Information regarding public health programs to improve patient outcomes, promote efficiency and accountability, ensure patient safety, encourage shared responsibility, and work toward high-value health care
c. Culturally competent quality health care for uninsured, underserved, vulnerable, older, and special needs populations

Youth, Violence, and Mental Health

The early identification of mental illness in youngsters is important for youth, their families, and their communities. Multiple resources are available that suggest an integrated approach to proactively identify and intervene with youth who are experiencing mental health problems and/or at high-risk for violent behavior. The following resources, and many others, can assist in providing safe and healthy school and community environments that reduce the incidence of youth violence and support the healthy development and general well-being, including mental health, of our youth.

General

The Asset-Based Community Development Institute

www.abcdinstitute.org

This institute serves as a resource to build skills of local residents, associations, and institutions to better their capacity to build stronger, more sustainable communities.

Centers for Disease Control and Prevention (CDC), Division of Violence Prevention (DVP)

www.cdc.gov/violenceprevention/youthviolence/schoolviolence/index.html

DVP's mission is to stop violence before it begins. The group does various types of work:

a. Provides resources and information on violence-related injuries
b. Conducts research on factors that put people at risk and factors that protect people from violence
c. Creates and evaluates the effectiveness of violence prevention programs
d. Helps state and local partners plan, implement, and evaluate prevention programs
e. Conducts research on the effective adoption and dissemination of prevention strategies

Collaborative for Academic, Social, and Emotional Learning (CASEL)

http://casel.org/social-and-emotional-learning

CASEL provides resources to advance the development of academic, social, and emotional learning, skills, and competence for all students from preschool through high school.

National School Safety Center

www.schoolsafety.us

Originally a joint program between the U.S. Departments of Education and Justice established in 1984, the Center now operates as an independent nonprofit organization serving schools and communities worldwide. This organization provides training and technical assistance in the areas of safe school planning and school crime prevention.

U.S. Department of Education, Office of Elementary and Secondary Education, Office of Safe and Healthy Students

www2.ed.gov/about/offices/list/oese/oshs/index.html

This federal office maintains resources, develops school safety policy, and provides financial assistance for violence prevention activities and other programs that promote student well-being.

U.S. Department of Health and Human Services (DHHS), Office of Adolescent Health: Mental Health

www.hhs.gov/ash/oah/adolescent-health-topics/mental-health

U.S. Department of Justice, Office of Justice Programs, Youth Violence Prevention

http://ojp.gov/programs/youthviolenceprevention.htm

Youth.gov

www.youth.gov

This Web site provides an overview of information, strategies, tools, and resources for youth, families, schools, and community organizations. It includes specific local information about interventions designed to support youth. It also provides information and resources with regard to youth suicide prevention, preventing gang involvement, substance abuse, reconnecting youth, preventing youth violence, bullying, and youth mental health.

Youth Violence Project (YVP)

http://curry.virginia.edu/research/labs/youth-violence-project

Based at the University of Virginia, the YVP has developed manuals for and conducted research on threat assessment and other safety interventions.

Youth Trauma Services

National Child Traumatic Stress Network

http://nctsn.org

This Web site includes resources to raise the standard of care and improve access to services for traumatized children, their families, and communities throughout the United States.

Suicide and Violence

Many of these resources provide information for the general public and training materials and opportunities for professionals.

General

American Association of Suicidology

www.suicidology.org

American Foundation for Suicide Prevention

www.afsp.org

Centers for Disease Control and Prevention, Injury Prevention & Control: Division of Violence Prevention

www.cdc.gov/violenceprevention/suicide

Means Matter, Harvard T.H. Chan School of Public Health

www.hsph.harvard.edu/means-matter

National Institute of Mental Health (NIMH), Suicide Prevention

www.nimh.nih.gov/health/topics/suicide-prevention/index.shtml

National Medical Council on Gun Violence (NMCGV)

www.nmcgv.org

Prevention Institute

www.preventioninstitute.org/services.html

Substance Abuse and Mental Health Services Administration (SAMHSA), Suicide Prevention

www.samhsa.gov/tribal-ttac/resources/suicide-prevention

Substance Abuse and Mental Health Services Administration (SAMHSA), Violence Prevention

www.samhsa.gov/tribal-ttac/resources/violence-prevention

Suicide Prevention Resource Center

www.sprc.org

Violence Risk Assessment

American Academy of Forensic Psychology

www.aafp.ws

Historical Clinical Risk Management–20, Version 3 (HCR-20V3)

http://hcr-20.com

University of Virginia's Institute of Law, Psychiatry, and Public Policy

http://cacsprd.web.virginia.edu/ILPPP

Suicide Risk Assessment

American Association of Suicidology, Training and Accreditation

www.suicidology.org/training-accreditation/rrsr

Suicide Prevention Resource Center Training Institute

www.sprc.org/training-institute/amsr

Firearm Injury Prevention and Research Programs

Although research on firearms and firearms injury prevention is limited, some research centers have conducted scientifically rigorous studies that have produced an evidence base referred to in multiple chapters throughout this volume. The resources listed here provide information regarding the different levels of intervention needed to prevent firearm injuries, which are frequently fatal, and the research evidence that supports the efficacy of these interventions.

General

Association of State and Territorial Health Officials, Preventing Firearm Injury and Death

www.astho.org/Prevention/Preventing-Firearm-Injury-and-Death

Harvard T.H. Chan School of Public Health, Injury Control Research Center, Firearms Research

www.hsph.harvard.edu/hicrc/firearms-research

Johns Hopkins Bloomberg School of Public Health, Center for Gun Policy and Research

www.jhsph.edu/research/centers-and-institutes/johns-hopkins-center-for-gun-policy-and-research

The Joyce Foundation, Gun Violence Prevention

www.joycefdn.org/programs/gun-violence-prevention

University of California, Davis, Violence Prevention Research Program

www.ucdmc.ucdavis.edu/vprp/publications

Firearm Regulation and Policy

Individuals who want to learn more about or find ways to prevent gun violence should contact local, state, or national gun violence prevention groups that support research and initiatives for commonsense gun laws. The following resources provide information on federal and state firearm regulation and policy.

General

Federal Bureau of Investigation National Instant Criminal Background Check System (NICS)

www.fbi.gov/about-us/cjis/nics

This Web site provides information on and links for all aspects of NICS, including NICS state participation and the appeals process.

GunPolicy.org—International Firearm Injury Prevention and Policy

www.gunpolicy.org

This University of Sydney Web site provides evidence-based, country-by-country intelligence from a broad range of official and academic sources. This site is for researchers, officials, journalists, and advocates who need accurate citations and rapid access to credible sources, although the organization has been criticized for an advocacy bias.

Law Center to Prevent Gun Violence

http://smartgunlaws.org/mental-health-reporting-policy-summary

This Web site provides a current, detailed, and comprehensive summary of federal and state firearm legislation enacted throughout the United States. This site also has summaries of state law by policy, including mental health reporting policy summaries (http://smartgunlaws.org/mental-health-reporting-policy-summary/). Advocacy bias is present.

National Rifle Association Institute for Legislative Action

http://home.nra.org/nraila/list/ila-feature

This Web site provides current information regarding state and federal firearm legislation. Advocacy bias is present.

U.S. Department of Justice, Bureau of Alcohol, Tobacco, Firearms and Explosives (ATF)

www.atf.gov

The ATF provides information regarding national firearm legislation and regulation.

Index

Page numbers printed in **boldface** *type refer to tables or figures.*